Practical Issues in Geriatri

Series Editor

Stefania Maggi
Aging Branch
CNR-Neuroscience Institute
Padua, Italy

This practically oriented series presents state of the art knowledge on the principal diseases encountered in older persons and addresses all aspects of management, including current multidisciplinary diagnostic and therapeutic approaches. It is intended as an educational tool that will enhance the everyday clinical practice of both young geriatricians and residents and also assist other specialists who deal with aged patients. Each volume is designed to provide comprehensive information on the topic that it covers, and whenever appropriate the text is complemented by additional material of high educational and practical value, including informative video-clips, standardized diagnostic flow charts and descriptive clinical cases. Practical Issues in Geriatrics will be of value to the scientific and professional community worldwide, improving understanding of the many clinical and social issues in Geriatrics and assisting in the delivery of optimal clinical care.

More information about this series at http://www.springer.com/series/15090

Paolo Falaschi · David Marsh

Editors

Orthogeriatrics

The Management of Older Patients with Fragility Fractures

Second Edition

In Collaboration with
Stefania Giordano

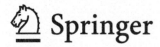 Springer

Editors
Paolo Falaschi
Geriatrics Department
Sapienza University of Rome
Roma
Italy

David Marsh
Department of Orthopaedics
University College London
London
UK

In Collaboration with
Stefania Giordano
Assistant Geriatrician at Italian
Hospital Group
Guidonia (RM)
Italy

This book is an open access publication.
ISSN 2509-6060   ISSN 2509-6079   (electronic)
Practical Issues in Geriatrics
ISBN 978-3-030-48128-5   ISBN 978-3-030-48126-1   (eBook)
https://doi.org/10.1007/978-3-030-48126-1

This Springer imprint is published by the registered company Springer Nature Switzerland AG
The registered company address is: Gewerbestrasse 11, 6330 Cham, Switzerland

Preface to the Second Edition

The first edition of *Orthogeriatrics* [1] stressed that the key feature of older patients with fragility fractures is that they often have the dual problem of *fragility* (of the bone) and *frailty* (of their entire physiology). Therefore, the appropriate mode of management in the acute phase is orthogeriatric co-management, bringing to bear the relevant skillsets for dealing with these two problems simultaneously. We asserted that this is true in all parts of the planet but that card-carrying geriatricians are not essential—geriatric *competencies* can be acquired by other physicians in countries where the discipline of geriatric medicine is not well established—and we tried to show what these competencies are. This second edition takes that attempt further, in the context of two significant developments that have occurred over the last 3 years.

The first was the publication of *A global call to action to improve the care of people with fragility fractures* [2]. The writing of this paper was led by the Fragility Fracture Network (FFN), with input from five other international organisations (EFORT, EuGMS, ICON, IGFS and IOF). It was then endorsed, prior to publication, by a further 75 organisations from the relevant disciplines, some global, some regional and some national from the larger countries of Brazil, China, India, Japan and the United States of America. Since publication, a steady stream of other national professional associations has been adding their endorsement.

However, this uniquely broad base of support is not the only special feature of this statement. It not only covers (i) the multidisciplinary management of the acute post-fracture period but also encompasses (ii) the rehabilitation phase, starting immediately post-op but continuing for the rest of the patient's life and (iii) the vital business of secondary prevention—stopping the next fracture by addressing both osteoporosis and falls risk. We have come to refer to these as the three 'Clinical Pillars' of the Call to Action (CtA). To these, a fourth pillar was added—the *political* pillar of creating national multidisciplinary alliances between the relevant mainstream professional associations, which can push for the policy change and multi-professional education needed to give impetus to the first three. The CtA has brought home the fact that these four elements are all essential to tackle the problem of fragility fractures going forward. Their linkage has effectively enlarged the meaning of 'the orthogeriatric approach' to encompass all the four pillars.

The second significant development was the development of the Regionalisation Policy of the FFN. This is specifically aimed at stimulating the creation of National

FFNs (nFFNs), who have the mission to promote the implementation of the four pillars of the CtA in their country. It was devised to address the fact that the ageing trajectory, and hence the predictions of fragility fracture incidence, are worst in the emerging economies of Asia Pacific, Latin America and the Middle East, where the FFN was least well established and from where health professionals could least afford to come to meetings in Europe, where the FFN was strong and the concept of orthogeriatrics better established. However, the fact that healthcare policy can only be changed at a national level means that the rationale for nFFNs is just as valid in the mature economies of Europe, North America and elsewhere.

This strategy has been accelerated by organising the so-called Regional Expert Meetings, starting in the Asia Pacific region and continued in Latin America and Europe. By March 2020, there were 14 nFFNs, 8 of them in Asia Pacific.

At a meeting held in Oxford, following the 2019 Global Congress, the authors of the chapters in this book got together with other fragility fracture activists to consider how the second edition needed to be modified to properly take into account these developments. The conclusions reached, including the grouping of chapters in accordance with the pillars of the Call to Action, are described in Chap. 1, which functions as a guide to the book as a whole.

This edition is open access and planned to be translated into several languages; we hope that this will increase the impact of the book in stimulating positive change on the ground, to the benefit of patients.

References

1. Falaschi P, Marsh DR (2017) Orthogeriatrics. Springer, Geneva
2. Dreinhöfer KE et al (2018) A global call to action to improve the care of people with fragility fractures. Injury 49(8):1393–1397

London, UK   David Marsh
Rome, Italy   Paolo Falaschi

Contents

Part I
Background

The Multidisciplinary Approach to Fragility Fractures Around the World: An Overview

1

David Marsh, Paul Mitchell, Paolo Falaschi,
Lauren Beaupre, Jay Magaziner, Hannah Seymour,
and Matthew Costa

1.1 Introduction

The opening chapter of the first edition of this book [1] told the story of the early evolution of orthogeriatric co-management in the UK and the beginnings of its spread around the world. It covered evidence accumulated up to 2016. That history will not be repeated here. Instead, this chapter aims to provide a guide to the book as a whole, which—as well as reviewing the more recent evidence—will consider the basic competencies that an effective orthogeriatric approach should deliver and propose how they might be supplied in health economies with fewer resources, in particular fewer geriatricians.

We are considering the orthogeriatric approach in its wider sense, covering the entire post-fracture pathway, including rehabilitation and secondary prevention, as well as multidisciplinary co-management of the acute fracture episode.

Already in 2015, a significant number of published studies showed better outcomes and improved cost-effectiveness with orthogeriatric co-management [2]. As Fig. 1.1 shows, the accumulation of further evidence since then has accelerated and there have now been almost 3500 publications in the decade beginning 2010, albeit not all uniformly positive in their assessment of the approach.

This chapter is a component of Part 1: Background.
An explanation of the grouping of chapters in this book is given in this chapter.

D. Marsh (✉) · P. Mitchell · P. Falaschi · L. Beaupre · J. Magaziner · H. Seymour · M. Costa
Fragility Fracture Network, Zurich, Switzerland
e-mail: d.marsh@ucl.ac.uk; paul.mitchell@synthesismedical.com;
paolo.falaschi@fondazione.uniroma1.it; lauren.beaupre@albertahealthservices.ca; jmagazin@epi.umaryland.edu; hannah.seymour@health.wa.gov.au; matthew.costa@ndorms.ox.ac.uk

© The Author(s) 2021
P. Falaschi, D. Marsh (eds.), *Orthogeriatrics*, Practical Issues in Geriatrics,
https://doi.org/10.1007/978-3-030-48126-1_1

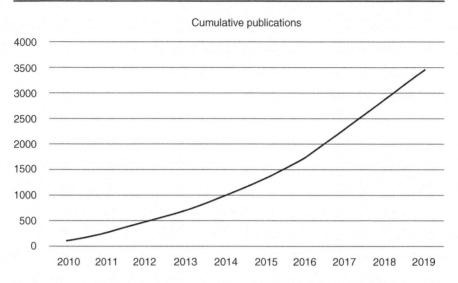

Fig. 1.1 Cumulative numbers of citations for keyword 'orthogeriatrics' in Google Scholar

One important publication in 2017 was the UN report on World Population Prospects [3]. Among other things, this gives—for each country—the **Old-Age Dependency Ratio**: *The number of people aged 65 years or older per 100 persons of working age (15–64)*. As Fig. 1.2 shows (giving Thailand as a somewhat extreme example), nothing illustrates more dramatically the suddenness of the demographic change the world will experience.

The curves are a little less steep in the developed healthcare economies because the ageing of the population has already been progressing in those territories for longer. In Africa, the ratio does not rise so high in the current century but otherwise, in most regions, levels of 40–60 are expected by 2100. Thus—at this moment in history—humankind is en route to a new demographic era.

The challenge of the ageing population, in terms of predicted population incidence of fragility fractures, is described in Chap. 2. However, the Old-Age Dependency Ratio adds a further dimension, stressing the societal consequences of ageing. The implications include:

• Society will need older people to be independent for much longer in the future. Prevention of fragility fractures and restoration of function after those fractures that do occur can make a significant contribution to that independence
• Mere survival after fracture is not going to be enough; we have to provide much more effective rehabilitation, so that 'dependency' is reduced/postponed: quality of life being more important to patients than longevity *per se*
• The change, and thus the pressure on health and social care services, is going to be extremely rapid; we have to start adapting and adopting measures immediately

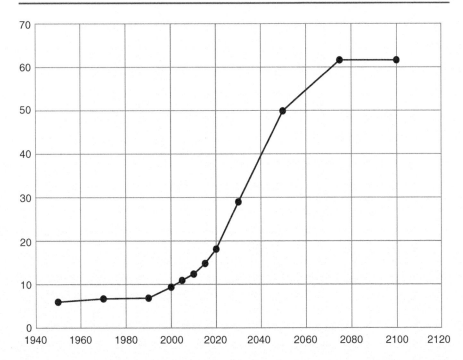

Fig. 1.2 The previous and projected Old-Age Dependency Ratio for Thailand (see text). (Data from [3], with permission)

1.2   General Developments Since 2016

The explosion of data generation indicates that clinical leaders all over the world are recognising the challenge and rising to it. However, it was also accompanied by other positive developments.

1.2.1   The Global Call to Action

At the conclusion of the 6th Global Congress of the Fragility Fracture Network (FFN) in Rome in 2016, five other organisations[1] joined with FFN in laying out their vision for the following decade of work in fragility fractures. This led to the collaborative writing of a Global Call to Action, which was published in 2018

---

[1] The European Federation of National Associations of Orthopaedics and Traumatology (EFORT), European Union Geriatric Medicine Society (EuGMS), International Collaboration of Orthopaedic Nursing (ICON), International Geriatric Fracture Society (IGFS) and the International Osteoporosis Foundation (IOF).

[4]—after it had been endorsed by 81 relevant professional associations, either international or from the countries with the largest populations (Brazil, China, India, Japan and USA). The recommendations in this paper can be summarised as four 'pillars':

1. Multidisciplinary care of the acute fracture episode along orthogeriatric lines
2. Excellent rehabilitation to recover function, independence and quality of life, starting immediately but continued long term
3. Reliable secondary prevention after every fragility fracture, addressing falls risk as well as bone health
4. Formation of multidisciplinary national alliances to promote policy change that enables the above three

Following publication, invitations to relevant national professional associations to endorse the Call to Action have been made; the total extent of global endorsement can be followed on the FFN website (www.fragilityfracturenetwork.org).

This succinct description of the entire sequence that should be triggered by a fragility fracture, plus the fourth—enabling—pillar, has effectively expanded the meaning of 'the orthogeriatric approach' to encompass the total response, not just the first phase. This integrated concept is well described by Pioli et al. [5], arguing that all elements are required in order to optimise patients' recovery from their fracture.

1.2.2   The Formation of National FFNs

The fourth pillar, multidisciplinary national alliances, took some time to achieve in the UK and other pioneer countries. Now, clinical leaders in countries wishing to take this path can speed up the process considerably by creating National FFNs. The National FFN is not the multidisciplinary national alliance *per se*—it is the catalyst to achieve it; the alliance has to be between the mainstream national professional associations, which the National FFN must never try to replace. The Memorandum of Understanding between the British Orthopaedic and Geriatrics organisations—described in the first edition [1]—is an early example of this approach.

The creation of National FFNs is considered the most effective method for ensuring that the Call to Action is actually implemented, rather than gathering dust on a shelf. The FFN is, therefore, promoting their formation, through a series of Regional Expert Meetings, where leaders from neighbouring countries can share experience, strategies for clinical and policy implementation, and encouragement. This approach constitutes the FFN's Regionalisation Strategy and its current status can also be found on the FFN website (www.fragilityfracturenetwork.org). A Guide to Formation of National FFNs is available at https://www.fragilityfracturenetwork.org/regionalisation/.

1.2.3   Initiation of New Hip Fracture Registries

A number of countries have adopted the approach pioneered in Sweden and then the UK, where a consensus agreement on quality standards for hip fracture care was accompanied by the creation of a patient-level audit tool for measurement of compliance with those standards. There is increasing evidence (reviewed in Chap. 19) that good quality audit data linked to quality indicators reduces mortality and improves the quality of life.

However, ensuring the completeness and quality of the data requires dedication and appropriate resources. Ideally, this involves the employment of clinically-trained coordinators who can advise data-entry personnel in busy fracture units. Such advisors are also ideally placed to promote the philosophy behind the quality standards and the logic of orthogeriatric co-management as the best way to deliver them. In the absence of clinical advisors, a critical analysis of the quality of data that is accumulated is needed, along with an assessment of the potential harm done by relying on data that is subsequently demonstrated to be unreliable. Certainly, the idea that the installation of a registry/audit system is some kind of magic wand—that will automatically raise the quality of care—needs to be resisted.

1.2.4   Implications of These General Developments for the Design of This Second Edition

At a meeting held in Oxford, following the 2019 Global Congress, the authors of the chapters in this book got together with other fragility fracture activists to consider how the second edition needed to be modified to properly take into account these developments. The main conclusions were:

- The chapters should be grouped according to the three clinical pillars of the Call to Action described earlier, with comprehensive cross-referencing between chapters to avoid too much repetition. The fourth pillar will be covered in other publications from the FFN
- There should be a background section covering epidemiology, osteoporosis, frailty and sarcopenia
- There should be a cross-cutting section for the role of nurses, audit and nutrition, which are relevant in all three phases
- For each of the pillars, there should be:
  - up-to-date evaluation of the current evidence for the best practice where resources are available
  - an analysis of what is really fundamental and critical to achieve in each pillar, that can be put in place even where resources are scarce
  - advice on how to progress from a minimalist implementation to a more extensive one, as experience accumulates and resources become available

- Although the book necessarily has to emphasise the *principles* within each pillar, allowing readers to shape the implementation in their healthcare system, where possible a sequence of essential practical steps towards implementation should be recommended

1.3 Background: Chaps. 2–4

1.3.1 Epidemiology of Fractures and Social Costs: Chap. 2

In addition to the re-shaping of society in terms of the Old-Age Dependency Ratio described earlier, the ageing population also has a direct effect on the population incidence of fragility fractures. This is particularly true of hip fractures, for which increasing age is a powerful risk fracture, independent of bone mineral density, and which tend to occur at later ages. Even in countries where the age-specific incidence of hip fractures is static or falling, the ageing population completely overwhelms that, so that population incidence is climbing everywhere. Chapter 2 explores that issue across the world and describes the very heavy costs of the condition, for patients, their carers and the health services.

The remaining two background issues are the underlying drivers of fragility fractures that stem from ageing: osteoporosis, which causes bone fragility (Chap. 3) and frailty, linked to sarcopenia (Chap. 4).

1.3.2 Osteoporosis in Older Patients: Chap. 3

Chapter 3 describes the basic biology of bone and how and why it deteriorates in osteoporosis. However, this does not lead to symptoms *per se*, until there is a fracture. The risk factors for fracture are manifold, in addition to the loss of bone mineral density, but there is a consistent increase in fracture risk as the T-score diminishes. Age plays a powerful role—independently of BMD, as do a history of previous fracture and a family history of fracture. The various modalities for estimating bone quality and fracture risk are discussed in this chapter (but also in Chap. 14). Similarly, the principles of treatment aimed at reducing fracture risk are covered in Chap. 3, but also in more detail in Chap. 15.

1.3.3 Frailty and Sarcopenia: Chap. 4

Frailty is a syndrome that affects the whole of an older person's physiology. As described below (Sect. 1.4), the existence of frailty in many patients presenting with fragility fractures is the prime reason for the need of orthogeriatric co-management, since the discipline of geriatric medicine specialises in it. This chapter, written by two leading European experts, defines its nature, its epidemiology and aetiology and its implications for clinical care. The prominent role of sarcopenia in frailty (analogous to that of osteoporosis in fragility) is explained.

The practical implications of frailty and sarcopenia for falls, fractures and recovery after fractures are explored, including the planning of rehabilitation and discharge from the hospital.

There are close links epidemiologically, biologically and clinically between frailty, sarcopenia, poor bone health and the geriatric syndrome of falls. Older people who have had a fall and/or a fracture should be assessed for frailty and sarcopenia to better develop a care plan. This calls for an integrated clinical approach to the prevention and treatment of fragility fractures.

1.4 Pillar I: Co-Management in the Acute Episode— Chaps. 5–11

The basic point about patients presenting with fragility fractures, especially older patients with hip fractures, is that most of them are suffering from two separate issues. The first is the *fragility* of their bone, due to osteoporosis or osteopenia, which has allowed the fracture to occur with minimal trauma. The second is *frailty*— of their whole body, which as Chap. 4 explains, weakens their capacity to respond to stress and is associated with comorbidities. It is unfortunate that several languages use the same word to describe these two entities, since they are totally different; the first being a biomechanical issue, the second physiological.

Orthopaedic surgeons are trained to deal with the fragility; geriatricians are trained to address frailty (other medical disciplines can also learn to do so). The older patients with fragility fractures, therefore, need the application of both skillsets if they are to emerge from the experience with good health and function. That is the basic argument for orthogeriatric co-management. It is expanded by the need to include other disciplines in a multidisciplinary team, particularly anaesthetists, nurses and physiotherapists.

The operative and non-operative treatment of incident fractures is clearly an enormous subject by itself, and one that is more appropriately dealt with in other publications. In this book, we have chosen two examples that illustrate important principles. The first is hip fracture, which we have chosen because (i) it is the index fracture for fragility fractures generally in much of the epidemiological and health economic literature, (ii) it accounts for the majority of in-patient costs of fragility fractures generally and (iii) it was historically, and remains, the prime setting for orthogeriatric co-management. The second is a proximal humeral fracture, which illustrates the paucity of solid evidence, in many fracture types, that operative fixation, with the maximal restoration of skeletal anatomy, leads to a better clinical result.

1.4.1 Establishing an Orthogeriatric Service: Chap. 5

Chapter 5 tackles the challenge of putting such a multidisciplinary service into practice, using a well-attested change-management methodology. It is as much a political as a medical challenge since it inescapably involves sharing between disciplines the care of patients traditionally under the sole care of one discipline—orthopaedic surgery. Diplomacy is required. This chapter describes an approach, based on eight steps:

1. Process mapping the hip fracture pathway
2. Identify a core multidisciplinary team and form a steering group
3. Analyse and review the patient pathway
4. Evaluate the resources required to drive change within the organisation
5. Develop the business case for the orthogeriatric service
6. Implementing and sustaining the service
7. Collect evidence of service improvement—Audit
8. Embrace the support of regional, national and international organisations

The sequence of chapters after that follows the patient journey in the acute episode: pre-hospital—pre-operative—anaesthetic—surgery—post-operative.

1.4.2 Pre-hospital Care and the Emergency Department: Chap. 6

Chapter 6 covers the period between the patient's injurious fall and their admission to the hospital. It is consistent with the well-developed methodology that is applied to high energy trauma victims and other emergencies, with prioritised primary and secondary surveys. There is an emphasis on rapid transfer, but with due regard to minimising pain through gentle immobilisation of the limb and gentle driving of the ambulance. History-taking at the scene and on the journey is a valuable contribution to the holistic picture of the patient and their circumstances that will guide future management and discharge. Pain relief is paramount but must not be gained at the expense of opiate overdosing. Paramedic-administered pre-hospital fascia iliaca compartment blockade can be seen on the horizon but, for the most part, that is currently something to be done once the Emergency Department has been reached.

The situation in developed countries, with short journeys in modern vehicles with highly-trained crews, is radically different from that in many low-resource settings in developing countries. There, it may be a difficult and prolonged journey to get the patient to the hospital, but the principles and goals of safety, pain-relief and adequate fluid management are universal. So the challenge is to implement effective protocols that deliver those goals as completely as possible in each setting. In some areas, every effort is made to minimise the time spent in A&E as this is a busy and often chaotic area where an immobile patient with frailty may come to harm with delirium and pressure damage. However, appropriate triage with recognition and management of acute inter-current conditions must not be missed. In contrast, in some countries, A&E physicians may take the lead in pre-operative optimisation.

1.4.3 Perioperative Orthogeriatric Care: Chaps. 7 and 11

The substantial meat of orthogeriatric wisdom and experience is to be found in Chaps. 7 and 11, covering respectively pre- and post-operative medical management. These chapters have been written by authors working in developed countries where there has been a drive to identify and proactively manage patients with frailty with the development of the specialty of geriatric medicine. Orthogeriatrics has evolved as a sub-specialty, with orthogeriatricians working closely with orthopaedic surgeons and anaesthetists, in addition to the multidisciplinary team.

These chapters are written aiming to describe gold standard management. It is important to acknowledge that many countries, and particularly those with the most significant challenges, where an epidemic of patients with hip fracture is predicted, may not have geriatric medicine as a defined specialty, and solutions to orthogeriatric care need to be imaginatively devised. This requires that the role of the orthogeriatrician be analysed and understood so that every country can find a way to ensure that patients with hip fracture and other fragility fractures, particularly in those with significant frailty, are managed appropriately.

Orthogeriatricians have often led the development of local pathways and protocols to standardise and improve care and to ensure communication between all specialists involved. This leadership role may be taken on by any member of the team but requires a real understanding of frailty and all the roles in the multidisciplinary team.

However, we must face up to the fact that there is no way that sufficient numbers of card-carrying geriatricians can be generated in time to deal with the epidemic of hip fractures that is on its way. Orthogeriatric competencies, based on recognition and understanding of frailty, *must* be inculcated in other species of health workers. There needs to be a wide army of 'Frailty Practitioners' who may, in different settings, be derived from other types of physicians or other professions such as nursing/pharmacy/physiotherapy/occupational therapy, albeit led and taught by geriatricians wherever possible. This is going to require a substantial shift in culture in many countries, where the empowerment of nurses and other healthcare professionals is an anathema. But the alternative, when the epidemiological predictions become reality, is chaos and misery.

Some key areas of orthogeriatric competency that are transferable from the discipline of geriatric medicine are:

- Skills in pre-operative assessment and optimisation of comorbidities: There is now a reasonable evidence base, as covered in Chaps. 7 and 11, that can be protocol-driven and delivered by those with basic training (junior doctors, advanced nurse practitioners) liaising with anaesthetists
- Recognition of severe frailty with limited reversibility: About a quarter of patients presenting with hip fracture are in their last year of life. Patients with significant frailty and limited physiological reserve benefit most from an early

operation and early mobilisation, aiming to reduce their high risk of complications. Setting realistic expectations—and appreciating when an operation is purely about managing pain rather than restoring mobility/independence—is crucial

- Continuity of care: The orthogeriatrician often oversees the patient's journey from admission through to discharge. This advocate role, requiring excellent communication with the patient, their family and all members of the team, is increasingly being undertaken by specialist nurses or others

Sandwiched between Chaps. 7 and 11, as they are in clinical reality—are the anaesthetic episode and the surgical intervention.

1.4.4   Orthogeriatric Anaesthesia: Chap. 8

Chapter 8 covers a lot more than the techniques of anaesthesia *per se*. The role of the anaesthetist is considered alongside that of the orthogeriatrician; after all, both are primarily interested in the patient's physiology. The goal is not just to bring the patient safely through the surgical procedure but also (i) to expedite readiness for surgery, (ii) to use the intraoperative, intensely-monitored phase to normalise the patient's physiology as far as possible, to maximise their ability to mobilise early and rehabilitate and (iii) to assist in ensuring good control of pain in all phases of the in-patient episode.

A simple key step, which can be a liberation in many fracture units, is to include anaesthetic colleagues in the definition of the consensus protocols governing the multidisciplinary management of fragility fractures requiring admission for surgery. The prime purpose of this is to secure the agreement of anaesthetic colleagues to a set of standardised procedures covering readiness for surgery and, as far as possible, the anaesthetic and pain management techniques to be deployed. An example of an issue where standardised techniques, established in consultation with orthogeriatric colleagues, can improve safety and early mobilisation, is the agreement to use only low doses of the local anaesthetic in spinal anaesthesia, to minimise the induced hypotension.

Anaesthetic practice also varies enormously across the world with access to trained practitioners, drugs, equipment and electricity lacking in some areas. There is a huge amount of work to do but, again, Chap. 8 summarises the evidence from developed countries and makes recommendations towards gold standard practice.

1.4.5   Hip Fracture: The Choice of Surgery—Chap. 9

Chapter 9 focuses on how to achieve stable fixation in the different patterns of hip fracture. As described in the first edition of this book [1], the very first paper on orthogeriatric co-management of elderly hip fracture patients, presented to the British Orthopaedic Association in 1966 was from the original orthogeriatric unit of

Devas (a surgeon) and Irvine (a geriatrician) in Hastings, UK [6]. Already, from these first 100 cases, they asserted that a successful operation needs to make it possible for the patient to mobilise, fully weight-bearing, on the first post-operative day. The bed is a dangerous place for older patients! It is disappointing how many orthopaedic surgeons around the world, over 50 years later, still insist on prolonged bed rest for their hip fracture patients, as if maintaining the pristine beauty of the post-operative X-ray is more important than the functional recovery of the patient.

1.4.6 Proximal Humeral Fractures: The Choice of Treatment—Chap. 10

Many surgeons find operating on proximal humeral fractures enjoyable and satisfying. However, the recent clinical evidence suggests that their enthusiasm is not matched by improved outcomes following operative treatment. Neither operative nor conservative management leads to a great recovery of shoulder mobility and function and the relief of pain—overwhelmingly the top priority for the patients—seems to be at least as good after non-operative management. There might, however, be a place for evidence-based surgery in older patients with fracture-dislocations, articular surface fractures and fractures with no contact between the bony fragments. Evidence from clinical trials is not of the highest quality so far, with very heterogeneous cohorts, but better-designed studies are in the pipeline; perhaps 'big data' from registries may give further insights.

1.5 Pillar II: Rehabilitation—Chaps. 12 and 13

As pointed out in Sect. 1.1 of this chapter, one of the implications of the rapidly-increasing Old-Age Dependency Ratio is that we need to provide much more effective rehabilitation after a fragility fracture, so that 'dependency' is reduced/postponed. A complementary dimension is that, to the extent that post-fracture patients do become dependent, their care is going to devolve increasingly to family caregivers, since the volume of cases will overwhelm existing services in all countries.

1.5.1 Rehabilitation Following Hip Fracture: Chap. 12

As noted above, in Sect. 1.4.5, the most immediate goal after hip fracture surgery should be early—next-day—mobilisation. It will take time to convince surgeons in some countries that this is so. However, that is just the beginning; there needs to be a planned, individualised rehabilitation programme that starts in the hospital and carries on for an extended period—basically for the rest of the patient's life—after discharge. Ideally, this should be delivered by a multidisciplinary team, integrating physical therapy with social support, nutrition advice and so on. It is important that the team meets to review progress and gives the patient a sense of coordination—and optimism. Chapter 12 is an exhaustive review of the current evidence about what rehabilitative measures are effective.

Recognising that large rehabilitation teams will not be available in many low- and middle-income countries, implementation strategies for those settings, including input from families, are suggested.

The point is made that cognitively-impaired patients are among those who benefit most from robust programmes and must not be excluded from rehabilitation efforts.

1.5.2   The Psychological Health of Patients and Their Caregivers: Chap. 13

The physical and emotional burden of looking after an elderly relative with some degree of disablement is considerable. As might intuitively be expected, there is now good evidence that the physical and psychological health of post-fracture patients and their caregivers are interdependent. Chapter 13 addresses the issue of how their status can be assessed and how the orthogeriatric team can help.

1.6   Pillar III: Secondary Prevention—Chaps. 14–16

As most readers of this book will know: (i) having a fragility fracture increases the risk of another one—'fracture begets fracture'; (ii) half of all hip fractures have been preceded by a previous fragility fracture and (iii) the risk of recurrent fracture is greatest in the first year the 'imminent refracture'. The obvious consequence of these facts is that the response to a patient presenting with any fragility fracture is not complete until there has been a determined attempt to prevent another one. This must address both osteoporosis and falls risk and it must happen as quickly as possible after the incident fragility fracture.

If this is done reliably, given that current treatments reduce fracture risk by around 50%, there is the potential to prevent 25% of subsequent hip fractures; as treatments improve, this should increase. The fact that it is *not* done reliably—with a 'treatment gap' in the order of 80%—means that the burning issue right now is the need for reconfiguration of fracture services to capture every fragility fracture and link them to the appropriate bone health and falls prevention services.

1.6.1   Fracture Liaison Services: Chap. 14

The basic model for achieving this is very clear and well-documented—it is the Fracture Liaison Service. Chapter 14 focuses on how such a service should assess the magnitude of the risk of another fracture and initiate action to reduce that risk.

It explains how such a service can be created, whatever the level of resources in any given location. Like orthogeriatric co-management generally, it is more a matter of changing attitudes than spending money. This chapter is written by leading drivers of the Capture the Fracture® campaign of the International Osteoporosis Foundation.

1.6.2 Current and Emerging Treatment of Osteoporosis: Chap. 15

Chapter 15 focuses on the pharmacological treatment of osteoporosis: the indications for it and the prospects for more powerful treatments than we have previously enjoyed. Gold standards of assessment in developed economies include measurement of bone mineral density, in younger fracture patients, by DXA scan; this will not be available in many low-resource settings. The authors suggest that, in such settings, the fact that a fragility fracture has already occurred can be considered sufficient grounds for initiating anti-resorptive treatment—even in younger patients. This is controversial, but all would agree that the possibility should be considered, and the decision be made on clinical judgement.

1.6.3 How Can We Prevent Falls?—Chap. 16

Whatever the degree of fragility conferred on the bones by osteoporosis, the vast majority of fragility fractures are nonetheless precipitated by falls (vertebral fractures being the obvious exception). The evidence base for fracture prevention by falls risk reduction is meagre compared to that for osteoporosis treatment because there has so far not been the commercial imperative for the industry to fund large scale trials. This may change whenever a realistic anti-sarcopenia agent becomes available.

However, Chap. 16 summarises a gradually-accumulating body of evidence about how an individual's risk of falling may be classified as low, intermediate or high and what treatment programmes are effective for each category. This body of evidence is related to that exhaustively described in Chap. 12—rehabilitation after hip fracture.

There is understandably great concern about falls that occur in care settings and it is recommended that all in-patients over the age of 65 be considered and treated as high risk. Patients with cognitive impairment may require special attention in addition to the high-risk programme; in advanced dementia, recurrent falls indicate the need for palliative care.

In post-fracture cases, falls clinics and programmes need to be linked to the Fracture Liaison Service and fall risk and bone health should always be considered together.

1.7   Cross-Cutting Issues: Chaps. 17–19

The nursing role, nutrition and fracture audit systems are relevant in all three clinical pillars.

1.7.1   Nursing in the Orthogeriatric Setting: Chap. 17

Attitudes to nurses, and what they may be capable of, vary widely across the globe. In some developed economies, they have been significantly empowered, based on models of advanced training, protocol-driven care and supervision by appropriate medical specialists. This includes, in many locations, the ability to order investigations and treatments within protocols. By contrast, there are many countries where such autonomy would be anathema. What is very clear, and needs to be asserted as frequently as possible, is that the volume of fragility fracture-related work—already now but more so in the future—is such that it cannot realistically be delivered without enhanced nurse input. There is *no* prospect that there will be (i) enough geriatricians on the planet to deliver orthogeriatric surveillance of all older fracture inpatients on a daily basis or (ii) enough endocrinologists for every fragility fracture patient to be assessed for secondary prevention by a doctor.

This chapter explores the key nursing roles and interventions relating to orthogeriatric nursing care. It considers how nursing care quality, focused on nurse-specific indicators, skill, education, leadership and resources, can positively impact patient outcomes in all phases of the care journey. The central nursing role in preventing and managing complications is specifically outlined.

1.7.2   Nutritional Care of the Older Patient with Fragility Fracture: Chap. 18

Nutrition is a subject that can be very complex in the elderly. Chapter 18 opts for the SIMPLE approach:

S	Screen for nutrition risk
I	Interdisciplinary assessment
M	Make the diagnosis (es)
P	Plan with the patient
L	impLement interventions
E	Evaluate ongoing care requirements

The essence of this approach is that, rather than requiring a highly-specialised nutritionist, a systematic assessment on the part of all the disciplines that are interacting with the patients can achieve what is needed for the nutritional care of the older patient with a fragility fracture, regardless of setting or healthcare provider.

1.7.3   Fragility Fracture Audit: Chap. 19

Fragility fracture audit is key to understanding fragility fracture management, identifying areas for its improvement, and measuring the impact of clinical initiatives and service change. A hip fracture can be considered a marker for fragility fractures, and hip fracture audits indirectly show the strengths and weaknesses of fragility fracture care overall. Notably, where effective hip fracture care exists, this has a favourable impact on the care of other fragility fractures. Early established audits, clinically led, have used clinical standards and feedback on compliance with them to improve care and outcomes. Although data collection, analysis and feedback require investment, the cost per case amounts to only a very small fraction of the cost of care per case.

Because patients with fractures requiring surgical intervention, such as hip fractures, are available for some time in the hospital, it is relatively easy to collect the data needed for a registry or audit database. Capturing the necessary data for secondary prevention is a lot harder, between the fleeting outpatient clinic visits and the variable passage from secondary to primary care settings. It is also complex to link databases in such a way that recurrent fractures are reliably captured and matched with data describing secondary prevention interventions. Nonetheless, this problem must be solved, if we are ever to have the evidence needed to persuade healthcare funders to commission reliable Fracture Liaison Services for the long term. This is likely to be one of the main developments in the following phase of fragility fracture service evolution.

1.8   Concluding Remarks

Demographic change over the following decades presents significant challenges in many areas of medicine. However, the strong association between age, skeletal fragility and physiological frailty mean that fragility fractures will feature very prominently in that development. Furthermore, the need to extend the period of independence in people's longer lives drives us to realise that we need to (i) prevent as many fractures as possible—in which secondary prevention represents the lowest-hanging fruit and (ii) treat those that do occur in the most cost-effective way possible, with full regard to recovery of function.

Hopefully, the chapters of this book summarise the current (2020) state of these arts adequately. But equally hopefully, they will be out of date pretty soon, as progress is made.

While the book will remain as it is until a subsequent edition, the FFN will maintain, on its website www.fragilityfracturenetwork.org, two toolkits that will complement the book and be updated as experience grows. One is a Clinical Toolkit, which is concerned with the practical implementation of Pillars I–III, as described in most of the chapters of this book. The other is a Policy Toolkit, which expands Chap. 1—particularly Sect. 1.2—in other words the fourth pillar of the healthcare policy change and the work of the National FFNs.

References

1. Marsh D (2017) The orthogeriatric approach—progress worldwide. In: Falaschi P, Marsh D (eds) Orthogeriatrics. Springer International, Cham
2. Sabharwal S, Wilson H (2015) Orthogeriatrics in the management of frail older patients with a fragility fracture. Osteoporos Int 26:2387–2399
3. Department of Economic and Social Affairs, Population Division (2017) World Population Prospects: The 2017 Revision. Volume II: Demographic Profiles. United Nations, New York.
4. Dreinhöfer KE (2018) A global call to action to improve the care of people with fragility fractures. Injury 49:1393–1397
5. Pioli G et al (2018) Orthogeriatric co-management—managing frailty as well as fragility. Injury 49:1398–1402
6. Devas RE, Irvine MB (1967) The geriatric orthopaedic unit. J Bone Jt Surg 49:186–187

Epidemiology of Fragility Fractures and Social Impact

2

Nicola Veronese, Helgi Kolk, and Stefania Maggi

2.1 Introduction

Ageing is becoming the next public health challenge worldwide. According to WHO data, the proportion of the population more than 60 years will nearly double from 12% in 2015 to 22% in 2050. By 2050, this population age group is expected to increase from the current 900 million to 2 billion, 80% of these people living in low- and middle-income countries [1]. Understanding the trends of age-related diseases has an important role in healthcare policy. Musculoskeletal disorders are among the most common problems affecting the elderly, with osteoporosis and osteoporotic fractures leading the field [2].

This chapter is a component of Part 1: Background.
For an explanation of the grouping of chapters in this book, please see Chapter 1: 'The Multidisciplinary Approach to Fragility Fractures Around the World—An Overview'.

N. Veronese
National Research Council, Neuroscience Institute, Aging Branch, Padova, Italy

Geriatric Unit, Department of Internal Medicine and Geriatrics, University of Palermo, Palermo, Italy

H. Kolk
Geriatric Unit, Department of Internal Medicine and Geriatrics, University of Palermo, Palermo, Italy

Department of Traumatology and Orthopaedics, University of Tartu, Tartu, Estonia
e-mail: helgi.kolk@kliinikum.ee

S. Maggi (✉)
National Research Council, Neuroscience Institute, Aging Branch, Padova, Italy
e-mail: stefania.maggi@in.cnr.it

© The Author(s) 2021
P. Falaschi, D. Marsh (eds.), *Orthogeriatrics*, Practical Issues in Geriatrics,
https://doi.org/10.1007/978-3-030-48126-1_2

Osteoporosis, defined by WHO as bone densitometry (DXA) T-scores less than −2.5 at the lumbar spine or femoral neck and microarchitectural deterioration of bone tissue, is recognised as a major public health issue through its association with fragility fractures, particularly of the hip, vertebrae, wrist and upper arm. Sarcopenia is generally understood as an age-dependent decline in muscle mass combined with low muscle strength and/or low physical performance. The combination of osteoporosis and sarcopenia is known as osteosarcopenia, which contributes to frailty, poor balance, falls and fragility fractures [3]. Fragility fractures have been defined as fractures that occur after minimal trauma (falling from a standing height or less) or without considerable trauma. Several factors contribute to the development of fragility fractures, two major groups are those affecting/decreasing bone mineral density (BMD) and increasing the rate of falls. To provide comprehensive care to older adults, particularly with attention to musculoskeletal health, clinicians must assess and manage different aspects, including osteosarcopenia and falls.

Please refer to Chaps. 3 and 15 for the management of osteoporosis in older patients and to Chap. 16 for the prevention of falls.

Fragility fractures may have a negative impact on the quality of life of older people and their families due to loss of independence and may also lead to disability and death. Significant geographic variation occurs in the age-specific incidence in osteoporotic fractures worldwide (Fig. 2.1), with Western populations (Europe, North America and Oceania) reporting an increase in hip fracture incidence during the second half of the twentieth century and a decline since 2000 [4, 5]. However, even in these countries, the fall in age-specific incidence is far outweighed by the ageing demographic described earlier, so population incidence continues to rise [6]. Osteoporosis and sarcopenia are frequently underdiagnosed and thus undertreated, even persons with proven bone mineral density loss and previous fragility fracture do not receive appropriate treatment to prevent

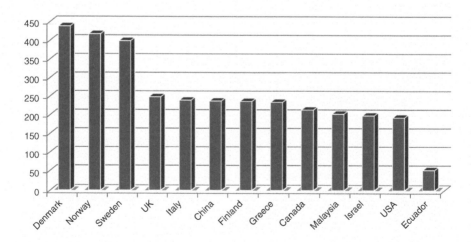

Fig. 2.1 Age-standardised hip fracture incidence rates (/100,000) for some representative countries

subsequent fractures. On the other hand, there is much current debate on what is the target population that may potentially benefit from treatments acting on bone metabolism [6].

The total costs of osteoporosis are difficult to calculate as cost estimates are based on many assumptions, making a comparison between countries and different healthcare systems challenging. In addition to direct medical costs in acute care of osteoporotic fractures and medications, these costs also include work-absence of family caregivers and long-term care of elderly fracture patients. The economic impact of hip fractures, the most detrimental of osteoporotic fractures, has been widely investigated, however, few studies have utilised the same instruments. Recovery from a fragility fracture can be influenced by social factors but might itself influence social activity and family relationships [7].

The objective of this chapter is to review and describe the epidemiology of osteoporosis and fragility fractures, highlighting the costs to society and the individual.

2.2 Prevalence of Osteoporosis

The WHO Osteoporosis Working Group and other international osteoporosis organisations have stated that the femoral neck is the only site that should be used in the estimation of osteoporosis prevalence at a population level. Osteoporosis is diagnosed using dual-energy X-ray absorptiometry (DXA), which measures bone mineral density (BMD) of the femoral neck. BMD is one of the most used tools for the management of osteoporosis, being used for diagnosis, fracture risk assessment, selection of patients for treatment and treatment monitoring [2]. According to the criterion set by a WHO Working Group, osteoporosis is diagnosed when the BMD at the femoral neck is 2.5 standard deviations or more below the average BMD of the young white female population. Accurate estimates of the prevalence of osteoporosis require country-specific data on the distribution of femoral neck BMD, for most studies, it is assumed that the mean femoral neck BMD is similar between countries at the age of 50 years and also the bone loss is similar [2]. Based on these estimates approximately 5.5 million osteoporotic men and more than 22 million osteoporotic women resided in the EU27 in 2010, that is, there were four times as many women with osteoporosis as there were men. Of all countries in the EU27, Germany was estimated to have the highest number of individuals with osteoporosis with approximately 1 million osteoporotic men and 4 million osteoporotic women. Overall the prevalence of osteoporosis was 6.6% and 22.1% in men and women aged 50 years or more and 5.5% in the general population of the EU. In males aged 50 years or more, the prevalence of osteoporosis varied from 5.7% in Slovakia to 6.9% in Greece, Italy and Sweden. The corresponding data for females were 19.3% in Bulgaria and 23.4% in Italy [2]. The prevalence of osteoporosis increased progressively with age, although the absolute number of individuals with osteoporosis increases less markedly. When stratifying the population between ages 50 and 80 in 5-year age groups, the highest number of women with osteoporosis (approximately 3.9 million) was observed in the 75–79 year age group, for men the highest estimated number was in the age group of 60–64 years (approximately 0.8 million) [2].

According to a review published in 2016, in East Asia (Hong Kong, Japan, Macau, Mongolia, North Korea, the People's Republic of China, South Korea and Taiwan) osteoporosis is recognised as a growing problem because of the rapidly increasing number of older people [8]. China has the largest aged population in the world, as the population aged more than 60 years will reach 400 million (approximately 30% of the total population) by 2050. In Japan, the percentage of the population aged more than 65 years rose from 10.3% in 1985 to 20.1% in 2005; this percentage is expected to double by 2050 [8]. Studies from the Chinese mainland, Hong Kong and Taiwan published between 1990 and 2017 have reported various prevalence rates of osteoporosis due to different reference values (US and Asian) and age groups; a clear tendency of increase in prevalence with age was recorded with osteoporosis affecting more than one-third of people aged 50 years and older. Variable osteoporosis prevalence was reported across Chinese cities before 2002: Jilin (15.5%) > Shanghai (14.2%) > Sichuan (11.3%) > Guangzhou (10.2%) > Beijing (5.2%). According to studies by Zhang et al., with a cut-off value of − 2.5 SD, osteoporosis prevalence increased from 6.37% in women aged 40–50 years to 76.74% in those aged 80–90 years [9]. A higher prevalence of osteoporosis was demonstrated in the female population and residents of northern China [9].

In Hong Kong, osteoporosis prevalence in women aged more than 50 years was 16% at the total hip, while in men the figure was 6% in 2005. In earlier studies (published in 1999) the prevalence of osteoporosis in Hong Kong was significantly higher than in the mainland at the same time. The prevalence of osteoporosis in Taiwan was comparable to that in the Chinese mainland [9].

The data on the prevalence of osteoporosis among women in India come from studies conducted in small groups spread across the country. The estimates suggested that out of the 230 million Indians expected to be over the age of 50 years in 2015, 20%, that is, ~46 million were women with osteoporosis. Thus, osteoporosis is a major public health problem in Indian women [10].

The reported prevalence of osteoporosis among postmenopausal women in Brazil varies from 15% to 33%, depending on the study methodology and the use of bone densitometry data or self-reporting by participants. However, recent studies using DXA report similar prevalence data to other countries [11].

Prevalence estimates of osteoporosis or low bone mass at the femoral neck or lumbar spine (adjusted by age, sex, and race/ethnicity to the 2010 Census, defined by WHO criteria) for the non-institutionalised population age 50 years and older were applied to determine the total number of older US residents with osteoporosis and low bone mass [12]. There were over 99 million adults 50 years and older in the US in 2010. Based on an overall 10.3% prevalence of osteoporosis, the estimated number of older adults having osteoporosis was 10.2 million in 2010, women and non-Hispanic Whites having the largest counts. The prevalence of osteoporosis was higher in men 80+ (10.9%) compared to men 50–59 years of age (3.4%); however, due to the decrease in male population counts by age, the estimated number of men with osteoporosis was lower by age: 0.7 million in the 50–59 group and 0.4 million in the 80+ group [12].

2.3   Factors Affecting Bone Mineral Density

Non-modifiable factors negatively affecting BMD and bone microstructure include older age, female sex, White race, personal and parental history of osteoporosis and fractures, and low body frame size. The known modifiable risk factors for osteoporosis include low calcium intake, reduced exposure to sunlight, prolonged immobility, excessive alcohol intake, smoking, eating disorders, long time immobility, low body mass index (BMI) and low physical activity. Several medications (glucocorticoids, PPI, anticonvulsants, chemotherapy of breast and prostatic cancer) require special attention: if these cannot be avoided, the length of treatment courses should be modified and measures to prevent the progression of osteoporosis need to be taken. The same risk factors are generally included in the FRAX model for the assessment of fracture probability [2, 13].

2.4   Osteosarcopenia

Prevalence rates of sarcopenia vary greatly due to different definitions, tools of diagnosis, and patient populations. Prevalence rates utilising the European Working Group on Sarcopenia in Older People (EWGSOP) definition vary from 1 to 29% in elderly community-dwelling populations and from 14 to 33% in long-term care populations [14]. Advanced age consistently appears to be a risk factor for sarcopenia. In most studies that reported gender, there was no significant association with sarcopenia prevalence. Nursing home residents, patients with hip fracture and these more than 80 years have higher rates of diagnosis [14].

Epidemiological measures of osteosarcopenia are fairly limited due to the recent origin of the term. A study of 680 elderly adults with a history of falls found an osteosarcopenia prevalence of 37%, with these patients having a higher frequency of comorbidities, impaired mobility and depression [15].

2.5   Falls

Age is one of the key risk factors for falls. Older people have the highest risk of death or serious injury arising from a fall and the risk increases with age. For example, in the US, 20 to 30% of older people who fall suffer moderate to severe injuries such as bruises, hip fractures, or head trauma (WHO). An estimated 95% of hip fractures are due to falls [16]. However, data on the prevalence and incidence of falls among the elderly are heterogeneous as there is no international consensus for assessing the fall risk profile of older people even for people at high risk of falls. People aged 75 or older, those who have fallen during the previous 12 months or those who have fear of falling or significant gait, muscle strength, or balance problems constitute the group of highest fall risk. The fall risk profile is also dependent on the setting and some other factors, including cognitive impairment. Even though a decline in balance, gait and muscle function increase the risk of falling, the relationship is not completely linear since those with most problems (i.e. bedridden) usually have a lower falls risk, similar to those without such problems, presumably due to low exposure to risk [2].

Knowledge of factors that predispose older persons to falls is important for tailoring appropriate preventive interventions. This is covered in more depth in Chap. 16.

2.6   Incidence of Fragility Fractures

Osteoporosis is clinically significant in the fractures that occur as a consequence of increased bone fragility. Although low BMD identifies individuals at increased risk of fracture, the majority of fragility fractures occur in individuals who have less marked reductions in bone mass or normal BMD, which means that other factors independent of BMD, such as the geometric and microarchitectural properties of the bone itself, and an individual's clinical risk factors, contribute to fracture risk [13]. The definition of an osteoporotic fracture is not straightforward, opinions differ concerning the inclusion or exclusion of different sites of fracture (most common are the forearm, hip, spine, proximal humerus) of fracture and also possible causative mechanisms [2]. One approach is to consider all fractures from low energy trauma as being osteoporotic. Low energy trauma is defined as a fall from a standing height or less, or trauma that in a healthy individual would not result in fracture [16]. The rising incidence of fractures with age might be caused by the rising incidence of falls and be multifactorial. The approach used in the report "Osteoporosis in the European Union" published by E. Hernlund and group in 2013 by and elsewhere is to characterise fracture sites as osteoporotic when they are associated with low bone mass and their incidence rises with age after of 50 years of age [2].

As hip fracture patients are treated in hospitals, the reports of incidence of hip fracture are more commonly available than reports of other sites of fractures [2]. Identifying the number of individuals at high fracture risk has value for future health resource allocation. Information on the incidence of fragility fractures varies between EU countries, as well as worldwide (Fig. 2.1). According to the calculations of the International Osteoporosis Foundation [2], there was marked heterogeneity in hip fracture risk between EU 27 countries: in women, the lowest annual incidences were found in Romania and Poland with the highest rates observed in Denmark and Sweden. There was an approximately three-fold range in hip fracture incidence which is somewhat lower than the tenfold range worldwide, but still substantial. The reason for the variation in hip fracture rates between countries is not known. Socio-economic prosperity seems to be one of the influencing factors, with higher hip fracture rates in countries with higher GDP.

In developing populations, however, particularly in Asia, the rates of osteoporotic fracture appear to be increasing [8, 13]. The lifetime risk for hip, vertebral and forearm (wrist) fractures has been estimated to be approximately 40%, similar to that for coronary heart disease.

It has been estimated that in 2010 there were 21 million men and 137 million women aged 50 years or more at high fracture risk and that this number is expected to double by 2040, with the increase predominantly borne by Asia [13].

2.7 Hip Fracture

Hip fractures are an important cause of disability and death around the world, especially amongst older people. Studies have shown heterogeneity in annual age-standardised hip fracture rates globally (Fig. 2.1). The systematic review, published in 2012, used a literature survey covering a 50-year period and UN data on population demography [4]. By this review, the highest annual age-standardised hip fracture incidences (per 100,000 person-years) were observed in Scandinavia: Denmark (574), Norway (563) and Sweden (539), also in Austria (501). The lowest rates were detected in Tunisia (58) and Ecuador (73). North-Western Europe, Central Europe, the Russian Federation and Middle-East countries (Iran, Kuwait, Oman), Hong Kong, Singapore and Taiwan were high-risk countries for the hip fracture. Low-risk regions included Latin America (except for Argentina), Africa, and Saudi Arabia. There was around a tenfold range in hip fracture incidence worldwide, with the overall age-standardised incidence in men being half that of women [4, 13].

The highest incidence of hip fracture was observed mainly in countries furthest from the equator and in countries with extensive coverage of the skin due to religious or cultural practices, suggesting that vitamin D status might be an important factor underlying this distribution [4].

The aforenamed systematic review reported the age-standardised annual incidence of hip fractures to be higher in Hong Kong, Japan, South Korea and Taiwan than in the United States and some European countries [4]. This is in contrast to a study two decades ago that showed the hip fracture incidence to be higher in the United States compared to Hong Kong [17]. For women, Taiwan was in the high-incidence category (incidence >300/100,000), ranking number 9 among 61 countries/regions. Hong Kong, Japan and South Korea were in the medium-incidence category (200–300/100,000), ranking 23, 32 and 34, respectively. China was in the low-incidence category (<200/100,000). For men, Japan, Korea and Taiwan were among the high-incidence countries (>150/100,000), while China and Hong Kong were in the moderate-incidence category (100–150/100,000) [4, 8].

The reasons for the large variation in age- and sex-adjusted hip fracture incidence worldwide are not clear. Genetic differences, environmental factors and treatment of osteoporosis might have a role. Interestingly, people living in the Mediterranean area have a lower incidence of fractures. This seems to be attributable to several factors, particularly higher serum 25-hydroxy vitamin D (25OHD) levels and healthier lifestyle [18]. Recent research highlights the role for a Mediterranean diet since the dietary pattern is associated with lower inflammation levels, lower adiposity and decreased risk of falls, all these factors being important for the development of hip fracture [19].

The total number of persons affected by hip fractures may be increasing over time in the following years, mainly due to the progressive ageing of the population. According to a conservative estimate, the annual number of hip fractures will increase from 1.66 million in 1990 to 6.26 million in 2050 [13]. Hip fracture rates appeared to have plateaued or decreased during the last one to two decades in many developed countries, following a rise in preceding years; however, in the developing world, age- and sex-specific rates are still rising in many areas [2, 8, 13]. In studies reporting a lower incidence of age- and sex-specific incidence hip fracture over time, possible explanations seem to be a higher adherence to anti-osteoporotic medications as well as increased use of calcium and vitamin D supplementation, avoidance of smoking and alcohol, and more efficacious strategies for the prevention of falls [20].

Technical reasons, such as inaccurate coding and recording of fractures and poor access to medical services in some regions might be part of the explanation of high variability in hip fracture incidence. According to the *Eastern European & Central Asian Regional Audit: Epidemiology, Costs and Burden of Osteoporosis in 2010*, in Georgia, 75% of patients with hip fracture are not hospitalised and, in Kazakhstan and Kyrgyzstan, 50% are not hospitalised due to poor access to surgical services and non-affordable medical care [13].

In summary, with a few exceptions, age-specific incidence rates of hip fracture significantly rose in Western populations until 1980 with subsequent stability or even a decrease. In Western countries, the trends seem to be more pronounced in women than in men [16]. However, confirmation is needed, by further longitudinal studies (particularly in non-white populations) to clarify in which direction we are moving. Moreover, the mean age of sustaining a hip fracture is increasing, meaning that this event is increasingly associated with disability and mortality, possibly because patients have more medical comorbidities.

2.8   Other Osteoporotic Fractures

From an epidemiological perspective, distal radius fractures are typical of the paediatric population, up to 25% of fractures in children involve the distal end of the radius, in older people up to 18% of all fractures involve the wrist [21]. The most common distal forearm fracture is a Colles' fracture. This fracture lies within 2.5 cm of the wrist joint margin and is associated with dorsal angulation and displacement of the distal fragment of the radius. It may be accompanied by a fracture of the ulna styloid process [2]. Forearm fractures account for a greater proportion in younger adults than the elderly. Conversely, hip fractures are rare at the age of 50 years but become the predominant osteoporosis fracture from the age of 75 years. In women, the median age for distal forearm fractures is around 65 years and for hip fracture, 80 years [2].

Vertebral fractures are the most common single osteoporotic fractures worldwide, these occur in 30–50% of people more than the age of 50 [22]. In contrast to hip fractures, many factors limit the availability of reliable information on their epidemiology: two-thirds to three-fourths of vertebral fractures are clinically silent and less than 10% require hospital admission, which itself may vary due to geographic differences in access to healthcare.

For example, in a study involving about 1000 hospitalised persons of older age, chest radiographs were assessed for various reasons. Of importance, moderate (25–40% height loss) or severe (>40% height loss) vertebral fractures were scored in 14% women by trained radiologists in a reference centre, but only half were reported in the X-ray report by the local radiologists [23]. This is often due to the scarce knowledge among radiologists in recognising asymptomatic vertebral fractures, the lack of any relevant signs or symptoms and/or the presence of other medical conditions for which a chest/abdomen X-ray was done that requires more attention (e.g. pneumonia or cancer) [23]. However, asymptomatic vertebral fractures are of importance since they represent a potential risk factor for symptomatic fractures and they are associated with a higher rate of disability and mortality, particularly in those having secondary forms of osteoporosis, such as glucocorticoid-induced osteoporosis [23].

In Europe, studies in men and women aged more than 50 years report that the incidence of clinical vertebral fracture is higher in men than women under 55 years, but that the risk rises in women after the age of 60 years [24]. The age-specific incidence of radiographic vertebral fracture (symptomatic or not) is estimated to be 2–2.5-fold higher in women than in men, being significantly higher in Scandinavia than in other European countries. It is reported that the incidence of vertebral fractures is highest at T12 and L1, second highest at L2 and L3, and third highest at T7 through T9 and at L4 [24]. However, the age-adjusted incidence may vary substantially from country to country. Some of these differences may be due to different patterns of clinical presentation and differences in vertebral fracture ascertainment in the studies that were used for calculating the incidence, rather than true differences in fracture incidence across countries. For example, symptomatic vertebral fracture rates seem to be particularly high in the United States, but the population-based study on which of these estimates are calculated included vertebral fractures discovered incidentally on lateral spine imaging obtained for other clinical reasons, not only for assessing vertebral fractures as was the case in European countries [25].

In terms of prevalence data, it is estimated that, in both men and women, prevalence linearly increases with age independently of country, with some data suggesting that almost half of very old people (i.e. ageing >85 years) are affected by a vertebral fracture [24].

2.9   The Burden of Fragility Fractures

Measurement of the burden of diseases and injuries is a crucial input into health policy. The burden of osteoporosis in the 27 EU countries in 2010 was characterised by 22 million women and 5.5 million men to have osteoporosis; and 3.5 million new fragility fractures were sustained, comprising 610,000 hip fractures, 520,000 vertebral fractures, 560,000 forearm fractures and 1,800,000 other fractures [2]. The greatest burden of hip fractures around the world is expected to occur in East Asia, especially China [8].

Information on the burden of osteoporosis in Latin American countries is limited. When analysing data in four Latin American countries [26] more than 840,000 osteoporosis-related fractures were predicted to occur in 2018, amounting to a total annual cost of ~1.17 billion USD. The total projected 5-year cost was ~6.25 billion USD. Annual costs were highest in Mexico (411 million USD), followed by Argentina (360 million USD), Brazil (310 million USD), and Colombia (94 million USD). The average burden per 1000 at risk was greatest in Argentina (32,583 USD), followed by Mexico (16,671 USD), Colombia (8240 USD), and Brazil (6130 USD). In the following 5 years, about four and half million fractures are anticipated to occur in these four countries.

To control and prevent these fractures, stakeholders must work together to close the care gap, particularly in secondary prevention. Indeed, all international scientific bodies agree upon the clinical recommendations to close the gap after a hip fracture, mainly: communicating with patients about their risks of future fractures and how to prevent them, by offering osteoporosis medications, improving long-term treatment persistence and assessing the risk of falls in routine follow-up visits [26].

2.10   The Costs and Social Impact of Hip Fracture

Hip fractures constitute a significant public health problem worldwide, and is associated with high rates of disability and mortality. Since hip fracture incidence increases linearly with advancing age and older people are expected to represent a growing proportion of the worldwide population in the near future, the costs of hip fracture will increase. Overall, hip fracture seems to be comparable to other disease groups, such as cardiovascular, in terms of hospitalisation and rehabilitation. However, other social costs, due to the onset of new comorbidities, sarcopenia, poor quality of life, disability and mortality are probably greater. Hip fracture and its surgical treatment predispose frail older persons to decompensation of chronic diseases, as well as complications such as anaemia, pneumonia, delirium, UTI and thromboembolic events.

Patients who have a hip fracture are at considerable risk for premature death. There has been no change in mortality rates for hip fractures since the last three decades, despite advancements in surgical solutions and the fact that the majority of patients in the developed economies are now operated on [27]. A report of osteoporosis in the European Union estimated that mortality related to low-impact trauma hip fracture is greater than road traffic accidents and equivalent to breast cancer [2]. The increased mortality risk after the hip fracture may persist for several years thereafter [28]. Patients experiencing hip fractures after low-impact trauma are at considerable risk for subsequent osteoporotic fractures and premature death [28].

In contrast to other types of fragility fracture (e.g. vertebral), hip fractures usually need immediate intervention and consequent hospitalisation. The mean duration of hospitalisation is highly variable dependent on local healthcare systems and populations studied.

A recent systematic review [29] has found that costs during the first year after the hip fracture ($43,669) are greater than equivalent estimates for the acute coronary syndrome ($32,345) and ischaemic stroke ($34,772). A systematic review of the costs of fragility hip fractures and key drivers of the differences in hip fracture costs between 1990 and 2015 analysed data of 670,173 patients from 27 different countries (mostly North America and Western Europe) [29]. The estimate for total health and social care costs in the first year following hip fracture was $43,669 per patient. High variability was found between regions but also inside the country: in the United States, the costs of medical care in the 12 months ranged from $21,259 to $44,200. Inpatient care was with the highest cost, estimated at $13,331. The mean length of stay for the index hospitalisation was 8.6 days and varied significantly by region. Studies from North America reported the shortest mean length of stay, whilst studies from Asia had the longest length of stay. Inpatient cost was followed by the cost of rehabilitation care, estimated at $12,020. The high costs of rehabilitation might be biased as a limited number of studies in this category were available with a very high cost from one study [29].

Comorbidities prior to fracture were associated with significantly higher costs in 80% of studies. Developing a complication after hip fracture was associated with significantly higher costs in 93% of studies assessing this variable. Gender, year of study, US studies and length of stay were significantly associated with costs. In studies outside the United States, the mean cost per patient was $3304 less per additional day of length of stay compared to the United States. On average, cases in females were found to be statistically significantly less expensive than in men, costing $134 less per patient. Studies published more recently were significantly associated with lower costs: authors suggested that this might represent changes in clinical practice and fewer complications, as well as methodological changes [29].

Saving hospital costs by reducing the length of stay could be an important factor to diminish the expenditure on hip fracture management. Data from the Swedish National Patient Register, published in 2015, indicate that shorter length of hospital stay was associated with an increased risk of death after discharge in older hip fracture patients (mean age 82 years) with the length of stay 10 days less. In this study, the discharge placement was not available, but the authors suggest that the quality of rehabilitation in the early postoperative period might have influenced the outcome as reductions in length of stay will probably result in more complications occurring after discharge. Furthermore, shorter length of stay reduces the time available for the comprehensive geriatric assessment (CGA) during hospital stay [30]. CGA has been shown to decrease the risks of complications and death after discharge in elderly hip fracture patients.

In contrast, a study in the United States by Nikkel et al. demonstrated that decreased length of stay was associated with reduced rates of early mortality [31]. A total of 188,208 patients admitted to hospital for hip fracture in New York state from 2000 to 2011, with 169,258 treated surgically and 18,950 treated non-surgically, were analysed. The average length of hospital stay was 8.1 days; during the study, the average length of stay decreased from 12.9 days in 2000 to 5.6 days in 2011. The 30-day mortality rate for surgically-treated hip fracture patients was 4.5%. A shorter hospital stay (<5 days and <10 days) was associated with decreased 30-day mortality. Factors associated with increased 30-day mortality were non-surgical treatment, male sex, being white, older age, longer time to surgery, blood transfusion, comorbid conditions, and discharge to hospice. The important factor in predicting early mortality is a longer time to surgery (more than 24/48 h after the fracture), which is also associated with a longer hospital stay, as has been described in earlier studies [32].

It has been estimated earlier that the expenditure needed for hip fracture exceeds that for breast and gynaecological cancers combined, but not those for cardiovascular disease in the United States [33]. The comparison of costs between hip fractures and cardiovascular diseases is intriguing. In Switzerland, osteoporotic hip fractures accounted for more hospital bed days than myocardial infarction and stroke and consequently led to higher costs [34], while in Italy the costs due to hip fractures were comparable to those of acute myocardial infarction.

As described in Chap. 12, rehabilitation is crucial for people after hip fracture [35]. However, the advanced age and the comorbidities affecting hip fracture patients often dictate that the completion of the rehabilitation programme takes place in long-term care (LTC) facility or a nursing home. The costs needed for a LTC seem to be almost double those required by a rehabilitation institute. However, the roles of these organisations for the rehabilitation of older patients are still debated. In a well-known study on this topic, hip fracture patients admitted to rehabilitation hospitals did not differ from patients admitted to nursing homes in their return to the community or disability rate [36]. Moreover, costs were significantly greater for rehabilitation hospital patients than for nursing home patients and the evidence about the value of these organisations in the elderly is still conflicting.

Poor recovery among older adults with hip fractures can occur despite successful surgical repair and rehabilitation, suggesting other factors might play a role in recovery, such as social factors [37]. In the review of the role of social factors in recovery after hip fracture, the majority of included studies have shown that both a higher level of social support and a better socioeconomic status has a positive effect on physical functional recovery post-hip fracture in individuals aged more than 65 years. Socioeconomic status was associated with both physical functional recovery and mortality from hip fractures. Income, employment, education skills and training are all socioeconomic factors that have been studied and found to influence recovery from hip fracture [7, 37].

Other consequences may be loss of muscle strength, increased postural sway and decline in walking speed that can lead to loss of functional muscle mass, sarcopenia and finally to disability. The impact on disability is striking: 1 year after fracturing a hip, 40% of patients are still unable to walk independently, 60% have difficulty with at least one essential activity of daily living, and 80% are restricted in instrumental activities of daily living, such as driving and grocery shopping [16].

A review published in 2016 included data from 32 cohort studies mostly from Western European and North American countries, but also included some studies from Australia, New Zealand, Japan and China [37]. The review provided clear evidence that people recovering from hip fractures experience ongoing limitations in mobility, basic activities of daily living (ADL), self-care, participation and quality of life. Between 40 and 60% of hip fracture survivors are likely to recover their pre-fracture level of mobility. Up to 70% of people may regain their pre-fracture level of independence for composite measures of basic ADL, but this proportion is likely to be lower for those with higher levels of dependence pre-fracture [37]. Only half or fewer people experiencing hip fracture may regain their pre-fracture level of independence in instrumental activities of daily living (IADLs). Most people who recover their ability to perform basic or instrumental ADLs do so within the first 6 months after discharge, although the time to recovery for individual ADLs ranges from approximately 4 to 11 months [37]. Studies in many countries world-wide have indicated that hip fracture has a significant impact on the quality of life in the medium to long term. In Western nations, between 10 and 20% of hip fracture patients are institutionalised within 6–12 months post-fracture [37].

Hip fracture seems to be associated with the onset of other co-morbidities with a high cost for society. Recent research has highlighted that people experiencing a hip fracture have a greater incidence of depression [38] and consequently a higher use of anti-depressant medications [39]. Another field of interest is the possible relationship between hip fracture and the onset of cardiovascular diseases. Hip fracture, in fact, seems to increase the risk of coronary heart disease, particularly during the first year after the event [40]. Since cardiovascular diseases are among the most expensive medical conditions, the impact of hip fracture in contributing to a huge increase in medical and social costs is highly relevant.

2.11   The Costs and Social Impact of Other Osteoporotic Fractures

Other osteoporotic/fragility fractures (e.g. wrist, spine, shoulder) are more common than hip fractures, but some of them (such as vertebral) are often asymptomatic and the others require less hospital stay than hip fractures. Limited data exist regarding the social costs of the other osteoporotic fractures. In a study including six different cohorts, the authors report that the adjusted mean first-year costs associated with hip, vertebral, and non-vertebral fractures were $26,545, $14,977, and $9183 for the 50–64 age cohort, and $15,196, $6701, and $6106 for patients ≥65 years, respectively [41]. However, after considering the prevalence rate of all major osteoporotic fractures, the proportion of the total fracture costs accounted for by non-vertebral, hip, and vertebral fractures were 66%, 21% and 13% in younger and 36%, 52% and 12% for in older people [41].

The importance of osteoporotic fractures, other than hip, from an economic point of view, was confirmed by a large study using administrative data and including almost all European countries. In this report, European countries report a marked difference in the LOS between men and women, with differences ranging from 0.32 days in Austria to 20.2 days in Spain [42]. The total cost of vertebral fractures in the European Union is enormous, being estimated at 377 million euros per year—about 63% of hip fractures [42]. However, more economic data are needed for non-femoral fractures, including data regarding asymptomatic fractures; this will require cohort studies designed to achieve this aim.

2.12 Conclusions

Hip fracture is a common and debilitating condition, particularly in older persons. Although the age- and gender-specific incidence is decreasing in some countries, the global incidence of hip fracture is rising worldwide, due to population ageing. More attention should be paid to prevention, given its great impact on social costs and quality of life. Other osteoporotic fractures, in particular those affecting spine and wrist, play an important role from an epidemiological point of view, but more data on their economic impact are needed. Thus, further epidemiological studies are needed to better verify the trends in the incidence of osteoporotic fractures and the strategies of effective prevention.

References

1. WHO. https://www.who.int/news-room/fact-sheets/detail/ageing-and-health. Approached February 1, 2020
2. Hernlund E, Svedbom A, Ivergård M, Compston J, Cooper C, Stenmark J, McCloskey EV, Jönsson B, Kanis JA (2013) Osteoporosis in the European Union: medical management, epidemiology and economic burden. A report prepared in collaboration with the International Osteoporosis Foundation (IOF) and the European Federation of Pharmaceutical Industry Associations (EFPIA). Arch Osteoporos 8:136
3. Zanker J, Duque G (2019) Osteoporosis in older persons: old and new players. J Am Geriatr Soc 67(4):831–840
4. Kanis JA, Oden A, McCloskey EV et al (2012) A systematic review of hip fracture incidence and probability of fracture worldwide. Osteoporos Int 23(9):2239–2256
5. Liu J, Curtis EM, Cooper C, Harvey NC (2019) State of the art in osteoporosis risk assessment and treatment. J Endocrinol Investig 42(10):1149–1164
6. Veronese N, Maggi S (2018) Epidemiology and social costs of hip fracture. Injury 49(8):1458–1460
7. Auais M, Al-Zoubi F, Matheson A, Brown K, Magaziner J, French SD (2019) Understanding the role of social factors in recovery after hip fractures: a structured scoping review. Health Soc Care Community 27(6):1375–1387
8. Cheung EYN, Tan KCB, Cheung CL, Kung AWC (2016) Osteoporosis in East Asia: current issues in assessment and management. Osteoporos Sarcopenia 2:118–133
9. Yu F, Xia W (2019) The epidemiology of osteoporosis, associated fragility fractures, and management gap in China. Arch Osteoporos 14(1):32
10. Khadilkar AV, Mandlik RM (2015) Epidemiology and treatment of osteoporosis in women: an Indian perspective. Int J Women's Health 7:841–850
11. Francisco L, Délio Marques C, Costa-Paiva L, Pinto-Neto AM (2015) The epidemiology and management of postmenopausal osteoporosis: a viewpoint from Brazil. Clin Interv Aging 10:583–591

12. Wright NC, Looker AC, Saag KG et al (2014) The recent prevalence of osteoporosis and low bone mass in the United States based on bone mineral density at the femoral neck or lumbar spine. J Bone Miner Res 29(11):2520–2526
13. Curtis EM, Moon RJ, Harvey NC, Cooper C (2017) The impact of fragility fracture and approaches to osteoporosis risk assessment worldwide. Bone 104:29–38
14. Cruz-Jentoft A, Landi F, Schneider FM et al (2014) Prevalence of and interventions for sarcopenia in ageing adults: a systematic review. Report of the International Sarcopenia Initiative (EWGSOP and IWGS). Age Ageing 43(6):748–759
15. Huo YR, Suriyaarachchi P, Gomez F, Curcio CL, Boersma D, Muir SW, Montero-Odasso M, Gunawardene P, Demontiero O, Duque G (2015) Phenotype of osteosarcopenia in older individuals with a history of falling. J Am Med Dir Assoc 16:290–295
16. Cooper C, Cole ZA, Holroyd CR, Earl SC, Harvey NC, Dennison EM et al (2011) Secular trends in the incidence of hip and other osteoporotic fractures. Osteoporos Int 22(5):1277–1288
17. Ho S, Bacon E, Harris T, Looker A, Maggi S (1993) Hip fracture rates in Hong Kong and the United States, 1988 through 1989. Am J Public Health 83:694–697
18. Haring B, Crandall CJ, Wu C, LeBlanc ES, Shikany JM, Carbone L et al (2016) Dietary patterns and fractures in postmenopausal women: results from the women's health initiative. JAMA Intern Med 176(5):645–652
19. Romero Pérez A, Rivas VA (2014) Adherence to Mediterranean diet and bone health. Nutr Hosp 29(5):989–996
20. Brauer CA, Coca-Perraillon M, Cutler DM, Rosen AB (2009) Incidence and mortality of hip fractures in the United States. JAMA 302(14):1573–1579
21. Nellans KW, Kowalski E, Chung KC (2012) The epidemiology of distal radius fractures. Hand Clin 28(2):113–125
22. Ballane G, Cauley JA, Luckey MM, Fuleihan GE (2017) Worldwide prevalence and incidence of osteoporotic vertebral fractures. Osteoporosis Int 28:1531–1542
23. Lems WF (2007) Clinical relevance of vertebral fractures. Ann Rheum Dis 66(1):2–4
24. Ensrud KE, Schousboe JT (2011) Vertebral fractures. NEJM 364(17):1634–1642
25. Amin S, Achenbach SJ, Atkinson EJ, Khosla S, Melton LJ III (2014) Trends in fracture incidence: a population-based study over 20 years. J Bone Miner Res 29(3):581–589
26. Aziziyeh R, Amin M, Habib M, Perlaza JG, McTavish RK, Lüdke A, Fernandes S, Sripada K, Cameron C (2019) A scorecard for osteoporosis in four Latin American countries: Brazil, Mexico, Colombia, and Argentina. Arch Osteoporos 14(1):69
27. Johansen A, Golding D, Brent L, Close J, Gjertsen J-E, Holt G, Hommel A, Pedersen AB, Röck ND, Thorngren K-G (2017) Using national hip fracture registries and audit databases to develop an international perspective. Injury 48(10):2174–2179
28. Abrahamsen B, van Staa T, Ariely R, Olson M, Cooper C (2009) Excess mortality following hip fracture: a systematic epidemiological review. Osteoporos Int 20(10):1633–1650
29. Williamson S, Landeiro F, McConnell T et al (2017) Costs of fragility hip fractures globally: a systematic review and meta-regression analysis. Osteoporos Int 28:2791–2800
30. Nordstrom P, Gustafson Y, Michaelsson K, Nordstrom A (2015) Length of hospital stay after hip fracture and short term risk of death after discharge: a total cohort study in Sweden. BMJ 350:h696
31. Nikkel LE, Kates SL, Schreck M, Maceroli M, Mahmood B, Elfar JC (2015) Length of hospital stay after hip fracture and risk of early mortality after discharge in New York state: retrospective cohort study. BMJ 351:h6246
32. Maggi S, Siviero P, Wetle T, Besdine RW, Saugo M, Crepaldi G (2010) A multicenter survey on profile of care for hip fracture: predictors of mortality and disability. Osteoporosis Int 21(2):223–231
33. Hoerger TJ, Downs KE, Lakshmanan MC, Lindroth RC, Plouffe L, Wendling B et al (1999) Healthcare use among U.S. women aged 45 and older: total costs and costs for selected postmenopausal health risks. J Womens Health Gend Based Med 8(8):1077–1089
34. Lippuner K, von Overbeck J, Perrelet R, Bosshard H, Jaeger P (1997) Incidence and direct medical costs of hospitalizations due to osteoporotic fractures in Switzerland. Osteoporosis Int 7(5):414–425

35. De Rui M, Veronese N, Manzato E, Sergi G (2013) Role of comprehensive geriatric assessment in the management of osteoporotic hip fracture in the elderly: an overview. Disabil Rehabil 35(9):758–765
36. Kramer AM, Steiner JF, Schlenker RE, Eilertsen TB, Hrincevich CA, Tropea DA et al (1997) Outcomes and costs after hip fracture and stroke. A comparison of rehabilitation settings. JAMA 277(5):396–404
37. Dyer SM, Crotty M, Fairhall N, Magaziner J, Beaupre LA, Cameron ID, Sherrington C (2016) Fragility Fracture Network (FFN) Rehabilitation Research Special Interest Group. A critical review of the long-term disability outcomes following hip fracture. BMC Geriatr 16(1):158
38. Cristancho P, Lenze EJ, Avidan MS, Rawson KS (2016) Trajectories of depressive symptoms after hip fracture. Psychol Med 46(07):1413–1425
39. Iaboni A, Seitz DP, Fischer HD, Diong CC, Rochon PA, Flint AJ (2015) Initiation of anti-depressant medication after hip fracture in community-dwelling older adults. Am J Geriatr Psychiatry 23(10):1007–1015
40. Veronese N, Stubbs B, Crepaldi G, Solmi M, Cooper C, Reginster J-Y et al (2017) Low bone mineral density and fractures are associated with incident cardiovascular disease: a systematic review and meta-analysis. Osteoporosis Int 28:180–181
41. Shi N, Foley K, Lenhart G, Badamgarav E (2009) Direct healthcare costs of hip, vertebral, and non-hip, non-vertebral fractures. Bone 45(6):1084–1090
42. Finnern HW, Sykes DP (2003) The hospital cost of vertebral fractures in the EU: estimates using national datasets. Osteoporosis Int 14(5):429–436

Osteoporosis and Fragility in Elderly Patients

Paolo Falaschi, Andrea Marques, and Stefania Giordano

3.1 Definition

Osteoporosis is a systemic bone disease characterised by a reduction and qualitative alterations of the bone mass leading to increased risk of fractures. There are two primary forms of osteoporosis (types I and II): postmenopausal osteoporosis and senile osteoporosis, which appears with advancing age. Secondary forms of osteoporosis are associated with a vast range of diseases and drugs [1].

According to the World Health Organisation, the diagnosis of osteoporosis rests on densitometry, as described below in Sect. 3.7.1, with a T-score diagnostic threshold of < -2.5 [1, 2].

This disease is progressive and if not diagnosed and treated (primary prevention) causes progressive fragility of the bones through a complex pathogenetic mechanism described in detail in Sect. 3.5. This acquired fragility of the skeleton increases the risk of fracture with low energy trauma or even spontaneously in the most severe

---

This chapter is a component of Part 1: Background.
For an explanation of the grouping of chapters in this book, please see Chapter 1: 'The Multidisciplinary Approach to Fragility Fractures Around the World—An Overview'.

P. Falaschi (✉)
Fragility Fracture Network, Zurich, Switzerland

Sapienza University of Rome, Rome, Italy
e-mail: paolo.falaschi@fondazione.uniroma1.it

A. Marques
RN at Rheumatology Department, Centro Hospitalar e Universitário de Coimbra, Coimbra, Portugal

School of Nursing, Coimbra, Portugal

S. Giordano
RSA Salus, Rome, Italy

© The Author(s) 2021
P. Falaschi, D. Marsh (eds.), *Orthogeriatrics*, Practical Issues in Geriatrics,
https://doi.org/10.1007/978-3-030-48126-1_3

cases. When a fragility fracture occurs a DEXA may not be necessary and the anti-osteoporotic treatment can be started to reduce the risk of further fractures (secondary prevention).

3.2   Epidemiology

Osteoporosis is a disease that impacts significantly on society. Its incidence increases with age; in fact, it affects most of the population which has entered the eighth decade of life [1]. Common sites of osteoporotic fractures are the spine, hip, distal forearm and proximal humerus. All told, osteoporotic fractures occur in 2.7 million in men and women in Europe with high direct costs [3]. A recent estimate (for 2010) calculated the direct cost at 29 billion in the five largest EU countries (France, Germany, Italy, Spain and the UK) [4] and 38.7 billion in the 27 EU countries of the time [5]. Hip fractures cause acute pain and loss of function, and nearly always lead to hospitalisation. Recovery is slow, and rehabilitation is often incomplete, with many patients permanently institutionalised in nursing homes. Vertebral fractures may cause acute pain and loss of function but may also occur without serious symptoms. Distal radial fractures also lead to acute pain and loss of function, but functional recovery is usually good, at times excellent. It is widely recognised that osteoporosis and the fractures it causes are associated with increased mortality, with the exception of forearm fractures [6]. In the case of hip fractures, most deaths occur during the first 3–6 months following the event, of which 20–30% are causally related to the fracture itself [7]. For an extensive description of the epidemiological distribution of osteoporosis, fragility fractures and costs, see Chap. 2.

3.3   The Anatomy of Bone

Eighty percent of the adult human skeleton is composed of cortical bone, 20% of trabecular bone. Cortical bone is dense and solid and surrounds the space occupied by the marrow, whereas trabecular bone is composed of a honeycomb-like network of trabecular plates and rods interspersed throughout the bone-marrow compartment. Both cortical and trabecular bone are composed of osteons. Cortical osteons are called Haversian systems. Haversian systems are cylindrical in shape, approximately 400 mm in length and 200 mm in width at their base and form a branching network within the cortical bone [8].

Bone tissue is composed of cells (Osteoclast, osteoblast and osteocytes) and matrix [8].

Osteoclasts are the only cells known to be capable of resorbing bone. Activated multinucleated osteoclasts are derived from mononuclear precursor cells of the monocyte-macrophage lineage [9].

Osteoblasts: Osteoprogenitor cells give rise to and maintain the osteoblasts that synthesise new bone matrix on bone-forming surfaces, the osteocytes within the bone matrix supporting the bone structure, and the protective lining cells that cover the surface of the quiescent bone. Within the osteoblast lineage, subpopulations of cells respond differently to various hormonal, mechanical or cytokine signals [8].

Osteocytes: Osteocytes represent terminally differentiated osteoblasts and function within syncytial networks to support bone structure and metabolism. Osteocytes lie in lacunae within mineralised bone and create extensive filopodial processes within the canaliculi in mineralised bone. Osteocytes express several matrix proteins that support intercellular adhesion and regulate the exchange of mineral in the bone fluid within the lacunae and the canalicular network. Osteocytes are active during osteolysis and may function as phagocytic cells because they contain lysosomes [8].

The bone extracellular matrix is composed of between 85% and 90% of collagenous proteins. Bone matrix is mostly composed of type I collagen, with trace amounts of types III and V and FACIT collagens at certain stages of bone formation. FACIT collagens are members of the family of Fibril-Associated Collagens with Interrupted Triple Helices, a group of nonfibrillar collagens that serve as molecular bridges important for the organisation and stability of extracellular matrices [10].

Bone is composed of 50–70% minerals, 20–40% organic matrix, 5–10% water, and <3% lipids. The mineral content of bone is mostly hydroxyapatite $[Ca_{10}(PO_4)_6(OH)_2]$, with small amounts of carbonate, magnesium, and acid phosphate, with missing hydroxyl groups that are normally present. Matrix maturation is associated with the expression of alkaline phosphatase and several non-collagenous proteins, including osteocalcin, osteopontin, and bone sialoprotein. Bone mineral provides mechanical rigidity and load-bearing strength to bone, whereas the organic matrix provides elasticity and flexibility [8].

The term 'bone quality' is used in two senses in the literature: in one bone quality represents the sum of all the characteristics of bone that affect its ability to resist fracture (i.e. all aspects of bone size, shape and its material properties); in the other, bone quality refers to the influence of factors that affect fracture but are not accounted for by bone mass or quantity [11, 12]. Regardless of one's preference regarding a general definition of bone quality, bone quality remains a skeletal trait and since it is important in determining fracture risk it must play a role in determining the mechanical properties of bone, and therefore cannot account for any non-skeletal factors that may also contribute to fracture incidence such as the risk of falling or limitations of commonly used measurements of bone mass [13].

Following the hierarchic structure of the bone we can recognise the following determinants for bone quality: whole bone morphology (size and shape), spatial distribution of bone density, microarchitecture, porosity, cortical-shell thickness, lacunar number/morphology, number, size and distribution of the remodelling cavity, mineral and collagen distribution/alignment, type, amount and distribution of microdamage structure and cross-linking of collagen, mineral type and crystal alignment and collagen–mineral interfaces [14].

3.4   The Physiology of Bone

Modelling is the process by which bones change their overall shape in response to physiological influences or mechanical forces, leading to a gradual adjustment of the skeleton to the forces it encounters [15].

Bone remodelling is the process by which bone is renewed to maintain bone strength and mineral homeostasis. Remodelling involves continuous removal of discrete packets of old bone, replacement of these packets with newly synthesised matrix, and subsequent mineralisation of the matrix to form new bone. The main functions of bone remodelling are preservation of the mechanical strength of bone by replacing the older, micro-damaged bone with newer, healthier bone and calcium and phosphate homeostasis [8].

The remodelling cycle comprises four sequential phases: activation, resorption, reversal, formation [16, 17]. Activation involves recruitment and activation of mononuclear monocyte-macrophage osteoclast precursors from the circulation, lifting of the endosteum containing the lining cells off the bone surface, and fusion of multiple mononuclear cells to form multinucleated preosteoclasts. Preosteoclasts bind to the bone matrix via interactions between integrin receptors in their cell membranes and RGD (arginine, glycine, and asparagine)-containing peptides in matrix proteins, to form annular sealing zones around bone-resorbing compartments beneath multinucleated osteoclasts [8].

Osteoclast-mediated bone resorption takes only approximately 2–4 weeks during each remodelling cycle. Osteoclast formation, activation, and resorption are regulated by the ratio of receptor activator of NF-κB ligand (RANKL) to osteoprotegerin (OPG) IL-1 and IL-6, colony-stimulating factor (CSF), parathyroid hormone, 1,25-dihydroxyvitamin D, and calcitonin [9, 18]. Resorbing osteoclasts secrete hydrogen ions via H+-ATPase proton pumps and chloride channels in their cell membranes into the resorbing compartment to lower the pH within the bone-resorbing compartment to as low as 4.5, which helps mobilise bone mineral. Resorbing osteoclasts secrete tartrate-resistant acid phosphatase, cathepsin K, matrix metalloproteinase 9, and gelatinase from cytoplasmic lysosomes to digest the organic matrix, resulting in the formation of saucer-shaped Howship's lacunae on the surface of trabecular bone and Haversian canals in cortical bone. The resorption phase is completed by mononuclear cells after the multinucleated osteoclasts undergo apoptosis [19]. Upon completion of bone resorption, resorption cavities contain a variety of mononuclear cells, including monocytes, osteocytes released from bone matrix, and preosteoblasts recruited to begin the formation of new bone. The coupling signals linking the end of bone resorption to the beginning of bone formation are not totally clear [20]. It has also been proposed that the reversal phase may be mediated by the strain gradient in the lacunae. As osteoclasts resorb cortical bone in a cutting cone, the strain is reduced in front and increased behind, and in Howship's lacunae, the strain is highest at the base and less in surrounding bone at the edges of the lacunae. The strain gradient may lead to sequential activation of osteoclasts and osteoblasts, with osteoclasts activated by reduced strain and osteoblasts by increased strain. It has also been proposed that the osteoclast itself may play a role during reversal [21]. Bone formation takes approximately

4–6 months to complete. Osteoblasts synthesise new collagenous organic matrix and regulate mineralisation of matrix by releasing small, membrane-bound matrix vesicles that concentrate calcium and phosphate and enzymatically destroy mineralisation inhibitors such as pyrophosphate or proteoglycans [22]. Osteoblasts surrounded by and buried within matrix become osteocytes with an extensive canalicular network connecting them to bone surface lining cells, osteoblasts, and other osteocytes, maintained by gap junctions between the cytoplasmic processes extending from the osteocytes [23]. At the completion of bone formation, approximately 50–70% of the osteoblasts undergo apoptosis, with the balance becoming osteocytes or bone-lining cells.

A critical advance in our understanding of skeletal biology of the last few years was the discovery of the role of Wnt/β catenin signalling in bone [24, 25]. Wnt/β catenin signalling is activated by binding of Wnt proteins to receptor complexes composed of frizzled receptors and co-receptors of the low-density lipoprotein receptor-related protein (LRP) family, LRP5 and 6. This event stabilises β catenin, induces its translocation to the nucleus, and activates gene transcription. This so-called canonical Wnt signalling pathway controls the differentiation of mesenchymal stem cells (MSC) restraining chondrogenic and adipogenic differentiation and favouring osteoblastic differentiation. Canonical Wnt signalling also promotes osteoblast maturation and survival of osteoblasts and osteocytes and inhibits osteoclast generation by increasing the expression in osteoblasts and osteocytes of osteoprotegerin (OPG), the decoy receptor of the receptor activator of Nfκb ligand (RANKL). Thus, activation of this pathway is critical for bone acquisition and maintenance through the increased bone formation and decreased resorption. Osteocytes are key players in the regulation of the canonical Wnt signalling pathway as producers and targets of Wnt ligands and as secretors of molecules that modulate Wnt actions [25, 26]. A potent antagonist of Wnt signalling secreted by osteocytes is sclerostin, a protein encoded by the SOST gene, primarily expressed by mature osteocytes but not by early osteocytes or osteoblasts [27]. Sclerostin binds to the Wnt co-receptors LRP5/6 antagonising downstream signalling [28]. Sclerostin also interacts with LRP4, another member of the LRP family of proteins, which acts as a chaperone and is required for the inhibitory action of sclerostin on Wnt/β catenin signalling [29]. Absence of sclerostin expression or secretion in humans causes inherited high bone mass conditions characterised by exaggerated bone formation, including sclerosteosis, van Buchem disease and craniodiaphyseal dysplasia [25].

Osteoprotegerin (OPG), the decoy receptor for RANKL and therefore the inhibitor of bone resorption, is a Wnt/β catenin target gene [30]. Thus, genetic manipulation of Wnt/β catenin signalling leads to marked changes in OPG expression with consequent effects on resorption. Specifically, inactivation of Wnt/β catenin in mature osteoblasts/osteocytes decreases OPG and increases osteoclast differentiation and bone resorption [31–33]. Conversely, activation of Wnt/β catenin in osteoblasts increases OPG expression and reduces bone resorption [31, 32]. Because sclerostin antagonises the Wnt/β catenin signalling pathway, it is not unexpected that changes in SOST/sclerostin expression might also modulate resorption by regulating OPG. In fact, neutralising anti-sclerostin antibodies increase bone formation and decrease bone resorption markers in experimental animals and humans, suggesting that the bone gain achieved results from the combination of enhanced bone formation and decreased bone resorption [34].

3.5   Pathogenesis

Peak bone mass is achieved between the ages of 16–25 in most people. After this age, bone mass decreases slowly but continuously [35].

There is epidemiologic evidence for substantial effects of nutrition and lifestyle on peak bone mass and fracture risk, not only during childhood and adolescence but even during gestation [36, 37].

Bone formation typically exceeds bone resorption on the periosteal surface, so bones normally increase in diameter with age. Bone resorption typically exceeds bone formation on the endosteal surface, so the marrow space normally expands as people age. Bone remodelling increases in perimenopausal and early postmenopausal women and then slows down with further ageing but continues at a faster rate than in premenopausal women. Bone remodelling is thought to increase mildly in ageing men [8].

Normal rates of bone loss are different in men and women. In men, bone mass is lost at a rate of 0.3% per annum, while in women this rate is 0.5%. By way of contrast, bone loss after menopause, in particular during the first 5 years after its onset, can be as high as 5–6% per annum [35].

Besides the difference in age at onset, types I and II osteoporosis have somewhat different effects on the kinds of bone lost. Type I appears to affect mostly trabecular bone, while type II affects both cortical and trabecular bone [35]. The cellular mechanism of type II osteoporosis is multifactorial. Factors involved are progressive dietary calcium deficiency, progressive inactivity [35, 38], and as in type I osteoporosis, decreases in oestrogen levels have been demonstrated in both elderly men and women to be an important cause of senile osteoporosis.

Normal cancellous bone is composed of both horizontal and vertical trabeculae. In the osteoporotic bone, there is a predisposition to loss of horizontal trabeculae. This leads to decreased interconnectivity of the internal scaffolding of the vertebral body. Without the support of crossing horizontal members, unsupported vertical beams of the bone easily succumb to minor loads [35].

3.6   Risk Factors for Fragility Fractures

Osteoporotic fractures are related to several risk factors (Table 3.1).

3.6.1   BMD

Several studies have demonstrated that the reduction of a single standard deviation in BMD corresponds to an increase in fracture risk of 1.5–3-fold [1]. However, fracture risk is not only related to BMD, consequently, T-score values alone are not

Table 3.1 Summary of clinical risk factors [1, 2]

Age
Female gender
Low body mass index
Previous fragility fracture, particularly of the hip, wrist and spine
Parental history of hip fracture
Glucocorticoid treatment (≥5 mg prednisolone daily or equivalent for 3 months or more)
Current smoking
Alcohol intake of three or more units daily
Premature menopause
Vitamin D deficiency
Reduced calcium intake
Drugs
Osteoporosis-related pathologies (see Table 3.2)
Organ transplant

For an extensive description of risk factors see Chap. 14

sufficient to define the probability of fracture and determine when a patient needs to be treated [39]. Moreover, the majority of fractures occur in patients presenting with osteopenia (T-scores of −2.5 to −1.0) [40].

An interesting situation is the diabetic patient since type 2 diabetes is usually associated with a 5–10% higher areal BMD than healthy subjects but despite that, they are at higher risk of fracture. It has been demonstrated that for a given T-score and age, the fracture risk was higher in type 2 diabetes patients than in those not presenting with type 2 diabetes [41].

3.6.2 Age

Age contributes, independently of BMD, to fracture risk; therefore, in the presence of the same BMD score, the risk of fracture will be higher for the elderly than for the young [39, 42]. Another major problem regarding the elderly is their reduced muscular functionality. This is an age-related condition, but it is often exaggerated by deficient nutrition and reduced mobility. Weakness is one of the five items that define frailty syndrome as proposed by Fried and colleagues [43]. Moreover, the 'frail phenotype' is associated with a very high risk of falls leading to fracture [44].

3.6.3 Previous Fractures

The presence of a previous fracture, regardless of its site, is an important risk factor for further fractures and is independent of BMD. The most common prognostic fractures are those of the vertebrae, hip, humerus and wrist. Moreover, risk of further fracture increases with the number of previous fractures: patients with three or more previous fractures have a ten times greater risk of fracture than patients who have never suffered from fractures [1].

Table 3.2 Pathologies relevant to fracture risk

Endocrine disorders	– Hypogonadism – Hypercortisolism – Hyperparathyroidism – Hyperthyroidism – Hyperprolactinaemia – Diabetes mellitus type I and II – Acromegaly – GH deficiency
Haematological disorders	– Myelo-lymphoproliferative diseases – Multiple myeloma and monoclonal gammopathies – Systemic mastocytosis – Thalassemia – Sickle-cell anaemia – Haemophilia
Gastrointestinal disorders	– Chronic liver disease – Primary biliary cirrhosis – Celiac disease – Chronic inflammatory bowel diseases – Gastro-intestinal resection – Gastric bypass – Lactose intolerance – Intestinal malabsorption – Pancreatic insufficiency
Rheumatological disorders	– Rheumatoid arthritis – LES – Ankylosing spondylitis – Psoriatic arthritis – Scleroderma – Other forms of connectivitis
Renal disorders	– Renal idiopathic hypercalciuria – Renal tubular acidosis – Chronic renal failure
Neurological disorders	– Parkinson's disease – Multiple sclerosis – Paraplegia – Aftermath of stroke – Muscular dystrophies
Genetic disorders	– Osteogenesis Imperfecta – Ehlers-Danlos Syndrome – Gaucher Syndrome – Glycogenosis – Hypophosphatasia – Hemochromatosis – Homocystinuria – Cystic fibrosis – Marfan Syndrome – Menkes Syndrome – Porphyria – Riley-Day Syndrome
Other pathologies	– Chronic obstructive pulmonary disease – Anorexia nervosa – AIDS/HIV – Amyloidosis – Sarcoidosis – Depression

3.6.4 Family History of Fracture

Family history influences fracture risk independently of BMD. In particular, parental hip fracture is significantly related to a higher risk of hip fractures in offspring and, to a lesser extent, of all other kinds of osteoporotic fractures [1].

3.6.5 Comorbidities

A broad range of pathologies is related to increased rates of fracture risk (Table 3.2).

In some cases, the increased fracture risk is caused by a reduction in BMD, but other mechanisms are often involved: chronic inflammation, alteration of bone quality, general impairment of health conditions, reduction of mobility, sarcopenia, with a higher risk of falls and other complications. Vitamin-D deficiency, which often coexists with this pathology, is another negative factor [1].

3.6.6 Drugs

Several drugs increase the risks of fracture. The most important class of drugs is glucocorticoids that have a negative effect on bone, causing rapid bone-quality loss and BMD depletion. Among the more recent classes of drugs, hormone-blockade treatments (aromatase inhibitors for women operated for breast cancer and GnRH agonists for men with prostate cancer) also lead to a reduction of BMD but at a slower rate. Other drugs involved are SSRI, PPI, H2 inhibitors, anticonvulsants, loop diuretics, anticoagulants, excess of thyroid hormones and antiretroviral treatment.

3.6.7 Assessment of Fracture Risk

Although BMD acts as the cornerstone when diagnosing osteoporosis, as mentioned earlier, the use of BMD alone does not suffice to identify an intervention threshold. This is why a vast number of scores are drawn up to better identify fracture risks; the most widely used assessment tool is FRAX®. This is a web-based algorithm (www.shef.ac.uk/FRAX) which calculates the 10-year probability of a major fracture (hip, clinical spine, humerus or wrist) and a 10-year hip-fracture probability [45].

Despite the fact that international literature has demonstrated the validity of these instruments when evaluating the risk of fracture, the intervention thresholds for osteoporosis currently depend on regional treatment and reimbursement policies, which are increasingly based on cost-effectiveness evaluations [46–48].

For a more extensive discussion see Chap. 14.

3.7   Diagnosis

There is no universally accepted population-screening policy in Europe for the recognition of patients with osteoporosis or those at high risk of fracture. In the absence of such a policy, patients are identified opportunistically using a case-finding strategy based on previous fragility fractures or the presence of significant risk factors [2].

3.7.1   Instrumental Diagnosis

Bone Mineral Density (BMD) may be evaluated by means of several techniques generally described as bone densitometry. Densitometry permits accurate measurement of bone mass, which is the best predictor of risks of osteoporotic fracture. The result is expressed as a T-score, which is the difference between the subject's BMD value and the mean BMD value for healthy young adults (peak bone mass) of the same sex, expressed in standard deviations (SD). BMD can also be expressed by comparing the average value for subjects of the same age and sex (Z-score). The threshold required to diagnose the presence of osteoporosis, according to the WHO, is a T-score of < -2.5 SD.

3.7.1.1   Dual X-Ray Absorptiometry (DXA)

This is, at present, the technique preferred for bone-mass evaluation used to enable the diagnosis of osteoporosis, prediction of fracture risk and follow-up monitoring. The technique uses X-rays of two different energies, which allow the subtraction of soft tissue absorption and provide an estimate of the bone's calcium content. When projected onto a surface, this gives a parameter called bone mineral density (BMD g/cm^2), from which bone mineral content (BMC, g/cm^3) may be inferred. In general, measurement at a particular site provides a more accurate estimate of fracture risk for that site. Since the most clinically relevant osteoporotic fractures occur in the spine and hip, the most frequently measured sites are the lumbar spine and proximal femur. However, there are a number of technical limitations to the application of DXA to diagnosis. For example, the presence of osteomalacia will underestimate the total bone matrix because of decreased bone mineralisation while, on the other hand, osteoarthrosis or osteoarthritis of the spine or hip will contribute to density but not to skeletal strength [2]. In the latter case, the specific site involved must be excluded from the analysis; at least two lumbar vertebrae must be evaluated so that the densitometry result may be considered reasonably accurate. For this reason, femoral densitometric evaluation is probably preferable after the age of 65. Recently some software has been developed to enable DXA to measure, not only BMD but also some of the geometrical parameters related to bone strength, such as HSA (hip structure analysis) and TBS (trabecular bone score).TBS has emerged as a novel grey-level texture measurement that uses experimental variograms of 2D projection images, quantifying variation in grey-level texture from one pixel to the adjacent pixels [49]. TBS is not a direct measurement of bone microarchitecture but is related to 3D bone characteristics such as the trabecular number, the trabecular separation and the connectivity density [50, 51]. An elevated TBS appears to represent a strong, fracture-resistant microarchitecture, while a low TBS reflects a weak, fracture-prone microarchitecture. As such, there is evidence that TBS can differentiate between two three-dimensional (3D) microarchitectures that exhibit the same bone density and different trabecular characteristics. Lumbar TBS, like a BMD, is an age-dependent variable. Little change in TBS is observed between the ages of 30 and 45 years. Thereafter, a progressive decrease is observed with advancing age, which is more marked in women than in men. Although this device has been approved by the FDA, its everyday use in clinical practice is still limited [52].

3.7.1.2 Quantitative Computerised Tomography (QCT)

This technique, because it is able to separate the trabecular BMD from the cortical BMD, permits total and local volumetric BMD (g/cm^3) measurements at both vertebral and femoral levels. However, this method exposes patients to high radiation dose levels (about 100 Sv). As a technique, DXA is usually preferred to QCT because of its accuracy, shorter scan times, more stable calibration, lower radiation dose and lower costs [2].

3.7.1.3 Quantitative Ultra-Sound (QUS)

This technique provides two parameters (speed and attenuation) which are indirect indicators of bone mass and structural integrity; it is used mainly to carry out measurements in two sites, the phalanges and the calcaneus. It has been demonstrated that ultrasound parameters are capable of predicting the risk of osteoporotic fractures (femoral and vertebral) no less accurately than lumbar or femoral DXA, both in postmenopausal women and in men, but this technique does not provide direct bone-density measurements. Discordant results between ultrasonographic and DXA evaluations are neither surprising nor infrequent and they do not necessarily indicate an error, but rather, that the QUS parameters are independent predictors of fracture risk influenced by other characteristics of the bone tissue. It does mean, however, that QUS cannot be used for the diagnoses of osteoporosis based on WHO criteria. QUS can be useful when it is not possible to estimate a lumbar or femoral BMD with DXA and may be recommended for epidemiological investigations and first-level screening, considering its relatively low cost, easy transportability and absence of radiation [2].

3.7.2 X-Ray of the Dorsal and Lumbar Spine

The presence of a non-traumatic vertebral fracture indicates a condition of skeletal fragility, regardless of BMD, and is a strong indicator of the need to start treatment to reduce risks of further fractures. Since most vertebral fractures are mild and asymptomatic, the use of diagnostic imaging is the only way to diagnose them. Vertebral fractures are defined, applying Genant's semi-quantitative method (SQ), more than a 20% reduction in one vertebral body height [2].

3.7.3 Laboratory Tests

Laboratory tests are an indispensable step in the diagnosis of osteoporosis because they can distinguish between this condition and other metabolic diseases of the skeleton, which may present a clinical picture similar to that of osteoporosis. Moreover, they can identify possible causal factors, permitting the diagnosis of secondary osteoporosis and suggesting an aetiological treatment where one exists. First-level tests are blood count, protein electrophoresis, serum–calcium and phosphorus levels, total alkaline phosphatase, creatinine, the erythrocyte sedimentation rate and 24 h urinary calcium. Normal results for these tests exclude up to 90% of secondary forms of osteoporosis. Sometimes it is necessary to perform second-level tests too, such as ionised calcium, TSH, PTH, serum 25-OH-vitamin D, cortisol after a suppression test with 1 mg of dexamethasone, total testosterone in males, serum and/or urinary immunofixation for anti-transglutaminase antibodies and specific tests for associated diseases.

The specific markers of bone turnover, detectable in serum and/or urine, are divided into bone-formation (bone isoenzyme of alkaline phosphatase, osteocalcin, type I procollagen propeptide) and bone-resorption markers (pyridinoline, deoxypyridinoline, N or C telopeptides of collagen type I). In adult subjects, the increase in bone turnover markers indicates an accelerated bone loss or the existence of other primary or secondary skeletal disorders (osteomalacia, Paget's disease, skeletal localisations of cancer). Markers are overall indices of skeletal remodelling and they may be useful when monitoring the efficacy of and adherence to therapy. However, these markers are characterised by broad biological variability so, at present, they cannot be used for routine clinical evaluations [2].

3.8   Management of Osteoporosis

3.8.1   Lifestyle Modification

Giving up smoking and abuse of alcohol and choosing an active lifestyle is fundamental as a starting point for the management of a patient with osteoporosis.

Immobility is one of the most important causes of bone loss and should be avoided wherever possible. Weight-bearing exercises are optimal for skeletal health and are, therefore, an important component of the management of patients with osteoporosis [53].

3.8.1.1 Prevention of Falls
Risk factors for falls include a history of fracture/falls, dizziness and orthostatic hypotension, visual impairment, gait deficits, urinary incontinence, chronic musculoskeletal pain, depression, functional and cognitive impairment, low body mass index, female sex, erectile dysfunction (in male adults), and people aged over 80 [54]. Some of these factors are modifiable and it is important to act on them [55]. A programme of exercises may prevent falls by improving confidence and

coordination and by preserving muscle strength but there is no consensus concerning the most suitable programme for the 'oldest old' [55, 56].

For a more extensive discussion of this issue see Chap. 16.

3.9 The Importance of Vitamin D, Calcium and Protein Intake

3.9.1 Vitamin D

Vitamin D is involved in the intestinal absorption of calcium and phosphorus and is necessary for mineralisation of the bone and the maintenance of the muscle, while also having numerous beneficial effects on other organs. Most Vitamin D is synthesised through the skin during exposure to the sun but this capacity is reduced in older people, moreover, they tend to expose their skin less than younger adults. Therefore, the majority of older people suffer from hypovitaminosis D [57]. The threshold values for vitamin D are presented below in Table 3.3. Several trials have demonstrated lower fracture risk in patients with a plasma concentration of 25-hydroxy-vitamin D (25-OH-D) of at least 60 nmol/L [58]. It has been demonstrated that improvement in 25-OH-D levels leads to a lower incidence of falls in older people; other trials have demonstrated that vitamin D supplementation is associated with a reduction in all-cause mortality [59]. The Recommended Nutrient Intakes (RNI) are 800 IU of vitamin D per day in men and women over 50 [2]. Intakes of at least 800 IU of vitamin D can be recommended in the general management of patients with osteoporosis, especially in patients receiving bone-protective therapy [60]. Considering that hypovitaminosis D is an epidemic among the elderly, there is probably no strong necessity to measure circulating levels of 25-OH-D in patients with high fracture risk [57]. Vitamin D supplementation should start as soon as possible and should precede the administration of any drug used to treat osteoporosis [60]. Since the inactive form of vitamin D (cholecalciferol) is stored in fat tissue, it is sensible to saturate the stores with repeated small, loading doses and then to continue with maintenance doses.

3.9.2 Calcium

Calcium is an element necessary for the mineralisation of the bone. It is mainly contained in dairy products, which may have calcium and vitamin D added. The Recommended Nutrient Intakes (RNI) are a minimum of 1000 mg of calcium per

Table 3.3 Threshold values of vitamin D [1]

Serum vitamin D level (nmol/L)	Serum vitamin D level (ng/mL)	Definition
<25	<10	Severe deficiency
25–50	10–20	Deficiency
50–75	20–30	Insufficiency
75–125	30–50	Target

day for men and women aged more than 50 years [2]. It is fundamental to ensure correct calcium intake by means of a balanced diet, but when this is not possible, calcium supplements of 0.5–1.2 g a day are recommended, especially in patients receiving bone-protective therapy [4, 61]. Calcium and vitamin D supplements decrease secondary hyperparathyroidism thus reducing bone resorption. Although, in one meta-analysis, calcium supplementation seemed to increase the risk of myocardial infarction, although other studies contradict these results [62, 63].

For a more extensive discussion of this issue see Chap. 18.

3.9.3 Protein

Nutritional insufficiency—in particular protein-energy malnutrition—is frequent in the elderly. Adequate nutrition is very important for bone health [64]. The Insulin-like growth factor-I (IGF-I) mediates the effects of the growth hormone (GH) and has promoting effects on several body tissues, especially on skeletal muscle, cartilage and bone. Moreover, it plays a role in the regulation of phosphate reabsorption in the kidney and the active uptake of Ca2+ and phosphate from the intestine via renal synthesis of calcitriol. In view of impaired protein assimilation in older people, for them, the RDA should be increased from 0.80 g/kg body weight per day to 1.0 or 1.2 g/kg per day [56].

For a more extensive discussion on nutritional aspects see Chap. 18.

For the pharmacological treatment at issue see Chap. 15.

3.10 Therapeutic Adherence in Osteoporosis and the Role of Health Professionals

Compelling research confirms that the vast majority of patients with osteoporosis, worldwide, are not treated or even diagnosed, because the disease often fails to manifest itself before a fracture occurs [65]. Unfortunately, even after fractures take place only a minority of patients receive prescriptions for adequate preventive treatment, either upon discharge from the hospital or over the following years. Research also demonstrates that although patients may have a good knowledge of what osteoporosis is, they generally have a low level of understanding of the role of medication in reducing fracture risk, various concerns about its side effects, poor understanding of the causes and risk factors of osteoporosis, and uncertainty about how it can be controlled [66].

An important epidemiological study by Rabenda and colleagues demonstrated that the medication possession ratio (MPR) at 12 months was higher among patients taking weekly, as compared to daily, doses of alendronate [67]. Adherence to therapeutic regimens is challenging, particularly for the elderly, who generally have a long list of drugs to take. They are often rather forgetful; it seems, however, that most instances of non-adherence are intentional, due to elderly patients carrying out an (erroneous) risk/benefit analysis on their behalf [68].

This situation obviously needs to be changed if we want to curtail the continuous expansion of the burden of osteoporotic fractures. New strategies and services, involving an enlarged group of health professionals and reliable mechanisms to articulate, foster and monitor their actions are needed. Nurses are often appointed as the key to the success of these services, due to their role in coordinating and communicating with other health professionals.[66].

Health professionals should provide education based on patient-centred care and create a mechanism that allows involvement of patients and families in their care, with particular focus on caring, patient communication, sharing of control over decisions, and the integration into the decision-making process of guidance by nurses, physicians, and other providers. It is important to explain to patients who have experienced a fracture that this was due to 'fragility' caused by osteoporosis and show them how drug treatment can help. It is fundamental to understand their reasons and excuses for not adhering to their medication programme.

Many studies show that people who actively seek to learn about and manage their health are more likely to take preventive healthy behaviour measures, self-manage their health conditions, adhere to the treatments prescribed, have better care experiences, and achieve better health outcomes.

Health care professionals should define a plan with the patient and family and provide education on dietary and lifestyle.

In general, periodic follow-up visits are beneficial: during which the patients should be asked to describe how they take their medicines while avoiding any notion of judgment [56].

References

1. Adami S, Bertoldo F, Brandi ML, Cepollaro C, Filipponi P, Fiore E, Frediani B, Giannini S et al (2009) Guidelines for the diagnosis, prevention and treatment of osteoporosis. Reumatismo 61:260–284
2. Kanis J, McCloskey E, Johansson H, Cooper C, Rizzoli R, Reginster J et al (2013) European guidance for the diagnosis and management of osteoporosis in postmenopausal women. Osteoporos Int 24:23–57
3. Kanis J, Borgstrom F, De Leat C, Johansson H, Johnell O, Jonsson B, Odea A, Zethraeus N, Pfleger B, Khaltaev N et al (2005) Assessment of fracture risk. Osteoporos Int 16:581–589
4. Strom O, Borgstrom F, Kanis J, Compston J, Cooper C, McCloskey E, Jonsson B (2011) Osteoporosis: burden, healthcare provision and opportunities in the EU. A report prepared in collaboration with the International Osteoporosis Foundation (IOF) and the European Federation of Pharmaceutical Industry Associations (EFPIA). Arch Osteoporos 6:59–155
5. Kanis J, Compston J, Cooper C et al (2012) The burden of fractures in the European Union in 2010. Osteoporos Int 23:S57
6. Cooper C, Atkinson E, Jacobsen S, O'Fallon W, Melton L (1993) Population-based study of survival after osteoporotic fractures. Am J Epidemiol 137:1001–1005
7. Kanis J, Oden A, Johnell O, De Laet C, Jonsson B, Oglesby A (2003) The components of excess mortality after hip fracture. Bone 32:468–473
8. Clarke B (2008) Normal bone anatomy and physiology. Clin J Am Soc Nephrol 3(Suppl 3):S131–S139
9. Boyle WJ, Simonet WS, Lacey DL (2003) Osteoclast differentiation and activation. Nature 423:337–342
10. Brodsky B, Persikov AV (2005) Molecular structure of the collagen triple helix. Adv Protein Chem 70:301–339
11. Bouxsein ML (2003) Bone quality: where do we go from here? Osteoporos Int 14(Suppl 5):118–127

12. Felsenberg D, Boonen S (2005) The bone quality framework: determinants of bone strength and their interrelationships, and implications for osteoporosis management. Clin Ther 27:1–11
13. Jarvinen TL, Sievanen H, Jokihaara J, Einhorn TA (2005) Revival of bone strength: the bottom line. J Bone Miner Res 20:717–720
14. Hernandez CJ, Keaveny TM (2006) A biomechanical perspective on bone quality. Bone 39(6):1173–1181
15. Kobayashi S, Takahashi HE, Ito A, Saito N, Nawata M, Horiuchi H, Ohta H, Ito A, Iorio R, Yamamoto N, Takaoka K (2003) Trabecular minimodeling in human iliac bone. Bone 32:163–169
16. Burr DB (2002) Targeted and nontargeted remodeling. Bone 30:2–4
17. Parfitt AM (2002) Targeted and nontargeted bone remodeling: relationship to basic multicellular unit origination and progression. Bone 30:5–7
18. Blair HC, Athanasou NA (2004) Recent advances in osteoclast biology and pathological bone resorption. Histol Histopathol 19:189–199
19. Reddy SV (2004) Regulatory mechanisms operative in osteoclasts. Crit Rev Eukaryot Gene Expr 14:255–270
20. Hock JM, Centrella M, Canalis E (2004) Insulin-like growth factor I (IGF-I) has independent effects on bone matrix formation and cell replication. Endocrinology 122:254–260
21. Martin TJ, Sims NA (2005) Osteoclast-derived activity in the coupling of bone formation to resorption. Trends Mol Med 11:76–81
22. Anderson HC (2003) Matrix vesicles and calcification. Curr Rheumatol Rep 5:222–226
23. Burger EH, Klein-Nuland J, Smit TH (2003) Strain-derived canalicular fluid flow regulates osteoclast activity in a remodeling osteon: a proposal. J Biomech 36:1452–1459
24. Delgado-Calle J, Sato AY, Bellido T (2017) Role and mechanism of action of Sclerostin in bone. Bone 96:29–37
25. Baron R, Kneissel M (2013) WNT signaling in bone homeostasis and disease: from human mutations to treatments. Nat Med 19(2):179–192
26. Gori F, Lerner U, Ohlsson C, Baron R (2015) A new WNT on the bone: WNT16, cortical bone thickness, porosity and fractures. Bonekey Rep 4:669
27. Poole KE, Van Bezooijen RL, Loveridge N, Hamersma H, Papapoulos SE, Lowik CW et al (2005) Sclerostin is a delayed secreted product of osteocytes that inhibits bone formation. FASEB J 19(13):1842–1844
28. Li X, Zhang Y, Kang H, Liu W, Liu P, Zhang J et al (2005) Sclerostin binds to LRP5/6 and antagonizes canonical Wntsignaling. J Biol Chem 280(20):19883–19887
29. Leupin O, Piters E, Halleux C, Hu S, Kramer I, Morvan F et al (2011) Bone overgrowth-associated mutations in the LRP4 gene impair sclerostin facilitator function. J Biol Chem 286(22):19489–19500
30. Boyce BF, Xing L (2008) Functions of RANKL/RANK/OPG in bone modeling and remodeling. Arch Biochem Biophys 473(2):139–146
31. Glass DA, Bialek P, Ahn JD, Starbuck M, Patel MS, Clevers H et al (2005) Canonical Wnt signaling in differentiated osteoblasts controls osteoclast differentiation. Dev Cell 8(5):751–764
32. Holmen SL, Zylstra CR, Mukherjee A, Sigler RE, Faugere MC, Bouxsein ML et al (2005) Essential role of beta-catenin in postnatal bone acquisition. J Biol Chem 280(22):21162–21168
33. Kramer I, Halleux C, Keller H, Pegurri M, Gooi JH, Weber PB et al (2010) Osteocyte Wnt/beta-catenin signaling is required for normal bone homeostasis. Mol Cell Biol 30(12):3071–3085
34. Stolina M, Dwyer D, Niu QT, Villasenor KS, Kurimoto P, Grisanti M et al (2014) Temporal changes in systemic and local expression of bone turnover markers during six months of sclerostin antibody administration to ovariectomized rats. Bone 67:305–313
35. Bono CM, Einhorn TA (2003) Overview of osteoporosis: pathophysiology and determinants of bone strength. Eur Spine J 12(Suppl. 2):S90–S96
36. Grzibovskis M, Pilmane M, Urtane I (2010) Today's understanding about bone aging. Stomatologija 12:99–104
37. Raisz LG (2007) Maintaining the life-long vitality and integrity of skeletal tissue. Bone 40(Suppl 1):S1–S4
38. Eastell R, Lambert H (2002) Strategies for skeletal health in the elderly. Proc Nutr Soc 61:173–180

39. Kanis J, Johnell O, Oden A, Dawson A, De Laet C, Jonsson B (2001) Ten year probabili-
    ties of osteoporotic fractures according to BMD and diagnostic thresholds. Osteoporos Int
    12(12):989–995
40. Miller P, Barlas S, Brenneman S, Abbott T, Chen Y, Barrett-Connor E, Siris E (2004) An
    approach to identifying osteopenic women at increased short-term risk of fracture. Arch Intern
    Med 164:1113–1120
41. Ferrari SL, Abrahamsen B, Napoli N, Akesson K, Chandran M, Eastell R, El-Hajj Fuleihan G,
    Josse R, Kendler DL, Kraenzlin M, Suzuki A, Pierroz DD, Schwartz AV, Leslie WD, on behalf
    of the Bone and Diabetes Working Group of IOF (2018) Diagnosis and management of bone
    fragility in diabetes: an emerging challenge. Osteoporos Int 29(12):2585–2596
42. Hui S, Slemenda C, Johnston C (1998) Age and bone mass as predictors of fracture in a pro-
    spective study. J Clin Invest 81:1804–1809
43. Fried L, Tangen C, Walston J, Newman A, Hirsch C, Gottdiener J, Seeman T, Tracy R, Kop
    W, Burke G, McBurnie M (2001) Frailty in older adults: evidence for a phenotype. J Gerontol
    ABiol Sci Med Sci 56:M146–M156
44. Tom S, Adachi J, Anderson F Jr, Boonen S, Chapurlat R, Compston J, Cooper C, Gehlbach S,
    Greenspan S, Hooven F, Nieves J, Pfeilschifter J, Roux C, Silverman S, Wyman A, La Croix
    A (2013) Frailty and fracture, disability, and falls: a multiple country study from the global
    longitudinal study of osteoporosis in women. J Am Geriatr Soc 61:327–334
45. Kanis J, Johnell O, Oden A, Johansson H, McCloskey E (2008) FRAX and the assessment of
    fracture probability in men and women from UK. Osteoporos Int 19:385–397
46. Kanis J, Hans D, Cooper C et al (2011) Interpretation and use of FRAX in clinical practice.
    Osteoporos Int 22:2395–2411
47. Leslie W, Lix L, Johansson H, Oden A, McCloskey E, Kanis J (2011) Spine-hip discor-
    dance and fracture risk assessment: a physician-friendly FRAX enhancement. Osteoporos Int
    22:839–847
48. Hiligsmann M, Kanis J, Compston J, Cooper C, Flamion B, Bergmann P, Body J, Boonen S,
    Bruyere ODJ, Goemaere S, Kaufman J, Rozenberg S, Reginster J (2013) Health technology
    assessment in osteoporosis. Calcif Tissue Int 93:1–14
49. Harvey NC, Glüer CC, Binkley N, McCloskey MV, Brandi ML, Cooper C, Kendler D, Lamy
    O, Laslop A, Camargos BM, Reginster JY, Rizzoli R, Kanis JA (2015) Trabecular bone score
    (TBS) as a new complementary approach for osteoporosis evaluation in clinical practice: a
    consensus report of a European Society for Clinical and Economic Aspects of Osteoporosis
    and Osteoarthritis (ESCEO) Working Group. Bone 78:216–224
50. Hans D, Goertzen AL, Krieg M-A, Leslie WD (2011) Bone micro-architecture assessed by
    TBS predicts osteoporotic fractures independent of bone density: the Manitoba study. J Bone
    Miner Res 26:2762–2769
51. Winzenrieth R, Michelet F, Hans D (2013) Three-dimensional (3D) microarchitecture correla-
    tions with 2D projection image gray-level variations assessed by trabecular bone score using
    high-resolution computed tomographic acquisitions: effects of resolution and noise. J Clin
    Densitom 16:287–296
52. Simonelli C, Leib E, Mossman N, Winzenrieth R, Hans D, McClung M (2014) Creation of an
    age-adjusted, dual-energy x-ray absorptiometry-derived trabecular bone score curve for the
    lumbar spine in non-Hispanic US White women. J Clin Densitom 17:314–319
53. Howe T, Rochester L, Neil F, Skelton D, Ballinger C (2011) Exercise for improving balance in
    older people. Cochrane Database Syst Rev (11):CD004963. https://doi.org/10.1002/14651858
54. AGS/BGS/AAOS (2001) Guideline for the prevention of falls in older persons. American
    Geriatrics Society, British Geriatrics Society, and American Academy of Orthopaedic Surgeons
    Panel on Falls Prevention. J Am Geriatr Soc 49:664–672
55. Michael Y, Whitlock E, Lin J, Fu R, O'Connor E, Gold R (2010) Primary care-relevant inter-
    ventions to prevent falling in older adults: a systematic evidence review for the U.S. Preventive
    Services Task Force. Ann Intern Med 153:815–825
56. Rizzoli R, Branco J, Brandi M, Boonen S, Bruyère O, Cacoub P, Cooper C (2014) Management
    of osteoporosis of the oldest old. Osteoporos Int 25:2507–2529
57. Boucher B (2012) The problems of vitamin D insufficiency in older people. Aging Dis
    3:313–329

58. Bischoff-Ferrari H, Willett W, Orav E, Lips P, Meunier P, Lyons R, Flicker L, Wark J, Jackson R, Cauley J, Meyer H, Pfeifer M, Sanders K, Stahelin H, Theiler R, Dawson-Hughes B (2012) A pooled analysis of vitamin D dose requirements for fracture prevention. N Engl J Med 367:40–49

59. Bischoff-Ferrari H, Dawson-Hughes B, Staehelin H, Orav J, Stuck A, Theiler R, Wong J, Egli A, Kiel D, Henschkowski J (2009) Fall prevention with supplemental and active forms of vitamin D: a meta-analysis of randomised controlled trials. BMJ 339:b3692. https://doi.org/10.1136/bmj.b3692

60. Rizzoli R, Boonen S, Brandi N, Bruyer O, Cooper C, Kanis J, Kaufman J, Ringe J, Weryha G, Reginster J (2013) Vitamin D supplementation in elderly or postmenopausal women: a 2013 update of 2008 reccomandations from the European Society for Clinical and Economic Aspects of Osteoporosis and Osteoarthritis (ESCEO). Curr Med Res Opin 29:305–313

61. Bischoff-Ferrari H, Kiel D, Dawson-Hughes B, Orav J, Li R, Spiegelman D, Dietrich T, Willett W (2009) Dietary calcium and serum 25-hydroxyvitamin D status in relation to BMD among U.S. adults. J Bone Miner Res 24:935–942

62. Bolland M, Avenell A, Baron J, Grey A, MacLennan G, Gamble G, Reid I (2010) Effect of calcium supplements on risk of myocardial infarction and cardiovascular events: metaanalysis. BMJ 341:c3691

63. Burckhardt P (2011) Potential negative cardiovascular effects of calcium supplements. Osteoporos Int 22:1645–1647

64. Genaro P, Martini L (2010) Effect of protein intake on bone and muscle mass in the elderly. Nutr Rev 68:616–623

65. Eisman JA, Bogoch ER, Dell R, Harrington JT, McKinney RE Jr, McLellan A, Mitchell PJ, Silverman S, Singleton R, Siris E (2012) Making the first fracture the last fracture: ASBMR task force report on secondary fracture prevention. J Bone Miner Res 27:2039–2046

66. Conley RB, Adib G, Adler RA, Akesson KE, Alexander IM, Amenta KC, Blank RD, Brox WT, Carmody EE, Chapman-Novakofski K, Clarke BL, Cody KM, Cooper C, Crandall CJ, Dirschl DR, Eagen TJ, Elderkin AL, Fujita M, Greenspan SL, Halbout P, Hochberg MC, Javaid M, Jeray KJ, Kearns AE, King T, Koinis TF, Koontz JS, Kuzma M, Lindsey C, Lorentzon M, Lyritis GP, Michaud LB, Miciano A, Morin SN, Mujahid N, Napoli N, Olenginski TP, Puzas JE, Rizou S, Rosen CJ, Saag K, Thompson E, Tosi LL, Tracer H, Khosla S, Kiel D (2020) Secondary fracture prevention: consensus clinical recommendations from a multistakeholder coalition. J Bsone Miner Res 35:36–52. https://doi.org/10.1002/jbmr.3877

67. Rabenda V, Mertens R, Fabri V, Vanoverloop J, Sumkay F, Vannecke C, Deswaef A, Verpooten G, Reginster JY (2008) Adherence to bisphosphonates therapy and hip fracture risk in osteoporotic women. Osteoporos Int 19:811–818

68. Tafaro L, Nati G, Leoni E, Baldini R, Cattaruzza MS, Mei M, Falaschi P (2013) Adherence to anti-osteoporotic therapies: role and determinants of "spot therapy". Osteoporos Int 24(8):2319–2323

Frailty and Sarcopenia

4

Finbarr C. Martin and Anette Hylen Ranhoff

4.1 Frailty

Frailty is generally understood as a progressive age-related decline in physiological systems that results in decreased reserves, which confers extreme vulnerability to stressors and increases the risk of a range of adverse health outcomes. There are however two distinct concepts that emerge from the clinical and research literature. The first is of a syndrome associated with underlying physiological and metabolic changes that are responsible for driving progressive physical and cognitive impairments through to loss of functional capacity, often helped on the way by acute or chronic disease or injury. This can be encapsulated by the definition proposed some two decades ago and still valid [1]. As a result, the frail person is at increased risk of disability or death from minor external stresses.

The second concept underpins a pragmatic approach, which treats frailty as a collection of risk factors for future adverse events, whilst not necessarily bearing a direct pathophysiological relationship to these outcomes. As discussed later these positions are not incompatible. Either way, both epidemiologically and

---

This chapter is a component of Part 1: Background.
For an explanation of the grouping of chapters in this book, please see Chapter 1: 'The Multidisciplinary Approach to Fragility Fractures Around the World—An Overview'.

F. C. Martin (✉)
Population Health Sciences, King's College London, London, UK
e-mail: finbarr.martin@kcl.ac.uk

A. H. Ranhoff
Department of Clinical Science, University of Bergen, Bergen, Norway

Department of Medicine, Diakonhjemmet Hospital, Oslo, Norway

Norwegian Institute of Public Health, Oslo, Norway
e-mail: anette.ranhoff@uib.no

© The Author(s) 2021
P. Falaschi, D. Marsh (eds.), *Orthogeriatrics*, Practical Issues in Geriatrics,
https://doi.org/10.1007/978-3-030-48126-1_4

conceptually, frailty overlaps with but is distinct from multimorbidity and disability [2]. In cross-sectional studies, some frail individuals are neither multimorbid nor disabled, but multimorbid individuals are more likely than others to be frail, and frail individuals are by definition more likely to develop a new disability. Frailty could therefore be looked upon as a risk factor for functional decline, in line with more traditional risk factors such as hypertension, hypercholesterolemia, obesity and smoking [3].

4.1.1 The Nature of Frailty

There are several diagnostic definitions and measures of frailty, validated in various populations in terms of predicting an increased incidence of adverse outcomes such as new disability, hospitalisation and death. The two best-established approaches are the phenotype model developed by Fried's group in the United States [4] and the deficit accumulation model developed by Rockwood and Mitnitski in Canada [5]. Both have been validated subsequently in unrelated cohorts internationally.

The phenotype approach was generated empirically from a larger number of candidate features tested in a longitudinal dataset, and analysis resolved them into five components—unintentional weight loss, self-reported fatigue, low physical activity and impairment of grip strength and gait speed comparative to relevant population norms. Three or more abnormalities define frailty, with pre-frailty defined as the presence of one or two. The criteria for judging abnormality is illustrated in Fig. 4.1, but in practice, subsequent researchers have adapted criterion definitions to the data available.

The Fried Phenotype Model of Frailty

Weight loss	**Self-reported weight loss of more than 4·5 kg or recorded weight loss of "5% per year**
Exhaustion	Self-reported exhaustion on US Center for Epidemiological Studies depression scale73 (3–4 days per week or most of the time)
Low energy expenditure	Energy expenditure <383 kcal/week (men) or <270 kcal/week (women)
Slow gait speed	Standardised cut-off times to walk 4·57 m, stratified by sex and height
Weak grip strength	Grip strength, stratified by sex and body-mass index

Fig. 4.1 The frailty phenotype

This phenotype model, therefore, does not explicitly include cognitive or psychosocial features that are also well known to be predictive of adverse health outcomes, but these domains may impact any of the five dimensions, for example, a low mood may be associated with self-assessed fatigue, and cognitive impairment is associated with slower gait. Nevertheless, there is substantial evidence that this predominantly physical frailty phenotype has predictive power for adverse health outcomes in several cohorts of older people.

The deficit accumulation approach is quite different. It operationalises frailty as the sum total of age-related factors that may be regarded as detrimental ("deficits"). These could be symptoms, sensory impairments, abnormal clinical findings or laboratory test results, diseases, disabilities or lack of social support. Suitable parameters are those that are increasingly prevalent with advancing age but do not saturate and are credibly associated with health. Thus, grey hair is not suitable! Generally, each is regarded as present or absent and thus accorded a score of 0 or 1, although some variables lend themselves to be divided in three or occasionally more grades, so become fractions of one. The total score, termed the frailty index (FI), is calculated from the sum of all the deficit scores divided by the number of items included. The theoretical range of the FI is therefore between 0 (no deficits apparent, good health) to 1 (deficits in every item), but in practice, a number of studies have now shown that survival is rare with scores above about 0.7. The deficit accumulation model is an approach rather than a fixed tool and is therefore highly flexible. A FI can be constructed from suitable variables in any comprehensive dataset about an individual as long as it covers a broad range of these health-related domains and includes upwards of 30 items. Despite these two approaches to diagnosing frailty being quite distinct, they perform fairly similarly in identifying frailty when applied to a common dataset [6, 7].

4.1.2 Epidemiology of Frailty

Whatever approach is used to define frailty, it becomes more prevalent with increasing age. The prevalence in community versus institutional care settings is 12% (95% CI 10–15%) and 45% (95% CI 27–63%), respectively. When using broader definitions than the physical phenotype, the prevalence increases to 16% (95% CI 7–29%) [8]. Frailty prevalence rises to 20–50% by age 85+ [9] and is more common in women, but several studies suggest that women are more resilient to frailty than men. Geographical differences in frailty prevalence may be related to health inequalities, as rates are significantly associated with national economic indicators. Differences within countries may also be associated with socioeconomic factors including social deprivation [10]. Frailty is a dynamic syndrome and may be reversible—people move in and out of a frailty state [11]. However, there are few studies of frailty trajectories.

4.1.3   How Does Frailty Develop?

Frailty may be best understood from the standpoint of ageing and evolution. A universal result of living is the gradual and progressive process of acquiring deleterious changes to body structure and function, affecting all individuals to variable degrees and not associated with a specific external cause. These ageing-related impairments result from the lifelong accumulation of unrepaired molecular and cellular damage, which take multiple forms and impact cell survival, protein synthesis and the efficiency of damage detection and repair processes. The pathophysiological pathways that result from this damage are not fully elucidated, but candidates include cytokines and other components of the inflammatory response [12, 13]. The defence and repair mechanisms are generally good enough in earlier life to enable normal growth, development and reproduction, but did not evolve to provide indefinite protection in older age. There was no evolutionary pressure to do so and since all metabolic processes use energy (ultimately from food), it makes biological sense to develop enough but not surplus repair capacity. These age-related changes are accompanied by an increased chance of certain "degenerative" diseases, but these are not universal. Disability results from the critical impairment of specific attributes, such as strength or balance, these impairments arising from ageing or disease or more usually both.

4.1.4   Assessment of Frailty in Clinical Practice

The scope and detail of assessment needed and the choice of assessment tool should be tailored to the population being assessed and the purpose of the assessment. For example, many of the functional tests such as walking speed and the Timed Up and Go test are not feasible in patients with acute hip fractures. Neither the phenotype model nor the FI is particularly feasible in routine clinical practice, so simpler tools are more commonly used such as the Clinical Frailty Scale [14] or the Edmonton Frail Scale [15]. The Clinical Frailty Scale uses descriptors covering the domains of mobility, energy, physical activity, and function to enable a standard clinical assessment to characterise nine levels from very fit, healthy through very severely frail to terminally ill. (Fig. 4.2). This provides a feasible description based on routine clinical assessment but does not conceptually distinguish frailty from multimorbidity or disability. Its mortality prediction is comparable to that of the more detailed FI and it is useful in settings where a quick impression can help indicate what clinical decisions need to be considered.

The Edmonton scale requires a number of specific but fairly simple clinical measures to be performed, which would be additional to routine clinical practice. The domains included are cognition (the clock drawing test), general health status, functional ability, social support, medication use, nutrition, mood, continence and a mobility function test—the Timed Up and Go. Scores range from 0 to 17, scores of 8 or above usually being considered to be frail, but relevant cut-offs can be established empirically depending upon the purpose. For example, the prediction of

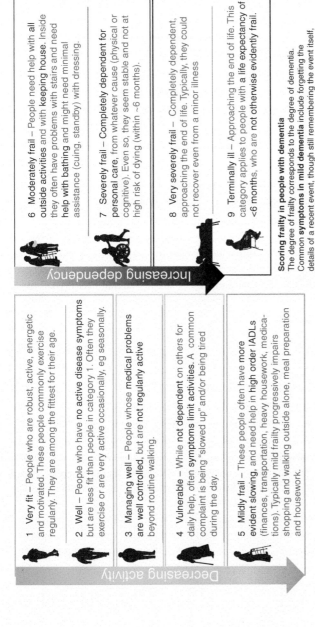

Decreasing activity

1   **Very fit** – People who are robust, active, energetic and motivated. These people commonly exercise regularly. They are among the fittest for their age.

2   **Well** – People who have no active disease symptoms but are less fit than people in category 1. Often they exercise or are very active occasionally, eg seasonally.

3   **Managing well** – People whose medical problems are **well controlled, but are not regularly active** beyond routine walking.

4   **Vulnerable** – While **not dependent** on others for daily help, often **symptoms limit activities**. A common complaint is being "slowed up" and/or being tired during the day.

5   **Mildly frail** – These people often have more evident slowing, and need help in high order IADLs (finances, transportation, heavy housework, medications). Typically, mild frailty progressively impairs shopping and walking outside alone, meal preparation and housework.

Increasing dependency

6   **Moderately frail** – People need help with all outside activities and with **keeping house**. Inside they often have problems with stairs and need **help with bathing** and might need minimal assistance (cuing, standby) with dressing.

7   **Severely frail** – **Completely dependent for personal care**, from whatever cause (physical or cognitive). Even so, they seem stable and not at high risk of dying (within ~6 months).

8   **Very severely frail** – Completely dependent, approaching the end of life. Typically, they could not recover even from a minor illness

9   **Terminally ill** – Approaching the end of life. This category applies to people with a life expectancy of **<6 months**, who are **not otherwise evidently frail**.

Scoring frailty in people with dementia
The degree of frailty corresponds to the degree of dementia.
Common **symptoms in mild dementia** include forgetting the details of a recent event, though still remembering the event itself, repeating the same question/story and social withdrawal.
In **moderate dementia**, recent memory is very impaired, even though they seemingly can remember their past life events well. They can do personal care with prompting.
In **severe dementia**, they cannot do personal care without help.

Fig. 4.2   The Clinical Frailty Scale. This reproduces the descriptive text from the Clinical Frailty Scale. Readers are advised to refer to the original that includes schematic drawings and this explanation about people with dementia. "The degree of frailty corresponds to the degree of dementia. Common symptoms in mild dementia include forgetting the details of a recent event, though still remembering the event itself, repeating the same question/story and social withdrawal. In moderate dementia, recent memory is very impaired, although they seemingly can remember their past life events well. They can do personal care with prompting. In severe dementia, they cannot do personal care without help"

1	Are you more than 85 years?	Yes = 1 point
2	Male?	Yes = 1 point
3	In general, do you have any health problems that require you to limit your activities?	Yes = 1 point
4	Do you need someone to help you on a regular basis?	Yes = 1 point
5	In general, do you have any health problems that require you to stay at home?	Yes = 1 point
6	In case of need, can you count on someone close to you?	No= 1 point
7	Do you regularly use a stick, walker or wheelchair to get about?	Yes = 1 point
	Total	

Fig. 4.3 The PRISMA score

likely higher rates of postoperative complications may be associated with lower scores. In contrast to some other tools, the Edmonton scale identifies potential targets for intervention across a number of clinically important domains.

In community or primary care settings, the issue may be to identify a target group for health-promoting interventions such as optimising nutrition and increasing physical activity levels. Here a more simple screening approach may be needed. A recent systematic review assessing available tools suggested that PRISMA-7 may be the most accurate [16], a score of 3 or more suggesting the increased likelihood of incident disability [17] (Fig. 4.3).

4.1.5 Incorporating Frailty into Treatment Plans and Service Design

In general, there is not sufficient evidence for screening programmes for frailty [18]. Case finding in clinical settings could be carried out in two phases, using a short screening test and then confirming the diagnosis using a comprehensive geriatric assessment (CGA) if a geriatric service is available, or at least an assessment of nutrition and muscle function. The need then is to provide intervention or package of interventions for those deemed to be pre-frail or frail to prevent, slow or reverse frailty [19]. Patients with fragility fractures could be assessed for frailty in the acute setting by using, for example, the Clinical Frailty Scale based on information from the patient and next-of-kin about the pre-fracture status. In a rehabilitation phase, the Edmonton scale or á full CGA would enable an individually tailored programme to be applied.

4.2 Sarcopenia

Sarcopenia was the term suggested by Rosenberg for the well-recognised loss of muscle with ageing [20]. It is a major component of frailty. The diagnosis, treatment and prevention of sarcopenia is recommended to become part of routine clinical practice [21]. Skeletal muscle accounts for a third or more of total body mass. As well as movement, muscle plays a key role in temperature regulation and metabolism. Low muscle mass is associated with poor outcomes from acute illness, probably because of the reduced metabolic reserve, as muscle is a reservoir for proteins and energy that can be used for the synthesis of antibodies and gluconeogenesis.

4.2.1 The Nature of Sarcopenia

Sarcopenia is characterised by motor neurone loss, reduced muscle mass per motor unit, relatively more loss of fast-twitch fibres and reduced strength per unit of cross-sectional area. Muscle fibres are lost by drop-out of motor neurones. Reinnervation of fibres by sprouting from surviving neurones cause less even distribution of fibre types cross-sectionally and a relatively greater loss of type II fibres that are associated with the generation of power (the product of force generation and speed of muscle contraction) [22].

Muscle mass and strength are of course related but not linearly [23]. Function is more important than mass for physical performance and disability [24] Leg power accounts for 40% of the decline in functional status with ageing [25]. Men who maintain physical activity into their 80s show compensatory hypertrophy of muscle fibres to compensate for the decrease in fibre number. Loss of efficiency also results from an accumulation of fat within and between fibres and an increase in non-contractile connective tissue material. Muscle strength and function also depend on neuromuscular integrity and muscle performance as well as muscle characteristics. Indeed, the force produced by external electrical stimulation to large muscle groups such as quadriceps exceeds that which can be achieved by maximal voluntary contraction, emphasising the importance of non-muscle factors.

4.2.2 Epidemiology

A systematic review on the prevalence of sarcopenia by the European Working Group on Sarcopenia in Older People (EWGSOP) criteria reported a variable prevalence from 1 to 29% in persons living in the community, 14–33% in those living in long-term care institutions and 10% for those in acute hospital care [26]. A higher prevalence at 30% was reported from a Norwegian population of hospitalised older persons [27]. In most of these studies, the prevalence of sarcopenia increased with age, but the effect of sex varied. A study from Iceland found an increase in the prevalence of sarcopenia from 7 to 17% from age 75 to 80. In older (65+) hip fracture patients sarcopenia is found in 17–74%, the highest prevalence in Chinese male patients. In a selected population of previously home-dwelling older hip fracture patients, mean age 79 years old, 38% had sarcopenia according to the EWGSOP 2010 definition [28].

4.2.3 How Does Sarcopenia Develop?

Muscle fibre development occurs before birth but fibres enlarge during childhood reaching a peak in early adulthood. Mass and function then gradually decline into older age [29]. Peak mass is affected by intra-uterine, genetic and early life influences. The decline is affected by physical activity, nutrition and sex. It is more pronounced in women from menopause onwards. Adding to the inevitable moderate decline of some 15–25% by old age is the impact of acute illness or chronic conditions, which have generally negative effects through the mechanisms of catabolic stress, reduced food intake and physical inactivity. The loss of muscle mass is thought to be multifactorial with potential factors illustrated in Fig. 4.4.

The factors implicated in sarcopenia overlap with those for frailty. A central feature of sarcopenia is a decrease in the rate of muscle protein synthesis. This leads to reduced protein levels including mitochondrial oxidative enzymes responsible for enabling work intensity. The age-related shift of the hormonal balance towards low testosterone, growth hormone and IGF-I contributes to the lower muscle protein synthesis rates, which also limits the structural recovery from muscle damage or apoptosis and possibly reduces the synthetic stimulus of exercise [30]. The role of cytokines such as interleukins IL-1β and IL-6 and TNF-α is less certain. They play

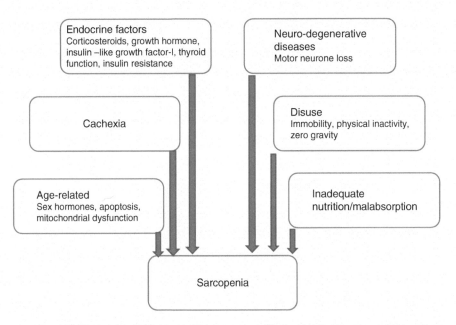

Fig. 4.4 Aetiological factors and mechanisms of sarcopenia (Adapted from Cruz-Jentoft AJ, Baeyens JP, Bauer JM, Boirie Y, Cederholm T, Landi F, Martin FC, Michel JP, Rolland Y, Schneider SM, Topinková E, Vandewoude M, Zamboni M. Sarcopenia: European consensus on definition and diagnosis: Report of the European Working Group on Sarcopenia in Older People. *Age Ageing*. 2010 Jul;39(4):412–23)

a role in the catabolic processes of acute illness and chronic inflammatory conditions, but whether the small differences in circulating levels associated with frailty reported from some population studies are relevant to the age-related sarcopenia is not established.

4.2.4 Assessing Sarcopenia in Clinical Practice

There are several different diagnostic definitions resulting in the range of prevalence rates reported earlier from community-dwelling populations of older people. A consensus definition and approach to screening and classification has been proposed by EWGSOP established by the European Geriatric Medicine Society, first in 2010, and with a revised version in 2018 [31]. This is shown in Fig. 4.5. Measuring gait speed of ambulant people is feasible in almost any community setting and is a useful global indicator of health, slower gait being associated with a greater likelihood of incident disability, falls, institutionalisation and death [32]. Grip strength was

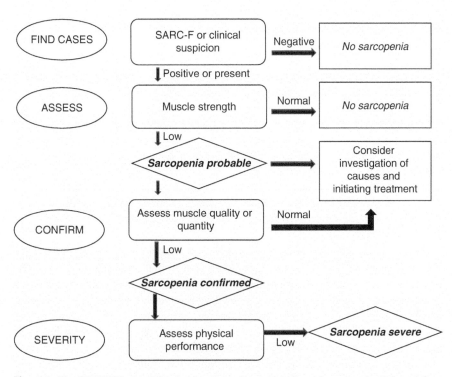

Fig. 4.5 The EWGSOP algorithm for the diagnosis and grading of sarcopenia (Adapted from Cruz-Jentoft AJ, Bahat G, Bauer JM, et al. (2019) Sarcopenia: revised European consensus on definition and diagnosis: Age Ageing; 48(1):16–31). Further details on how to apply this algorithm can be found in this paper, with suggestions for feasible and reliable methods to assess muscle strength, quality and quantity, and physical performance

chosen as it is a portable, simple, reliable and valid proxy measure of body strength, and has a good correlation with lower limb physical performance. Low grip strength of community-dwelling older people is associated with falls, increased incident disability and earlier mortality. It also predicts slower and less complete functional recovery from illness in men [33].

Measurement of muscle mass can be done with CT scan or, less accurately, with impedance techniques or anthropometry (measurements of upper mid-arm circumference, estimation of upper mid-arm muscle cross-sectional area, measurement of mid-calf circumference) [31]. Ultrasound is a promising emerging technique but not yet in routine use. Assessment of sarcopenia with the above-mentioned methods may not be feasible in clinical populations such as after lower limb fractures, and measurement of muscle function is more important than measurement of muscle mass in clinical practice. An indication of pre-fracture severe sarcopenia can be obtained, using the Sarc-F tool, which is a brief questionnaire about muscle function (mobility and ability to carry a certain weight). The Sarc-F tool is available in many languages [34].

4.2.5   Incorporating Sarcopenia into Treatment Plans and Service Design

Sarcopenia has recently been recognized as a clinical diagnosis with a corresponding code in the ICD system. For the diagnosis of sarcopenia, either the definitions from EWGSOP or the Foundation for the National Institutes of Health (FNIH) are recommended. But for rapid screening and special patient groups, such as hip fracture patients, rapid screening with the SARC-F is recommended. All health personnel working with older patients should be aware of sarcopenia.

4.3   The Implications of Frailty and Sarcopenia on Falls, Fractures and the Recovery After Fractures

With the exception of the vertebra, most fractures in older people are related to falls. Poor bone health makes a fracture more likely, but from the population perspective, risk of falling is more predictive of fractures than bone mineral density [35], leading to the suggestion that the focus of primary fracture prevention must rest with identifying those at risk of falls rather than those with osteoporosis [36]. After a fragility fracture, however, it is imperative to consider falls prevention and bone health as described in detail in Chapters 14–16 of the IIIrd Pillar.

There are common risk factors and overlap in the biology of frailty, sarcopenia and osteoporosis. Frailty predicts lower bone mineral density, an increased likelihood of falls, vertebral and hip fractures [37, 38]. Sarcopenia and osteoporosis often co-exist and shared risk factors have given rise to the notion of osteosarcopenioa [39]. The typical hip fracture sufferer is a frail woman more than 80 years, so prevention requires a multicomponent approach embracing frailty.

For older people with osteoporosis, a consensus panel recommended a multi-component exercise programme including resistance and balance training [40]. In general, physical exercise programmes are shown to be effective for reducing or postponing frailty with benefits more likely if conducted in groups. Physical exercise with nutritional supplementation, supplementation alone, cognitive training and combined treatment do also show a favourable effect on frailty outcomes [41]. Recognition of frailty is also key in the management of those who have fractured. For example, frailty, as assessed with the FI, was associated with longer hospital length of stay and reduced chance of returning home within 30 days after hip fracture [42].

4.4 Concluding Statement

There are close links epidemiologically, biologically and clinically between frailty, sarcopenia, poor bone health and the geriatric syndrome of falls. Older people who have had a fall and/or a fracture should be assessed for frailty and sarcopenia to better develop a care plan. This calls for an integrated clinical approach to the prevention and treatment of fragility fractures.

References

1. Campbell AJ, Buckner DM (1997) Unstable disability and the fluctuations of frailty. Age Ageing 26(4):315–318
2. Fried LP, Ferrucci L, Darer J, Williamson JD, Anderson G (2004) Untangling the concepts of disability, frailty, and comorbidity: implications for improved targeting and care. J Gerontol Med Sci 59(3):255–263
3. Cesari M, Pérez-Zepeda MU, Marzetti E (2017) Frailty and multimorbidity: different ways of thinking about geriatrics. J Am Med Dir Assoc 18(4):361–364
4. Fried LP, Tangen CM, Walston J et al (2001) Frailty in older adults: evidence for a phenotype. J Gerontol A Biol Sci Med Sci 56:M146–M156
5. Rockwood K, Song X, MacKnight C, Bergman H, Hogan DB, McDowell I, Mitnitski A (2005) A global clinical measure of fi tness and frailty in elderly people. Can Med Assoc J 173(5):489–495
6. Romero-Ortuno R (2013) The frailty instrument for primary care of the Survey of Health, Ageing and Retirement in Europe predicts mortality similarly to a frailty index based on comprehensive geriatric assessment. Geriatr Gerontol Int 13:497–504
7. Rockwood K, Andrew M, Mitnitski A (2007) A comparison of two approaches to measuring frailty in elderly people. J Gerontol A Biol Sci Med Sci 62(7):738–743
8. O'Caoimh R, Galluzzo L, Rodríguez-Laso Á, Work Package 5 of the Joint Action ADVANTAGE et al (2018) Prevalence of frailty at population level in European ADVANTAGE Joint Action Member States: a systematic review and meta-analysis. Ann Ist Super Sanita 54(3):226–238
9. Collard RM, Boter H, Schoevers RA, Oude Voshaar RC (2012) Prevalence of frailty in community- dwelling older persons: a systematic review. J Am Geriatr Soc 60(8):1487–1492
10. Lang IA, Hubbard RE, Andrew MK, Llewellyn DJ, Melzer D, Rockwood K (2009) Neighborhood deprivation, individual socioeconomic status, and frailty in older adults. J Am Geriatr Soc 57(10):1776–1780

11. Xue QL, Bandeen-Roche K, Varadhan R, Zhou J, Fried LP (2008) Initial manifestations of frailty criteria and the development of frailty phenotype in the Women's Health and Aging Study II. J Gerontol A Biol Sci Med Sci 63(9):984–990

12. Clegg A, Young J, Iliffe S, Rikkert MO, Rockwood K (2013) Frailty in elderly people. Lancet 381(9868):752–762

13. Puts MTE, Visser M, Twisk JWR, Deeg DJH, Lips P (2005) Endocrine and inflammatory markers as predictors of frailty. Clin Endocrinol 63:403–411

14. National Institute for Health and Care Excellence (2016) Multimorbidity: assessment, prioritisation and management of care for people with commonly occurring multimorbidity. NICE guideline. http://www.nice.org.uk. Accessed 12 Sept 2019

15. Rolfson DB, Majumdar SR, Tsuyuki RT et al (2006) Validity and reliability of the Edmonton Frail Scale. Age Ageing 35:526–529

16. Hoogendijk EO, Van Der Horst HE, Deeg DJH et al (2013) The identification of frail older adults in primary care: comparing the accuracy of five simple instruments. Age Ageing 42:262–265

17. Raiche M, Hebert R, Dubois MF (2008) PRISMA-7: a case-finding tool to identify older adults with moderate to severe disabilities. Arch Gerontol Geriatr 47:9–18

18. Dent E, Martin FC, Bergman H, Woo J, Romero-Ortuno R, Walston JD (2019) Management of frailty: opportunities, challenges, and future directions. Lancet 394:1376–1386

19. Rodríguez-Laso Á, O'Caoimh R, Galluzzo L, Carcaillon-Bentata L, Beltzer N, Macijauskiene J, Albaina Bacaicoa O, Ciutan M, Hendry A, López-Samaniego L, Liew A, Work Package 5 of the Joint Action ADVANTAGE (2018) Population screening, monitoring and surveillance for frailty: three systematic reviews and a grey literature review. Ann Ist Super Sanita 54(3):253–262

20. Rosenberg IH (1989) Summary comments. Am J Clin Nutr 50:1231–1233

21. Cruz-Jentoft AJ, Sayer AA (2019) Sarcopenia. Lancet 393(10191):2636–2646

22. Lexell J (1995) Human aging, muscle mass, and fiber type composition. J Gerontol A Biol Sci Med Sci 50:A11–A16

23. Goodpaster BH, Park SW, Harris TB et al (2006) The loss of skeletal muscle strength, mass and quality in older adults. J Gerontol A Biol Sci Med Sci 61:1059–1064

24. Metter EJ, Talbot LA, Schrager M, Conwit R (2002) Skeletal muscle strength as a predictor of all-cause mortality in healthy men. J Gerontol A Biol Sci Med Sci 57(10):B35

25. Foldvari M, Clark M, Laviolette LC et al (2000) Association of muscle power with functional status in community-dwelling elderly women. J Gerontol A Biol Sci Med Sci 55A:M192–M199

26. Cruz-Jentoft AJ, Landi F, Schneider SM, Zuniga C, Arai H, Boirie Y et al (2014) Prevalence of and interventions for sarcopenia in ageing adults: a systematic review. Report of the International Sarcopenia Initiative (EWGSOP and IWGS). Age Ageing 43(6):748–759

27. Jacobsen EL, Brovold T, Bergland A, Bye A (2016) Prevalence of factors associated with malnutrition among acute geriatric patients in Norway: a cross-sectional study. BMJ Open 6(9):e011512

28. Steihaug OM, Gjesdal CG, Bogen B, Kristoffersen MH, Lien G, Hufthammer KO et al (2018) Does sarcopenia predict change in mobility after hip fracture? a multicenter observational study with one-year follow-up. BMC Geriatr 18(1):65

29. Janssen I, Heymsfield SB, Wang ZM, Ross R (2000) Skeletal muscle mass and distribution in 468 men and women aged 18–88 yr. J Appl Physiol 89(1):81–88

30. Giannoulis MG, Martin FC, Nair KS, Umpleby AM, Sonksen P (2012) Hormone replacement therapy and physical function in healthy older men. Time to talk hormones? Endocr Rev 33(3):314–377. https://doi.org/10.1210/er.2012-1002

31. Cruz-Jentoft AJ, Bahat G, Bauer J et al (2019) Sarcopenia: revised European consensus on definition and diagnosis. Age Ageing 48(1):16–31. Erratum in: Age Ageing. 48(4):601, 2019

32. Vermeulen J, Neyens JC, van Rossum E, Spreeuwenberg MD, de Witte LP (2011) Predicting ADL disability in community-dwelling elderly people using physical frailty indicators: a systematic review. BMC Geriatr 11:33

33. Roberts HC, Syddall HE, Cooper C, Aihie Sayer A (2012) Is grip strength associated with length of stay in hospitalised older patients admitted for rehabilitation? Findings from the Southampton grip strength study. Age Ageing 41(5):641–646
34. Bahat G, Yilmaz O, Oren M et al (2018) Cross-cultural adaptation and validation of the SARC-F to assess sarcopenia: methodological report from European Geriatric Medicine Society Sarcopenia Special Interest Group. Eur Geriatr Med 9:23–28
35. Kaptoge S, Benevolenskaya LI, Bhalla AK et al (2005) Low BMD is less predictive than reported falls for future limb fractures in women across Europe: results from the European Prospective Osteoporosis Study. Bone 36(3):387–398
36. Järvinen TL, Sievänen H, Khan KM, Heinonen A, Kannus P (2008) Analysis—shifting the focus in fracture prevention from osteoporosis to falls. BMJ 336:124–126
37. Sternberg SA, Levin R, Dkaidek S, Edelman S, Resnick T, Menczel J (2014) Frailty and osteoporosis in older women – a prospective study. Osteoporos Int 25(2):763–768
38. Ensrud KE, Ewing SK, Taylor BC et al (2007) Frailty and the risk of falls, fracture, and mortality in older women: the study of osteoporotic fractures. J Gerontol A Biol Sci Med Sci 62:744–751
39. Hassan EB, Duque G (2017) Osteosarcopenia: a new geriatric syndrome. Aust Fam Physician 46(11):849–853
40. Giangregorio LM, Papaioannou A, MacIntyre NJ (2014) Too fit to fracture: exercise recommendations for individuals with osteoporosis or osteoporotic fracture. Osteoporos Int 25:821–835
41. Apóstolo J, Cooke R, Bobrowicz-Campos E et al (2018) Effectiveness of interventions to prevent pre-frailty and frailty progression in older adults: a systematic review. JBI Database System Rev Implement Rep 16(1):140–232
42. Krishnan M, Beck S, Havelock W, Eeles E, Hubbard RE, Johansen A (2014) Predicting outcome after hip fracture: using a frailty index to integrate comprehensive geriatric assessment results. Age Ageing 43(1):122–126

Part II

Pillar I: Co-management in the Acute Episode

Establishing an Orthogeriatric Service

5

Terence Ong and Opinder Sahota

5.1 Introduction

Older people with fragility fractures do not present with the acute problem of the fracture only. Alongside their broken bone, many present concurrently with medical illnesses, frailty, multi-morbidity and disability. They are at risk of future falls and/or fractures, have a challenging peri-operative period, are at risk of medical complications and many do not return to their pre-fracture level of function. Orthogeriatric care is an adaption of the Comprehensive Geriatric Assessment (CGA) [1, 2], which is a multidimensional, interdisciplinary assessment and treatment of an older person. This co-management model of care with CGA principles, bringing together the relevant multidisciplinary expertise in fragility fracture management, has been shown to be the most effective way to address the complex healthcare needs of these patients and deliver improved outcomes [1, 3, 4]. Orthogeriatric care is now established as the ideal model of care for hip fracture management and is recommended in several national guidelines (see Fragility Fracture Network website—select a region and then choose Fragility Fracture Care Guidelines option) [5].

This chapter is a component of Part 2: Pillar I.
For an explanation of the grouping of chapters in this book, please see Chapter 1—"The Multidisciplinary Approach to Fragility Fractures Around the World—An Overview".

T. Ong (✉)
Faculty of Medicine, University of Malaya, Kuala Lumpur, Malaysia
e-mail: terenceong@doctors.org.uk

O. Sahota
Department of Healthcare for Older People,
Nottingham University Hospitals NHS Trust, Nottingham, UK
e-mail: opinder.sahota@nuh.nhs.uk

© The Author(s) 2021
P. Falaschi, D. Marsh (eds.), *Orthogeriatrics*, Practical Issues in Geriatrics,
https://doi.org/10.1007/978-3-030-48126-1_5

Different models of hip fracture orthogeriatric services have been described depending on how the different orthopaedic and geriatric medicine services interact with each other [3, 6]. The most integrated model of co-management has demonstrated the best outcome in time to surgery, hospital length of stay and survival [3, 4, 7]. This chapter focuses on the framework required to establish such an orthogeriatric service. The steps detailed here are not prescriptive but should provide the guidance required to either start the service or develop parts of the existing service.

5.2 Designing the Orthogeriatric Service

5.2.1 Step 1: Process Mapping the Hip Fracture Pathway

An orthogeriatric service needs to consider the entire journey of the patient with a hip fracture, from their presentation to the Emergency Department all the way through to their rehabilitation and recovery. Hence, an important initial step to understand the local hip fracture pathway and how the future orthogeriatric service can be delivered locally is by performing a mapping exercise. The mapping exercise has to be a detailed assessment of each phase of care during the patients' hospital journey from what happens in the Emergency Department, pre-operatively, during the operation, after the operation and rehabilitation period. In each phase, the mapping exercise needs to specify what the treatment goals are (principles of care) and how these goals can be delivered (explicit care delivered) (Table 5.1).

Another benefit of mapping the hip fracture pathway is that it facilitates information gathering to justify an orthogeriatric service locally. Orthogeriatric care is still not a routine practice in many parts of the world. Moving hip fracture care from the traditional model of an orthopaedic team overseeing care with reactive medical input, to a co-management model will require justification that such a service is required. This is especially important in places where musculoskeletal health is not part of a national agenda and receives little attention. Extracting information and translating clinical evidence generated from other units or countries may not suffice. Healthcare managers would also be more receptive to establishing a service with local data. Hence, this mapping exercise should also attempt to generate data to serve two important purposes:

Table 5.1 An example of a mapping exercise of an orthogeriatric service across the different phases of care and components of care delivered that need to be delivered

Phases of care	Principles of care	Care delivered
Emergency Department (ED)	1. Prompt fracture identification 2. Pain relief 3. Transfer to trauma/orthopaedic wards	1. Early clinical and radiological identification of a hip fracture 2. Prompt assessment of pain and analgesia appropriate to pain severity 3. Minimise delay in transferring patient to orthopaedic or trauma units

Table 5.1 (continued)

Phases of care	Principles of care	Care delivered
Pre-operative phase	1. Multidisciplinary team involvement 2. Pre-operative assessment and optimisation of co-pathology/co-morbidities 3. Risk stratification for adverse outcomes	1. Early involvement of orthogeriatric care team to agree surgical, anaesthesia and medical plan 2. Clear documentation and information sharing between specialties, e.g., using a joint admission clerking trauma booklet 3. Adequate pain management before surgery and appropriate use of nerve blocks 4. Optimisation of co-pathology and co-morbidities (e.g., fluid status, delirium, anaemia, glycaemic control, anticoagulation) 5. Implementation of standardised guidelines in commonly encountered problems (e.g., anticoagulation reversal, blood transfusion, delirium management) 6. Utilise validated hip fracture risk stratification tool (e.g., Nottingham Hip Fracture Score) and agree to appropriate ceilings of care 7. Agreed pathways to a specialist investigation (e.g., magnetic resonance imaging for occult fracture, echocardiogram to assess cardiac function)
Operative phase	1. Timely surgery 2. Choice of anaesthesia and surgical technique as appropriate for the patient	1. Minimise wait for an operation 2. Adequate staff and theatre capacity 3. Agreed prophylactic antibiotic treatment 4. Surgical and anaesthetic plan in place delivered by adequately skilled clinicians 5. Clear post-operative instructions, including weight-bearing status 6. Identification of those that require more intense post-operative monitoring 7. Target haemoglobin and criteria for transfusion
Post-operative phase	1. Mobilisation 2. Minimising hospital complications 3. Nutrition support 4. Continence care 5. Prevention of pressure sores 6. Planning for post-hospital care	1. Routine review by orthogeriatric team members to identify complications early and facilitate recovery 2. Early mobilisation and identification of barriers (e.g., pain, delirium, hypovolaemia, anaemia) 3. Identification of those at risk of malnutrition and nutrition supporting strategies 4. Bowel and continence care 5. Regular review of pressure areas 6. Identifying those that would require extended venous thromboprophylaxis

(continued)

Table 5.1 (continued)

Phases of care	Principles of care	Care delivered
Rehabilitation	1. Transfer of care out of the hospital with the right support in place 2. Information sharing with patient and primary care providers 3. Falls and fracture risk assessment and treatment	1. Routine and regular multidisciplinary team meetings to discuss recovery and plan for post-hospital care 2. Minimise delay and wait for community rehabilitation 3. Identification of risk factors for falls and fractures Implementing individualised falls and fracture prevention plan 4. Fall and fracture prevention followed up by a relevant clinical team 5. Clear sharing of information with the primary care provider

- Convincing people that there is a problem—gather data on local hip fracture epidemiology with an idea of absolute numbers presenting to the local hospital, and if available, how this has changed over time.
- Convincing people that orthogeriatric co-management is the solution—demonstrate the characteristics and outcomes of this patients that would require orthogeriatric co-management, that is, fragility fracture and frailty needs.

5.2.2 Step 2: Identify a Core Multidisciplinary Team and Form a Steering Group

Many healthcare professionals with different discipline backgrounds have important contributions to make to high-quality care for older patients with hip fractures. Mapping the pathway allows identification of these key members of the interprofessional multidisciplinary team (MDT). These key members usually include:

- Orthopaedic surgeon
- Physician with expertise in older people, frailty, trauma and bone health (e.g., ortho-geriatrician)
- Anaesthetist
- Nurse
- Physiotherapist
- Occupational therapist

This is not an exhaustive list as many successful services are supported by other health professionals such as social workers, clinical pharmacists, dieticians, fracture liaison services and radiology. The key to efficient multidisciplinary working has to be coordination and communication between the various team members. Responsibility is shared across the pathway depending on the patient's clinical need. For instance, the operative procedure is the responsibility of the surgeon and managing medical barriers to early mobilisation is better led by the geriatrician.

Table 5.2 Geriatric medicine competencies in the management of hip fractures. Adapted from training requirements for UK specialist trainees in Geriatric Medicine in Orthogeriatrics [9]

Orthogeriatric medicine competencies
Awareness of the different models of orthogeriatric care and the evidence base of their evaluation
Understanding the impact of hip fracture on the older person
Understanding of surgical and anaesthetic issues related to hip fracture care
Preoperative optimisation of acute illnesses and chronic medical conditions
Management of postoperative care and complications (delirium, continence issues, tissue viability, pneumonia, thromboembolism, anaemia, acute kidney injury and cardiovascular complications)
Recognising the role of palliative and end of life care
Nutritional assessment and intervention
Knowledge of appropriate assessment tools for mobility, daily living and function
Planning rehabilitation goals and transfer of care (discharge planning)
Knowledge of the causes and management of falls and fragility fractures
Knowledge of the role of the Fracture Liaison Service and its evidence-base
Ability to work in a multidisciplinary team and value the role of different team members
Leadership and management skills in interdisciplinary and multi-agency working
Understanding of the role of quality improvement, audit and morbidity/mortality reviews

Appropriate organisation of ward rounds and the use of a common admission/assessment proforma can support much of this MDT working. Many admission/assessment proformas are available for download from sites such as the UK National Hip Fracture Database (NHFD) in its resources section [8].

However, in many countries the input from geriatricians, i.e., physicians with expertise in managing frail older people, is limited because either the number of practising geriatricians is small, or that geriatric medicine is still not recognised as its own medical specialty. In such a situation, geriatric medicine competencies can be acquired by other physicians, such as hospital internists or general physicians, to support the care of older patients with hip fractures. An example of geriatric medicine competencies in orthogeriatric care is listed in the table below (Table 5.2).

5.2.3 Step 3: Analyse and Review the Patient Pathway

The key MDT members identified in the earlier step will also form the steering group that will review the whole hip fracture pathway, determine the overall strategy (short, medium and long term aims), review quality improvement work and discusses clinical governance issues through regular meetings. In practice, the initiation and leadership of such a steering group require the existence of just a few champions—people who have realised how much better and more cost-effective the multidisciplinary approach can be, especially for hip fracture patients, which are the most numerous and costly patient group. Although the steering group itself needs to be kept to a manageable size in order to have efficient meetings, it is important that the wider healthcare workers involved in the whole hip fracture pathway are engaged on an occasional basis. This helps to raise the general level of knowledge and foster commitment among the wider MDT.

The steering group needs to decide how to operationalise the orthogeriatric service and how each phase of care should be delivered. This is determined by research, consensus of good clinical practice and clinician experience (subsequent chapters of this book describe these good practices in more detail in each phase of care). Even at this planning stage, there needs to be engagement with healthcare managers and relevant stakeholders.

When analysing and addressing gaps in care, there are two managerial strategies that have been recognised to support this process. One, the "five whys," [10] is a sequential means of addressing the superficial, symptomatic problems that are immediately obvious and then breaking them down in stages to get to the real underlying issues. Asking the question "why?" five times often reveal problems that the service user was previously unaware of. The second strategy is to perform a SWOT (strengths, weaknesses, opportunities and threats) analysis [11]. This allows the organisation to concentrate on internal factors (strengths and weaknesses of the existing service) and external factors (opportunities and threats that the new service provides). This gives a very clear global view of the situation and often reveals issues that were previously not considered. Both analyses rely on the steering group brainstorming, which circumvents the bias of a single proponent.

5.2.4   Step 4: Evaluate the Resources Required to Drive Change Within the Organisation

The resource required is more than just the finances needed to establish the service. Devised in 1980 by Waterman and colleagues, the "Seven S" model (Fig. 5.1) is a way of thinking holistically about the resources required to drive change within the organisation to achieve the components of optimal hip fracture care [12]. Each "S" must be addressed in order to meet management criteria:

- *Staff*—Are the right staff members in place to facilitate the introduction of the new orthogeriatric service? Are more or fewer staff required? Means of appropriate recruitment need to be considered.
- *Skills*—Do the staff have the necessary expertise? Do they require more training?
- *Structure*—Does the existing organisational structure lend itself to supporting this venture? The answer in most acute hospitals is "yes" as most surgical departments are already performing hip surgery. This is a natural evolvement of an existing service.
- *Shared values*—All parties involved in the change have to truly believe in the process in order for it to be implemented smoothly. Management, ward, theatre staff, and surgeons all need to back the venture, and this will only happen if all parties are involved in the whole process from its conception to its execution. There must be an opportunity for discussion and debate.

Fig. 5.1 The seven S
model developed by Peters,
Philips and Waterman.
(Adapted from Business
Horizons [12])

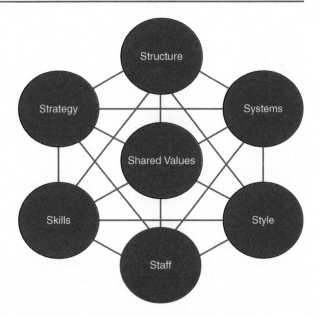

- *Style of management*—Is the current management style appropriate to oversee this? The orthogeriatric service needs to be driven predominantly by the core MDT with management as willing co-partners; a management autocracy here is not appropriate.
- *Strategy*—Are the steps in place to facilitate change? All staff providing hip fracture care need to know about the patient pathway; patients need to be informed about new services, and ward staff have to change existing care protocols to make them more specific. A global, long-term strategy is required to ensure success.
- *Systems*—This encompasses all aspects from information technology to patient support. Existing systems may need to be adapted.

5.2.5 Step 5: Develop the Business Case for the Orthogeriatric Service

The previous steps and information gathered up to this point should provide the basis for the business case for the planned orthogeriatric service. The business case is a concise document that will take the recipient, usually the relevant healthcare managers, on a journey from conception of the idea (justify why it is required) to delivery of the service (how it can be delivered). It aims to persuade those in charge of finances and service provision how an orthogeriatric service can benefit the patient, department, hospital and wider organisation. It must leave no stone unturned and be subjected to intense scrutiny. The business case also has to match with what is feasible and can be realistically delivered. The business case should be broken down into several subheadings and should include:

- Project title
- Summary statement
- Background
- Description of the service
- Benefits analysis
- Project planning

The United Kingdom National Hip Fracture Database website has a resource section (NHFD) [8], which includes an orthogeriatric care handbook and contains:

- Suggested job plans for ortho-geriatricians and specialist nurses in orthogeriatrics
- Links to publications describing different models of orthogeriatric care
- Model business cases and links to publications demonstrating cost-effectiveness

5.2.6   Step 6: Implementing and Sustaining the Service

When the business case has been approved by the hospital board, which will include executive and non-executive members, managers, clinicians and financial representatives, the service may be started as either a small pilot of the whole orthogeriatric pathway or implementation of certain phases of the pathway (Table 5.1). The service, overseen by the steering group, aims to implement the good practice that will be further described in subsequent chapters of this book.

The process does not stop with the implementation of the orthogeriatric service. It has to be followed by constant evaluation of the service and quality improvement work led by the steering group to sustain and develop it. The Plan, Do, Study, Act (PDSA) cycle, is a widely accepted and used framework for developing, testing and implementing change [13] (Fig. 5.2).

> **Example of a PDSA Cycle Used to Improve Care**
> *Plan*
> Patients with hip fracture on anticoagulation waited longer to go to theatre compared to those not on an anticoagulant. A quality improvement project was performed to report on the scale of the problem and identify potential solutions.
> *Do*
> An analysis was conducted using hospital service level data and patient case notes retrospectively. Data collected on how much longer patients waited, its clinical impact and where these delays occurred.

Study

Patients on vitamin K antagonists (warfarin) waited almost 24 h longer and those on direct oral anticoagulants (DOACs) waited over 48 h longer than those not on any anticoagulation. These patients had a longer length of stay. There were delays in identifying these patients, administering vitamin K to reverse the effects of warfarin, delays in repeating the coagulation profile post-reversal, uncertainty over when the DOAC was last taken and variation in surgeons' instructions on how long to wait for surgery after the last dose.

Act

A guideline on anticoagulation management in the peri-operative hip fracture period was written which addressed the reversal of warfarin and DOACs, monitoring of coagulation profile and when it is safe to operate. The admission documentation was altered to explicitly ask if the patient is on anticoagulation and when it was last taken. The steering group sought consensus on time to theatre. These steps standardised anticoagulation management and reduce variation in practice. An audit was embedded into the guideline to benchmark clinical practice with published standards.

It is important to remember that a successful implementation of an orthogeriatric service does not guarantee its success. It needs to be sustained and developed. This has to be paced appropriately with constant re-evaluation of the pathway to ensure resources match the provision of service. The steering group and leadership within it need to drive this. There is a wealth of literature that has reported on sustainability

Fig. 5.2 PDSA cycle. (Adapted from NHS Improvement [13])

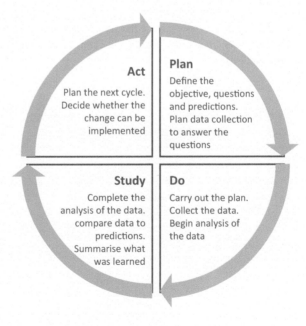

Act
Plan the next cycle. Decide whether the change can be implemented

Plan
Define the objective, questions and predictions. Plan data collection to answer the questions

Study
Complete the analysis of the data. compare data to predictions. Summarise what was learned

Do
Carry out the plan. Collect the data. Begin analysis of the data

and improvement in healthcare [14–16]. In a report by the health service body, NHS Improvement, they highlighted six key factors to sustainability [14].

1. Supportive management structure
2. Structures (e.g., IT systems and infrastructure) to foolproof change so that embedding takes place
3. Improvement supported by robust, transparent feedback systems + PDSA cycles
4. Effective collaboration across many levels from managers to front line staff and a shared sense of the systems to be improved
5. Culture of improvement with engaged staff and patients
6. Formal capacity building programs through formal and informal training

5.2.7   Step 7: Collect Evidence of Service Improvement: Audit

The audit is a way of measuring what is being delivered against a defined quality standard. National audits such as the United Kingdom Scottish Hip Fracture Audit and the National Hip Fracture Database (NHFD) across England, Wales and Northern Ireland have allowed individual hospitals to continuously audit their care based on agreed quality standards and benchmark it against other units. These audits have been very useful in sustaining and driving improvement in hip fracture within hospitals and across the country overall. National audits exist in countries where orthogeriatric service is delivered routinely; however, in places where this is not the case, regular review of what is delivered using robust audit processes across the pathway still needs to be embedded into the service. Agreed audit standards by the steering group need to measure what is delivered (process and service outcomes) by the whole orthogeriatric service. These quality standards need to be important and realistically deliverable within the time frame allocated. This is different from clinical outcome measures, such as length of stay, mortality and medical complications.

An Example of Audit Standards: Adapted from the Scottish Standards of Care for Hip Fracture Patients [17]
1. Patients with a hip fracture are transferred from the Emergency Department to the orthopaedic ward within 4 h.
2. Within 24 h of admission
   (a) Screening for delirium
   (b) Assessment of nutrition
   (c) Falls assessment
   (d) Pressure area assessment

3. Patients undergo surgical repair of their hip fracture within 36 h of admission.
4. No patients repeatedly fasted in preparation for surgery. Clear oral fluids offered up to 2 h prior to surgery.
5. Cemented hemiarthroplasty implants are standard unless clinically indicated otherwise.
6. An older patient receives a review by a geriatrician within 72 h of admission.
7. Mobilisation has begun by the end of the first day after surgery.
8. Every patient has a documented occupational therapy assessment commenced within 72 h of admission.
9. Every patient has an assessment or a referral for their bone health within 60 days.
10. Multidisciplinary team meeting during their acute orthopaedic admission.

Figure 5.3 below illustrates the use of an audit cycle to measure and improve the assessment of delirium in patients with hip fractures [18].

Besides audit, all orthogeriatric services need to have a robust governance process, where learning from harms, morbidity and mortality reviews happen regularly. This promotes a culture of open learning to improve care. Furthermore, hip fracture

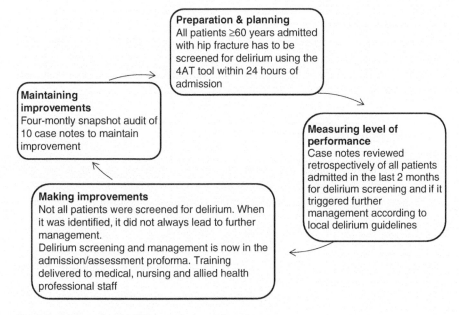

Fig. 5.3 Audit cycle of delirium screening and management

management continues to develop and remains a subject of tremendous research interest. Thus, continuing professional development and training in this area is required to keep up to date with all its developments. Information sharing, networking and specialist conferences provide an opportunity to utilise new information and good practice developed elsewhere to address specific clinical problems, for example, reversal of anticoagulation and management of direct oral anticoagulants peri-operatively.

5.2.8 Step 8: Embrace the Support of Regional, National and International Organisations

In many countries, there is no national musculoskeletal agenda or policy. Hence, it is important to seek support elsewhere to highlight the importance of better fragility fracture care. The World Health Organisation's report on ageing and health highlighted the importance of musculoskeletal health and preventing fractures as part of its strategy towards healthy ageing [19]. Many national and international orthopaedic and geriatric medicine societies have adopted orthogeriatric co-management as a way of delivering better care for older people with hip fractures. These societies have come together to support the work of the Fragility Fracture Network (FFN) and more recently its Global Call to Action [20]. The FFN's annual Global Congress and Regional Expert Meetings are excellent opportunities to get good ideas and advice from colleagues tackling similar problems in different countries. In addition, the role of patient or public advocates can be a powerful tool in delivering the message of orthogeriatric care and needs to be encouraged. Many lay members already sit on national boards such as the UK's Falls and Fragility Fractures Audit Programme panel. Hence, a way of sustaining an orthogeriatric service is by aligning local initiatives to a much larger national and international initiative.

5.3 Conclusion

This chapter has described a framework through eight steps to establish an orthogeriatric service for hip fractures. Establishing such a service is challenging, involving a high level of dedication, management and clinical staff coming together, and a great deal of commitment towards improving patient care. The growth in orthogeriatric services internationally has shown that setting this up is possible with the right approach and appropriate level of support. Orthogeriatric services have consistently delivered better care and outcomes for hip fracture patients and should be part of routine hip fracture management.

Box
Eight steps to establishing an orthogeriatric service

1. Process mapping the hip fracture pathway
2. Identify a core multidisciplinary team and form a steering group
3. Analyse and review the patient pathway
4. Evaluate the resources required to drive change within the organisation
5. Develop the business case for the orthogeriatric service
6. Implementing and sustaining the service
7. Collect evidence of service improvement—Audit
8. Embrace the support of a regional, national and international organisation

References

1. Ellis G, Whitehead MA, Robinson D, O'Neill D, Langhorne P (2011) Comprehensive geriatric assessment for older adults admitted to hospital: meta-analysis of randomised controlled trials. BMJ 343:d6553
2. Eamer G, Taheri A, Chen SS, Daviduck Q, Chambers T, Shi X, Khadaroo RG (2018) Comprehensive geriatric assessment for older people admitted to a surgical review. Cochrane Database Syst Rev 2018(1):CD012485. https://doi.org/10.1002/14651858.CD012485.pub2
3. Kammerlander C, Roth T, Friedman SM, Suhm N et al (2010) Ortho-geriatric service—a literature review comparing different models. Osteoporos Int 21(supple 4):s637–s646
4. Grigoryan KV, Javedan H, Rudolph JL (2014) Ortho-geriatric care models and outcomes in hip fracture patients: a systematic review and meta-analysis. J Orthop Trauma 28(3):e49–e55
5. Fragility Fracture Network. http://fragilityfracturenetwork.org/global-regions/. Accessed 31 Oct 2019
6. Giusti A, Barone A, Razzano M, Pizzonia M, Pioli G (2011) Optimal setting and care organization in the management of older adults with hip fracture. Eur J Phys Rehabil Med 47(2):281–296
7. Patel JN, Klein DS, Sreekumar S, Liporace FA, Yoon RS (2020) Outcomes in multidisciplinary team-based approach in geriatric hip fracture care: a systematic review. J Am Acad Orthop Surg 28:128–133. https://doi.org/10.5435/JAAOS-D-18-00425
8. National Hip Fracture Database. http://www.nhfd.co.uk/20/hipfractureR.nsf/ResourceDisplay. Accessed 31 Oct 2019
9. British Geriatrics Society. https://www.bgs.org.uk/resources/clarification-of-training-requirements-for-higher-specialist-trainees-in-geriatric-0. Accessed 31 Oct 2019
10. Pojasek RB (2000) Asking "Why" five times. Environ Qual Manag 10(1):79–84
11. Cranfield S, Ward H (2006) Managing change in the NHS: making informed decisions on change. NCCSDO, London
12. Peters TJ, Waterman RH, Phillips JR (2006) The seven S model—a managerial tool for analysing and improving organizations. NCCDSO, London
13. NHS Improvement. https://improvement.nhs.uk/documents/2142/plan-do-study-act.pdf. Accessed 31 Oct 2019
14. NHS Institute for Innovation and Improvement. https://www.england.nhs.uk/improvement-hub/wp-content/uploads/sites/44/2017/11/ILG-1.7-Sustainability-and-its-Relationship-with-Spread-and-Adoption.pdf. Accessed 31 Oct 2019

15. NHS Scotland Quality Improvement Hub. http://www.qihub.scot.nhs.uk/media/596811/the%20spread%20and%20sustainability%20ofquality%20improvement%20in%20health-care%20pdf%20.pdf. Accessed 31 Oct 2019
16. Lennox L, Maher L, Reed J (2018) Navigating the sustainability landscape: a systematic review of sustainability approaches in healthcare. Implement Sci 13(1):27
17. Scottish Standards of Care for Hip Fracture Patients. https://www.shfa.scot.nhs.uk/_docs/2019/Scottish-standards-of-care-for-hip-fracture-patients-2019.pdf. Accessed 31 Oct 2019
18. Healthcare Quality Improvement Partnership. https://www.hqip.org.uk/wp-content/uploads/2018/02/developing-clinical-audit-patient-panels.pdf. Accessed 31 Oct 2019
19. World Health Organization. World report on ageing and health. https://www.who.int/ageing/events/world-report-2015-launch/en/. Accessed 31 Oct 2019
20. Dreinhofer KE, Mitchell PJ, Begue T, Cooper C et al (2018) A global call to action to improve the care of people with fragility fractures. Injury 49(8):1393–1397

Pre-hospital Care and the Emergency Department

6

Alex Ritchie, Andrew Imrie, Julia Williams, Alice Cook, and Helen Wilson

6.1 Pre-hospital Care

Hip fractures are considered a major global healthcare challenge [1] especially in older people with frailty, and this is likely to increase in the next few decades with estimates of the size of the problem being predicted conservatively at 4.5 million cases worldwide by 2050 [2]. The Healthcare Quality Improvement Partnership [3] estimate that in the United Kingdom around 76,000 hip fractures occur every year, and it is reasonable to assume that most of these patients will present through ambulance services; this is a significant number of people requiring assessment, management and treatment from ambulance staff. Whilst there may be differences in scope of clinical practices between (or within) countries relating to pre-hospital care of patients with hip fracture depending on differences in healthcare systems, skill mix of available clinical staff, and use of drugs and technology, the essential principles of management and treatment are likely to be similar.

In the United Kingdom, the first ambulance crew on scene may not include a paramedic. A non-paramedic crew will request paramedic back-up if required for a structured assessment and management of the patient including intravenous drug administration where required.

This chapter is a component of Part 2: Pillar I.
For an explanation of the grouping of chapters in this book, please see Chapter 1: 'The Multidisciplinary Approach to Fragility Fractures Around the World—An Overview'.

A. Ritchie · A. Imrie · J. Williams (✉)
University of Hertfordshire, Hertfordshire, UK
e-mail: alex.ritchie@nhs.net; a.imrie@herts.ac.uk; j.williams@herts.ac.uk

A. Cook · H. Wilson
Royal Surrey County Hospital NHS Foundation Trust, Guildford, UK
e-mail: Alicecook1@nhs.net; hwilson6@nhs.net

© The Author(s) 2021
P. Falaschi, D. Marsh (eds.), *Orthogeriatrics*, Practical Issues in Geriatrics,
https://doi.org/10.1007/978-3-030-48126-1_6

This chapter will focus on principles of management of a patient with suspected hip fracture once any immediate time-critical life-threatening events have been dealt with. This is not to dismiss the severity of a hip fracture in an older person with frailty, as mortality rates within the first year are high (often due to multiple co-morbidities) [4]. Pre-hospital management of a patient with an isolated hip fracture, from the point of assimilation of the information gained during the secondary survey, is summarised in Fig. 6.1. This systematic assessment of the patient occurs after completion of a dynamic risk assessment of the scene and a primary survey.

6.1.1   Clinical Assessment: Primary Survey

To provide context and clarity, a primary survey in a pre-hospital trauma patient uses a systematic approach such as the R < C > ABCDE [3, 5] framework. This involves assessing the patient in a stepwise approach, correcting any complications that present themselves, before moving on to the next stage in the sequence:

- Response level
- Catastrophic Haemorrhage
- Airway (consider c-spine injury at this stage)
- Breathing
- Circulation
- Disability
- Exposure and environment

If the patient is presenting with areas of concern during the primary survey, the ambulance staff will attempt to correct those deficit areas. If this is not possible on scene, they may decide to undertake a time-critical transfer with a pre-alert to an appropriate receiving facility whilst continuing patient treatment en route if it is safe to do so and in accordance with local policies. This may mean that definitive treatment of a patient's hip fracture is delayed, whilst other interventions take a higher priority in, for example, a patient with an acute myocardial infarction or an acute stroke. A systematic primary survey usually takes an experienced paramedic around one minute to complete if no interventions are required during this assessment [5].

6.1.2   Clinical Assessment: Secondary Survey

Once it has been established from the primary survey that there is no immediate threat to life, the paramedic (or other attending ambulance staff) will complete a comprehensive secondary survey whilst still being mindful of the need for this patient to get to definitive care in a timely manner. This process includes acquiring a patient history as well as undertaking a 'head to toe' physical assessment and documenting a full set of vital signs. The latter will contribute to the assessment of

Pre-hospital Management of Suspected Fractured Neck of Femur

Based on in-depth history and full secondary assessment, the crew identifies some or all of the following:
• Moderate or severe pain
• Shortened and/or externally rotated leg and/or deformity
• Pain to hip &/or referred pain to knee
• Unable to straight leg lift
• Unable to weight bear
• Clinician suspects hip fracture

Cautions:
• Has this patient fallen?
• Has this patient had a long-lie prior to assessment?
• Is this patient on anti coagulant or anti platelet theraphy?
• Has this patient had a previous fracture or prosthesis to affected hip?
• Does this patient have a diagnosis of osteoporosis and/or arthritis and/ or malignancy?

Management: Non Paramedic Crew
• Management of haemorrhage if present
• Check presence and quality of pedal and popliteal pulses
• Monitor vital signs
• Regular assessment of pain levels
• Entonox (or appropriate analgesia within local scope of practice)
• Request Paramedic assistance
• Assess for compromised skin integrity and manage accordingly
• Splinting and/or immobilisation of affected limb
• Optimise patient for surgery, consider as Nil By Mouth
• Extricate patient supine, on a orthopaedic scoop or vacuum mattress

Management: Paramedic Crew
Continue with management identified above, additional elements to consider:
• IV Access
• IV Paracetamol (consider IV Morphine, if pain connot be controlled via other methods)
• IV Fluid (250ml bolus Initially)
• Consider Oxygen therapy, to target 94-98% or 88-92% in COPD patients - post Morphine
• ECG Monitoring - post Morphine

No Specialist Fast-track Pathway Available

Transportation:
• Patient supported effectively with immobilisation of affected limb
• Pre-Alert Trauma Unit/Emergency Department
• Smooth transportation of patient
• Ensure patient comfort is considered throughout journey
• Effective and structured handover the patient to trauma Unit/ED staff

Local Specialist Fast-track Pathway Available

Transportation:
• Patient supported effectively with immobilisation of affected limb
• Pre-Alert to Local Fast-track pathway receiving unit - this may involve bypassing Trauma Unit/ED and going direct to an alternative specified destination (e.g. ward or radiology) OR the Fast-track may be initiated within the Trauma Unit/ED
• Smooth transportation of patient
• Ensure patient comfort is considered throughout journey
• Effective and structured handover the patient to Fast-track receiving staff

Analgesia Guidelines:

Refer to local policies

Mild - Moderate Pain
• Endonox, PRN - IH
• Methoxyflurane, 3ml - IH
• Paracetamol, 1g - IV

Severe Pain
• Morphine, 2-10mg - IV
• Ondansetron, 4mg - IV (or alternative anti-emetic for prophylactic prevention of nausea)

NSAIDs are not recommended

REMEMBER

Reassess patient's pain at all stages of treatment. Consider non-pharmacological pain management techniques such as positioning and physical support of limbs

Would this patient be suitable for Fascia Iliaca Compartment Block [1] (FICB)?

Contraindications of FICB:

• Patient declines
• Allergy to local anaesthetic
• Infection at injection site
• Previous femoral vascular surgery
• Patient connot report complications (eg. severe dementia, confusion)
• High risk of compartment syndrome

If FICB contraindicated, consider IV Morphine - as per local policy

[1] At the time of writing, paramedic administered FICB is not standard practice in the UK

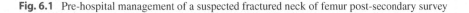

Fig. 6.1 Pre-hospital management of a suspected fractured neck of femur post-secondary survey

the patient's National Early Warning Score 2 (NEWS2) which will provide baseline information for the hospital to monitor any changes in the patient's condition.

6.1.3 Patient History

As part of the secondary survey, gaining a patient history as soon as possible after the fall is likely to give the most accurate account. History taking should be structured and include details of the fall and events leading up to it, the past medical history, allergies and medications and a social history [5, 6]. Global characteristics of the patient and their environment are noted, including general appearance, living arrangements and level of independence. This information is essential to support subsequent discharge planning.

Patients with a fall and a 'long lie' [7], which is considered anything in excess of one hour, are at risk of hypothermia, compromised skin integrity due to unrelieved pressure, rhabdomyolysis and aspiration pneumonia [7–9].

Early pain assessment and management is a key role for ambulance staff [10]. Classically, in patients with a hip fracture, there is pain on movement of the leg, in the groin and/or thigh, with pain referred to the knee [11].

Establishing a list of current medications and any known drug allergies is important for ongoing management. Recognition of anti-platelet or anticoagulant therapy is essential. Ambulance staff need to establish whether the patient has taken any analgesics recently, before administration of further doses.

6.1.4 Physical Assessment and Vital Signs

Early establishment of the patient's vital signs is recommended to identify possible intercurrent illness, monitor the patient's progress and recognise any deterioration in their clinical status. Basic observations should include blood glucose testing to rule out hypoglycaemia. The assessment of the limb should include inspection and palpation, comparing it to the uninjured side [6], examining for irregularities/deformities, swelling or bruising. Classically, with a hip fracture there is shortening and external rotation of the leg. Undisplaced hip fractures may have no signs, but patients may complain of pain on internal rotation and will be unable to straight-leg raise the affected limb [12]. Patients may be able to get up but then are unable to weight bear due to pain. In older people presenting with these signs and symptoms, ambulance crews should have a low threshold for transferring the patient to definitive care for radiological assessment.

If the emergency call relates to a fall where no clear extrinsic reason can be identified, then a 12-lead ECG should be performed, and a brief neurological assessment such as FAST (Face/Arm/Speech Test) should be undertaken to exclude stroke/TIA [7].

This information will provide the paramedic with relevant information to develop differential diagnoses and formulate a management plan whilst always being mindful that time is a factor for these patients and extended time on scene if they have a hip fracture may not be beneficial to their overall outcomes.

6.1.5   Management of Pain

Pain management should include non-pharmacological options such as splinting, immobilisation and positioning in addition to the use of pharmacological agents, always with continual assessment of the level of the patient's pain.

Consideration needs to be given to both static pain (when the patient is at rest) and dynamic pain (when the patient is moving or being moved). Adequate analgesia should be given prior to moving the patient when transferring them from the scene of the injury to the ambulance and during transportation to hospital. Pain rating scales may be used to assess the efficacy of any drugs or techniques used to control and reduce pain. There are many different pain scales available [5–7, 13], but broadly there are Numeric Rating Scales (NRS) where the patient is asked to score their pain between 0 and 10 with 10 being the 'worst level of pain'; Visual Analogue Scales (VAS) where patients choose any point on a line usually between 0 and 100 with 0 being 'no pain' and 100 being the 'worst level of pain'; Faces Pain Scale (frequently used with children and people with some level of cognitive impairment) where the faces at one end of the continuum are happy faces and then gradually change to faces in torment; and a Verbal Rating Scale (VRS) where people align with statements such as 'No Pain', 'Mild Pain' etc. [14].

Whatever scale is used, it is essential to assess pain levels both before and after intervention to ensure effective management.

Choice of analgesia may in the first instance depend on the skill mix of the ambulance crew. In the United Kingdom, if a non-paramedic crew is in attendance the most usual quick acting analgesic offered to the patient is likely to be Entonox which was introduced into UK ambulance services in 1970 [15]. Entonox is fast acting and rapidly excreted, but there can be some challenges to its use with older patients with frailty. The delivery device for Entonox is a mouthpiece and a demand valve which requires respiratory effort and coordination; this is not suitable for all patients. The alternative delivery route is via a face mask [16] which can be considered if patients struggle with the mouthpiece. Ideally, the patient should be able to hold the mask independently with Entonox being self-administered, but again this is not possible for all patients. If a paramedic is available, then intravenous paracetamol should be considered, as it has been shown to be comparable in analgesic effect to that of morphine when administered for pain control in isolated limb trauma [17]. It is important to ensure that intravenous paracetamol is given at appropriate doses in low-weight patients.

Another approach to managing pain in isolated hip fracture is paramedic-administered Fascia Iliaca Compartment Block (FICB) delivered in the pre-hospital setting. This is a new consideration in relation to paramedics' scope of practice and it is not yet routine in the United Kingdom. FICB is covered in more depth later in this chapter. A feasibility trial of paramedic-administered FICB has been carried out in Wales [18], and the early findings are positive; funding has been approved for a fully powered multi-centre randomised controlled trial of paramedic-administered FICB in pre-hospital settings starting in October 2020.

If the patient's pain is not controlled, and if there is a paramedic available, then intravenous morphine may be considered. This should be started at the lowest possible dose and titrated to therapeutic effect. It should be emphasised that opiates are often associated with significant side effects particularly in older patients with frailty and are not recommended as the drug of first choice in this age group [7]. Concurrent prophylactic use of an anti-emetic is recommended due to high incidence of nausea associated with opioids [5]. Careful observation of vital signs should be undertaken post administration of intravenous morphine, as it is a central nervous system suppressant. ECG and blood pressure monitoring are advised to detect any early changes. Additionally, the patient may need supplemental oxygen post-morphine administration, as it is a respiratory depressant. Target oxygen saturation in adults is between 94% and 98% [7] unless they are diagnosed with COPD when target saturations will usually range from 88% to 92% SPO_2.

Non-pharmacological techniques of pain management include positioning the patient carefully and ensuring limbs are well supported. Splinting and immobilisation can help to reduce pain as well as protect from further internal damage to blood vessels and/or nerves. Current recommendations are to use padding between the legs for the whole length of the leg and then to use broad fold bandages. The bandages should be applied in sequence with a figure of eight around the feet and ankles being placed first of all. This will help with gentle manual traction to straighten the leg and bring it into position. Then, there should be two broad fold bandages placed above the knee and two below the knee to securely keep the legs in alignment and minimise movement [7].

Successful pain management for these patients is likely to employ a combination of pharmacological and non-pharmacological approaches.

6.1.6 Fluid Replacement

Older patients with frailty are often dehydrated and should be given intravenous fluids. Caution needs to be exercised in patients with a history of heart failure. In the United Kingdom, the recommendations recommend a loading volume of 250 mls of crystalloids in the form of intravenous sodium chloride 0.9% [7] to improve tissue perfusion and combat dehydration, but each patient's needs will be different. Another indication for administration of intravenous fluids is related to trauma and possible haemorrhage. Paramedics need to be guided by local policies and practices relating to fluid replacement therapy, as these will determine what options they have in management of the haemodynamic status of the patient [5–7, 19].

Traditionally, patients have been kept nil by mouth in anticipation of surgery, but most units would now advocate feeding the patient until a definite time for surgery is confirmed, to avoid long periods of starvation.

6.1.7 Extrication

Ambulance staff must consider the best method of transferring the patient with a hip fracture into the ambulance and transporting them to a place of definitive care. A carry chair is not appropriate with the risk of further damage at the site of injury and is likely to be extremely painful for the patient [19]. An orthopaedic scoop stretcher is a good option to get a patient from the floor onto a trolley without the need to log-roll the patient. If the patient has to be taken downstairs, however, the scoop stretcher may be more difficult to use, and the crew may need to request additional staff to do this safely. Deployment of a vacuum mattress can also be considered as an adjunct to extrication, but, at times, there may be limited options [19].

6.1.8   Transportation

Fast-track hip fracture care has been developed in some countries, but there is no standardisation. Further research is required to identify which components, at what stage, and in what combination of the fast-track pathway have the most significant impact on patients' outcomes and experiences [20]. This should include research in pre-hospital care, involving paramedics and other ambulance staff.

In the United Kingdom, there are a growing number of fast-track pathways for patients who have a suspected hip fracture. In some regions, after a pre-alert call from the ambulance crew to the hospital, patients will by-pass the Emergency Department and go straight to radiology or a specialist ward to reduce time to definitive treatment. Other areas rely on the pre-alert call from the ambulance staff to the receiving unit to ensure the patient is fast-tracked through the Emergency Department [7].

Key principles of patient management during transportation revolve around continual monitoring of the patient's vital signs. Equally important is to re-assess pain levels and try to minimise exposure to protracted pain through a combination of appropriate pharmacological interventions in conjunction with effective splinting and immobilisation of the limb, comfortable positioning of the patient and, as far as is possible, a smooth, controlled approach to driving to avoid the patient being exposed to unnecessary sudden movements and jolts.

Effective handover to the receiving unit staff is essential and is frequently performed using various frameworks such as IMIST-AMBO [21] (Identification of patient, Mechanism of injury/medical complaint, Injuries/information relative to the complaint, Signs, vitals and GCS, Treatment/response to treatment, Allergies, Medications, Background history and Other (social) information), developed in Australia. It has been shown, amongst other things, to improve the quality of information, shorten the duration of handover and reduce the number of questions asked after the handover. In the United Kingdom, ATMIST (Age, Time of onset, Medical complaint/injury, Investigation, Signs and Treatment) is the recommended mnemonic [7] which contains the relevant clinical information for an effective handover. There is still a need for further evidence to establish whether standardised frameworks consistently achieve improved performance in this area and, if so, to what degree [22].

Pre-hospital clinicians have an important role in the management of patients with hip fracture. They are well placed to get a clear account of the patient's fall, comorbidities and circumstances and handover of this information to the hospital team can save time and repetition. Early appropriate management of pain and hydration can also influence peri-operative complications. It is important that pre-hospital staff and hospital staff work and learn together, to continually improve patient care.

6.2   The Emergency Department

As soon as a patient with suspected hip fracture arrives, triage assessment should ensure that the patient is cardiovascularly stable, using an early warning score. A brief review of the cause of the fall is essential to ensure that unstable medical conditions such as dehydration, sepsis, gastro-intestinal haemorrhage, stroke or cardiac syncope are not missed.

Most hospitals in the United Kingdom now have a fast-track pathway for patients with suspected hip fracture [23]. This enables patients who are stable at triage to be prioritised for X-ray. The current targets from the Royal College of Emergency Medicine are that 90% of X-rays completed should be within 60 minutes of arrival and 75% of patients with a hip fracture should be referred within 120 minutes of arrival [24].

For patients with frailty or those with a history of respiratory disease, a baseline chest X-ray should be performed at the same time. In patients with known malignancy or concerns about pathological fracture, a full-length femur view is required to assess for lytic lesions and plan surgery.

Blood should be taken early for routine testing, ideally with point-of-care testing of haemoglobin and lactate to dictate early management. A significant proportion of patients will require blood transfusion in the peri-operative period, and group-and-save samples should be sent routinely.

Those with complex fractures or those on anti-platelets or anticoagulants may bleed significantly into the fracture site, and resuscitation with intravenous fluids should be commenced early, with consideration of blood transfusion in appropriate cases.

6.2.1   Nutrition and Hydration

Patients should be encouraged to eat and drink if able, until 6 hours before planned surgery. For elective patients, there is evidence to suggest that it is safe to continue with clear oral fluids up until 2–3 hours pre-surgery [25]. Oral carbohydrate loading drinks are actively encouraged for elective patients with evidence from enhanced recovery programmes. However, care must be taken with frail older patients with fragility fractures, as some will have required opiates for pain control and may have delayed gastric emptying.

Most patients with frailty are at high risk of malnutrition and should not be kept nil by mouth unnecessarily. Those who have had a long lie after their fall, or who have intercurrent illness, are likely to be dehydrated, and this should be addressed with appropriate fluid resuscitation. Others with pain or delirium may not manage adequate oral fluids and should have maintenance intravenous fluids prescribed.

Caution must be taken in those with decompensated heart failure or fluid overload from other conditions.

6.2.2 Management of Pain

Pain from a fracture is best managed by initial immobilisation and fixation where possible to aid healing. Immobilisation in plaster or with traction without surgery has significant risks in frail patients, as skin integrity is often poor. Immobility often rapidly leads to poor oral intake, generalised muscle weakness, orthostatic pneumonia, thromboembolic disease, incontinence and skin breakdown. As such, a decision for early surgery is usually the best option.

6.2.3 Ongoing Analgesia

Pain leads to distress and is the symptom that people fear the most. It may be a key feature in the development of delirium in those at risk.

As previously discussed, it is important to monitor pain both at rest (static pain) and on movement (dynamic pain), as even those immobilised still experience pain during personal care and toileting. Pain should be measured, ideally using a validated score on admission and after 30 minutes of administering analgesia, to ensure effectiveness [26]. Ongoing review of pain should form part of routine nursing observations. Paracetamol should be continued every 6 hours. It is reported to have very few side effects and may also be effective in reducing delirium [27].

Opioids such as Codeine, Tramadol and others have significant side effects and are poorly tolerated by older people causing nausea, vomiting, constipation and confusion and should be avoided.

Opiates may be required but should be used in the lowest possible dose to avoid nausea, vomiting, sedation and respiratory depression. Older patients with poor renal function may not metabolise opiates effectively, and even small doses can cause prolonged side effects.

Non-steroidal anti-inflammatory drugs (NSAID) should only be used with extreme caution. Trauma and poor oral intake increase the risk of gastric irritation and bleeding and this may be exacerbated with the use of NSAIDs. Those on antihypertensive medication are at high risk of renal impairment with NSAIDs.

6.2.4 Local Nerve Blocks

Local nerve blocks are increasingly being used to manage both static and dynamic pain and to reduce the requirements for opiate analgesia.

NICE guidelines state that nerve blocks should be used where possible to limit the use of systemic analgesia [28]. For hip fracture, both femoral nerve blocks and fascia-iliaca compartment blocks (FICB) have been shown to be effective [29].

Single dose fascia-iliac a blocks given in the pre-operative period significantly reduce the post-operative and total analgesic requirements. These patients experience lower rates of delirium and those that manage to return directly home, do so more quickly, reducing the cost of inpatient stay but also lessening the burden of hip fracture on older comorbid patients [30].

Traditionally performed as part of the anaesthetic, these procedures are being used earlier to manage pre-operative pain in the first 8–16 hours. FICB is a low-skill, inexpensive procedure which may be performed by trained individuals including non-physician practitioners as outlined in a position statement by the Association of Anaesthetists of Great Britain and Ireland [31]. The fascia–iliaca compartment is a potential space containing the iliacus muscle, the femoral nerve and the lateral cutaneous nerve of the thigh. A single high-volume injection using 30 mls (for under 55 kg) to 40 mls (over 55 kg) of 0.25% levobupivacaine local anaesthetic, injected through the fascia lata and into the fascia iliaca compartment, will affect the femoral nerve, the lateral femoral cutaneous nerve and, to some extent, the obturator nerve. These supply the medial, anterior and lateral aspects of the thigh and the femoral head. Although this can be performed without ultrasound by trained practitioners with good effect, a small study suggests that ultrasound guidance, where available, may improve efficacy from 47% to 60% up to 82–95% [32].

Guidelines recommend that observations need to be performed for 30 minutes following a nerve block. As the fracture pain is relieved, the side effects of previously administered morphine may become apparent as respiratory depression, with fatal consequences [33].

6.2.5 Skin Care

Traction is rarely used in hip fracture, as it offers little benefit and is poorly tolerated in those with frail skin.

There is a high risk of skin breakdown and pressure ulcers in those who are immobile, particularly in those with low body weight, malnutrition, poor skin and incontinence. Patients with diabetes or neuropathy have an increased risk.

Pressure-relieving mattresses should be used where available to minimise risk of pressure damage.

Urinary catheters may be considered for short-term use pre-operatively to help to minimise skin damage and reduce the need for painful movement.

6.2.6 Referral for Early Surgery

An orthopaedic assessment should occur as soon as the X-rays are available, and if a fracture is confirmed, a proposed time for an early operation should be agreed.

6.3   Summary

In general, patients with hip fracture need early assessment and initial management of pain. This can be initiated in the pre-hospital setting to reduce distress associated with transfer to hospital. The principles of assessment, management and optimisation have an increasing evidence base, but the patient pathway may vary with different roles of healthcare practitioners in different healthcare systems.

References

1. Lu Y, Uppal HS (2019) Hip fractures: relevant anatomy, classification, and biomechanics of fracture and fixation. Geriatr Orthop Surg Rehabilit 10:2151459319859139. https://doi.org/10.1177/2151459319859139
2. Veronese N, Maggi S (2018) Epidemiology and social costs of hip fracture. Injury 49(8):1458–1460
3. Healthcare Quality Improvement Partnership. National Hip Fracture Database Annual Report. https://data.gov.uk/dataset/3a1f3c15-3789-4299-b24b-cd0a5b1f065b/national-hip-fracture-database-annual-report-2018. Accessed 23 Dec 2019
4. Riemann AHK, Hutchison JD (2016) The multidisciplinary management of hip fractures in older patients. Orthop Traumatol 30(2):117–122
5. Willis S, Dalrymple R (eds) (2020) Fundamentals of paramedic practice: a systems approach, 2nd edn. Wiley Blackwell, Oxford
6. Gregory P, Ward A (2010) Sanders' paramedic textbook. Mosby, Edinburgh
7. Joint Royal Colleges Ambulance Liaison Committee (2019) Association of Ambulance Chief Executives JRCALC Clinical Guidelines 2019. Class Professional Publishing, Bridgewater
8. Wongrakpanich S, Kallis C, Prasad P, Rangaswami J, Rosenzweig A (2018) The study of rhabdomyolysis in the elderly: an epidemiological study and single center experience. Aging Dis 9(1):1–7
9. Bledsoe BE, Porter RS, Cherry RA (2014) Paramedic care, principles & practice, 4th edn. Pearson Education Ltd, New York
10. Pilbery R, Lethbridge K (2016) Ambulance care practice. Class Professional Publishing, Bridgewater
11. LeBlanc KE, Muncie HL Jr, LeBlanc LL (2014) Hip fracture: diagnosis, treatment, and secondary prevention. Am Fam Physician 89(12):945–951
12. Greaves I, Porter K (2007) Oxford handbook of pre-hospital care. Open University Press, Oxford
13. Blaber AY, Harris G (eds) (2016) Assessment skills for paramedics, 2nd edn. Open University Press, Maidenhead
14. Ferreira-Valente MA, Pais-Ribeiro JL, Jensen MP (2011) Validity of four pain intensity rating scales. Pain 152(10):2399–2404
15. Baskett PJ, Withnell A (1970) Use of Entonox in the ambulance service. Br Med J 2:41–43
16. Gregory P, Mursell I (2010) Manual of clinical paramedic procedures. Wiley, Oxford
17. Craig M, Jeavons R, Probert J et al (2012) Randomised comparison of intravenous paracetamol and intravenous morphine for acute traumatic limb pain in the emergency department. Emerg Med J 29(1):37–39
18. Jones JK, Evans BA, Fegan G, Ford S, Guy K, Jones S et al (2019) Rapid Analgesia for Prehospital hip Disruption (RAPID): findings from a randomised feasibility study. Pilot Feasibil Stud 5(1):77
19. Eaton G (2012) Management of an isolated neck-of-femur fracture in an elderly patient. JPP 4(7):400–408

20. Pollmann CT, Røtterud JH, Gjertsen JE, Dahl FA, Lenvik O, Årøen A (2019) Fast track hip fracture care and mortality–an observational study of 2230 patients. BMC Musculoskelet Disord 20(1):248
21. Iedema R, Ball C, Daly B, Young J, Green T, Middleton PM, Foster-Curry C, Jones M, Hoy S, Comerford D (2012) Design and trial of a new ambulance-to-emergency department handover protocol: 'IMIST-AMBO'. BMJ Qual Saf 21(8):627–633
22. Fitzpatrick D, McKenna M, Duncan EA, Laird C, Lyon R, Corfield A (2018) Critcomms: a national cross-sectional questionnaire based study to investigate prehospital handover practices between ambulance clinicians and specialist prehospital teams in Scotland. Scand J Traum Resuscit Emerg Med 26(1):45
23. Audit Commission (2000) United they stand: co-ordinating care for elderly patients with hip fractures. HMSO, London
24. Royal College Emergency Medicine (2014) Clinical Standards for Emergency Departments. https://www.rcem.ac.uk/docs/Clinical%20Standards%20and%20Guidance/Clinical%20Standards%20for%20Emergency%20Departments.pdf
25. Brady M, Kinn S, Stuart P (2003) Preoperative fasting for adults to prevent peri-operative complications. Cochrane Database Syst Rev 2003(4):CD004423
26. NICE (2011) NICE clinical guideline 124. Hip Fracture: the management of hip fracture in adults. Guidance.nice.org.uk/cg124
27. Morrison R, Magaziner J, McLaughlin MA et al (2003) The impact of post-operative pain on outcomes following hip fracture. Pain 103(3):303–311. Management of Pain Reduces Delirium.
28. NICE Guidance: The Management of Hip Fractures in Adults (2017) Page 36. https://www.nice.org.uk/guidance/cg124/evidence/full-guideline-pdf-183081997
29. Foss NB, Kristensen BB, Bundgaard M et al (2007) Fascia iliaca compartment blockade for acute pain control in hip fracture patients: a randomized, placebo-controlled trial. Anesthesiology 106(4):773–778
30. Callear J, Shah K (2016) Analgesia in hip fractures: Do fascia-iliac blocks make any difference? BMJ Quality Improv Rep 5:u210130.w4147
31. Griffiths R, Tighe S (2013) Fascia iliaca blocks and non-physician practitioners. Aagbi Position Statement.   http://www.aagbi.org/sites/default/files/Fascia%20Ilaica%20statement%2022JAN2013.pdf
32. Dolan J et al (2008) Ultrasound guided fascia iliaca block: a comparison with the loss of resistance technique. Reg Anesth Pain Med 33(6):526–531
33. RCEM (2018) Safety alert: the importance of monitoring after Fascia-iliaca block. https://www.rcem.ac.uk/docs/Safety%20Resources%20+%20Guidance/RCEM_Fascia%20Iliaca%20Block_Safety%20Newsflash%20Feb%20(22022018)%20revised.pdf

Pre-operative Medical Assessment and Optimisation

7

Helen Wilson and Amy Mayor

7.1 Pre-operative Medical Assessment

Comprehensive Geriatric Assessment (CGA) has a strong evidence base in reducing mortality, increasing the number of patients discharged back to their own homes and reducing length of stay [1]. This approach should form the basis of assessment for any older person with frailty in hospital.

The pre-operative medical assessment forms part of an interdisciplinary review to understand the medical conditions that a patient may have in the context of their functional ability. The medical history can be evaluated by physicians, anaesthetists, peri-operative physicians, orthogeriatricians, or any frailty practitioner with skills in developing a clear understanding of the implications of co-morbidities on an individual's ability to function in addition to gauging the likely impact of trauma, anaesthesia and surgery.

In addition, therapists often conduct initial assessments to gather information about mobility, activities of daily living, cognition, mood, environmental and social circumstances.

This chapter is a component of Part 2: Pillar I.
For an explanation of the grouping of chapters in this book, please see Chapter 1: 'The Multidisciplinary Approach to Fragility Fractures Around the World—An Overview'.

H. Wilson (✉)
Royal Surrey County Hospital, Guildford, UK
e-mail: hwilson6@nhs.net

A. Mayor
Calderdale and Huddersfield Hospital, Huddersfield, UK
e-mail: Amy.mayor@cht.nhs.uk

© The Author(s) 2021
P. Falaschi, D. Marsh (eds.), *Orthogeriatrics*, Practical Issues in Geriatrics,
https://doi.org/10.1007/978-3-030-48126-1_7

95

7.2   Information Gathering

This can be more complex than it seems with older patients often unaware of their personal medical history, previous investigations or reasons for prescribed medications. A significant proportion also has cognitive impairment and is unable to provide information. Collateral history from carers, the primary care physician, previous hospital medical notes, previous imaging and pathology results are key to piecing together a complete picture.

Having a standardised clerking proforma can help to ensure that all necessary information is captured, including a pre-operative assessment of cognition. This together with collateral from family/friends/carers can identify those with established dementia in addition to those with likely undiagnosed dementia. These patients are at particularly high risk of developing peri-operative delirium. Proactive orthogeriatric management has been shown to reduce the incidence of delirium after hip fracture by one-third and severe delirium by a half [2].

Studies have looked at using haloperidol routinely peri-operatively in those at risk of delirium. A randomised placebo-controlled trial of 430 patients given either placebo or haloperidol 1.5 mg/day showed no reduction in incidence of delirium, but it did reduce the severity and duration of delirium with a reduction in length of stay. Its routine use is not recommended [3].

The 4AT is a useful tool for recognising and monitoring delirium [4]. It is a simple score which can be performed with good reliability by all staff and requires no specific training. It has been validated in patients with hip fracture [5] and should be a routine part of hip fracture management.

A description of an individual's functional ability adds to an understanding of the impact and severity of co-morbidities, particularly with regard to cardiac and respiratory disease. This is often described in metabolic equivalents (METS) with one MET being defined as the amount of oxygen consumed while sitting at rest and is equal to 3.5 mL O_2/kg/min [6]. Those able to undertake activity such as easily managing a flight of stairs (four METs or more) are unlikely to have significant cardio-respiratory disease and have low cardiovascular risk (see Table 7.1).

Table 7.1 Metabolic equivalents

Physical activity	METs
Sitting reading/watching television	1.0
Washing and dressing independently	2.1
Walking slowly on flat	2.3
Gentle household activity, e.g., cooking/cleaning	2.5
Walking a small dog (3 km/h)	2.7
Light static cycling/bowling	3.0
Gardening or outdoor activity	3.6
Walking quickly (5 km/h)	3.6
Climb flight of stairs without stopping	4.0
Dancing	4.5
Playing tennis/racquet sports	8.5

Those with low levels of activity may have asymptomatic underlying cardiovascular disease or may be limited by musculoskeletal disorders including arthritis, osteoporosis with kyphosis, sarcopenia or indeed obesity.

7.3   Cardiovascular Disease

Patients with a history of ischaemic heart disease are clearly at risk of peri-operative cardiac events. Cardiovascular risk factors should also be considered including the presence of diabetes, hypertension and smoking.

The Goldman cardiac risk index [7] or the Revised Cardiac risk index [8] may be used to identify high-risk patients and predict the likelihood of peri-operative cardiac event or death.

A baseline electrocardiogram may give indications of asymptomatic cardiac disease with left bundle branch block or evidence of q waves or poor r-wave progression in the anterior leads.

An echocardiogram will give an indication of regional wall abnormalities from myocardial infarction, an estimate of left ventricular function and an indication of underlying valvular heart disease. This information can assist with risk stratification but should not delay surgery.

Patients with suspected coronary artery disease should be discussed with an anaesthetist. Unless a patient is symptomatic with cardiac chest pain, surgery should not be delayed to perform cardiac investigations. Routine troponin measurements are not helpful and do not correlate with early mortality [9]. Those already on beta blockers should continue their usual dose pre-operatively unless there is significant bradycardia or hypotension. Attention to haemoglobin levels is important, as peri-operative anaemia may increase cardiac strain and increase the risk of a cardiac event.

7.3.1   Valvular Heart Disease

Cardiac murmurs are often present in older people, with insignificant aortic sclerosis or mild mitral regurgitation being the most common. A large retrospective study showed that 6.9% of patients with hip fracture had previously undiagnosed significant aortic stenosis [10]. This may influence the type of anaesthetic and the need for invasive cardiac monitoring. Significant aortic stenosis is suspected if the patient has an ejection systolic murmur in the aortic area in combination with a history of angina on exertion, unexplained syncope or near syncope, a slow rising pulse clinically in the brachial artery and an absent second heart sound or LVH on the ECG without hypertension. Patients with significant aortic stenosis require careful fluid balance and are at high risk of pulmonary oedema. Echocardiography should not delay timing of operation but may be useful if readily available.

7.3.2 Heart Failure

Many older patients will have a history or symptoms in keeping with poor ventricular function on a background of hypertension, ischaemic heart disease, valvular heart disease or atrial fibrillation. The mainstays of medical treatment are diuretics, ACE inhibitors, angiotensin receptor blockers, beta blockers, aldosterone antagonists and a combination of hydralazine and nitrates. Increasingly, therapies for heart failure include electrophysiological interventions such as cardiac resynchronisation therapy (CRT), pacemakers with or without implantable cardioverter–defibrillators (ICDs). A recent echocardiogram can be useful to evaluate the severity of left ventricular dysfunction but should not delay operation. Severity can usually be gauged from the history, symptoms and required medication.

Those who are euvolaemic should undergo early surgery, omitting heart failure medication until 48–72 h post-operatively to reduce the incidence of symptomatic low blood pressure preventing mobilisation. Caution should be observed with administering intravenous fluid. Anaemia should be managed proactively to maintain haemoglobin levels above 100 g/L. Once able to transfer out of bed medication can be slowly re-introduced. These patients often develop increasing peripheral oedema 5–7 days post-operatively and may require an increased dose of diuretics for a period of time.

Patients with decompensated heart failure and fluid overload at presentation need careful attention. Those with acute left ventricular failure need stabilising before theatre. This is often associated with an acute ischaemic event. Anti-platelet and anti-coagulant therapy may cause increased blood loss at the fracture site and should only be started with caution for acute cardiac ischaemia. Discussion with cardiologists regarding appropriate intervention and an individualised decision about timing of surgery should be made.

Those with poor right ventricular function and fluid overload need high-dose diuretics with close monitoring of peripheral oedema, weight and renal function. This is often associated with hyponatraemia, hypotension and renal impairment and requires close observation. Correction to achieve a euvolaemic state often takes 5–10 days. It is usually better to proceed with surgery and manage the decompensated heart failure in the post-operative period. Significant peripheral oedema in the thigh however may increase the risk of wound breakdown.

7.3.3 Conduction Defects, Pacemakers and Implantable Cardiac Defibrillators (ICD)

Conduction defects seen on the 12-lead ECG are very common in older people. Temporary pacing is only indicated if a patient has complete heart block or has had syncope related to tri-fascicular heart block. First-degree heart block, bundle branch block and ectopics are of unlikely significance if asymptomatic and do not require pre-operative investigation.

Pacemakers have become increasingly sophisticated, and a basic knowledge of different devices and their indications is required to aid the acute management of patients with fragility fracture. All patients with pacemakers have routine annual checks, and a pre-operative check is only required if there is concern about malfunction or if it has not been checked within 12 months.

It is important to understand the reason for the device and whether the patient is pacemaker dependent. External pacing equipment and a defibrillator must be available during surgery. The use of surgical diathermy/electrocautery can give rise to electrical interference, and this can present additional risks when used in patients with pacemakers and ICDs. Energy can also be induced in heart lead systems causing tissue heating at lead tips through high-frequency current [11]. The manufacturers recommend avoiding surgical diathermy if surgery is occurring within 50 cm from the device. If diathermy is deemed essential, then the use of bipolar diathermy with short bursts of energy minimises the risk. Where available, the use of a harmonic scalpel should be considered.

If a cardiac technician is available, then an ICD can be turned onto monitor only mode to prevent shock delivery during surgery. Otherwise ICDs should be turned off by placing a magnet over the device which should be secured with micropore tape. Any sustained ventricular tachycardia or ventricular fibrillation intraoperatively should be managed with external defibrillation. Post-operatively, the magnet should be removed, and the patient monitored until the device has been checked.

7.3.4   Atrial Fibrillation (AF)

Public campaigns such as 'know your pulse' have increased public awareness of the risk of stroke from atrial fibrillation. Patients with permanent AF and a controlled ventricular rate should continue with rate control medication (usually a betablocker, dioxin or verapamil) pre-operatively, with their usual dose administered on the day of surgery. Some patients are known to have paroxysmal atrial fibrillation (PAF). Amiodarone, flecainide or beta blockers are often used to try and maintain sinus rhythm and prevent PAF. Periods of fast atrial fibrillation are commonly induced by trauma, anaesthesia and a stress response.

Those with new AF, persistent AF or PAF with a fast ventricular rate need review. Tachycardia may be due to pain, a cardiac event or sepsis and a 12-lead ECG, measurement of lactate and inflammatory markers is advised. Those with no evidence of inter-current illness may simply have new AF or poor rate control. Correction of dehydration and electrolyte imbalance should be initiated immediately. If the rate remains persistently above 110 bpm, then urgent rate control may be required pre-operatively. Digoxin loading often takes 24 h to establish rate control. New prescription of betablockers is not advised pre-operatively due to concerns about hypotension. Short-acting intravenous metoprolol may be used with caution. The most effective method for rapid rate control is with intravenous amiodarone. This is usually administered with a slow bolus of 300 mg over 1 h followed by a 24-h infusion of 0.5 mg/kg/h (450 mg in 500 mL normal saline). This must be administered through a large bore cannula and ideally into a central line with cardiac monitoring. Cardiology advice may be required for complex patients.

7.4   Management of Anticoagulants and Anti-platelets

Anti-platelets are mainly used for secondary prevention of stroke, in peripheral vascular disease and following cardiac events. Anti-platelet agents cause irreversible platelet dysfunction and recovery only occurs with production of new platelets over 7–10 days. However, delay for urgent surgery, such as fractured neck of femur fixation, is not recommended [12]. With regard to choice of anaesthesia, aspirin is usually of little consequence, and SIGN guidance supports central neuraxial blockade in aspirin monotherapy [12]. Clopidogrel monotherapy should not delay surgery [13] and indeed should not be a contraindication to spinal or epidural anaesthesia, with little evidence for increase in rates of vertebral canal haematoma [12]. General anaesthesia should be considered for patients taking dual anti-platelet therapy [12]. Prophylactic peri-operative platelet transfusions are not necessary and should only be considered if there is excessive surgical bleeding [12].

Up to 40% of patients admitted with a hip fracture will be anticoagulated [14]. Direct oral anticoagulants (DOACs), such as apixaban, rivaroxaban, edoxaban and dabigatran, are currently prescribed more commonly than warfarin in the United Kingdom [15]. They have the advantage of fewer drug interactions, do not require plasma level monitoring for dosing and are effective and relatively safe [16].

In patients taking warfarin, AAGBI guidance recommends proceeding with surgery under general anaesthesia when the INR has been reduced by intravenous vitamin K to less than 2.0 [17]. Spinal anaesthesia and surgery are considered safe with an INR < 1.5 [17].

Guidance for anaesthesia and surgery on patients with a hip fracture receiving DOACs is currently lacking. European and Scandinavian guidelines have advocated a pragmatic pharmacokinetic model with the passage of two half-lives between drug discontinuation and central neuraxial blockade [17].

The factor Xa inhibitors apixaban and rivaroxaban have a reversal agent, andexanet alfa, but it is only licenced for life-threatening bleeding and not routine use. The ANNEXA-4 study demonstrated effective clinical haemostasis with andexanet alfa, but thrombotic events occurred in 18% of patients during the 30-day follow-up [18].

Dabigatran, the direct thrombin inhibitor, has a licensed safe reversal agent, idarucizumab.

Traditional coagulation tests such as PT/INR and APTT are not sensitive in monitoring DOAC plasma activity [17]. Furthermore, the INR can be normal when clinically relevant plasma levels of DOAC are present. Therefore, traditional coagulation tests are not recommended. Plasma Xa assays are accurate but not commonly available in many hospital laboratories, and without an evidence base to guide the correlation of plasma levels to neuraxial performance safety, their use is limited. Conversely, clinical activity of dabigatran can be monitored easily and reliably through plasma thrombin time.

With the secondary analysis of the national audit project ASAP 1 showing no difference in 30-day mortality between patients who received a general anaesthetic versus a spinal anaesthetic for hip fracture surgery, for many patients general anaesthesia is an acceptable alternative to spinal anaesthesia [19]. However, this is not a straightforward decision and should be made on an individual basis depending upon type of anticoagulant, renal function, the type of surgery required, anticipated blood loss, pain control and risk of immobility.

Table 7.2 gives details of suggested management for different anticoagulant medications.

Table 7.2 Anti-platelets and anticoagulants in patients with fragility fracture

Drug	Elimination half-life	Management	Acceptable to proceed with spinal
Warfarin	4–5 days	5 mg vitamin K intravenously and repeat INR after 4–6 h. This can be repeated or consider Beriplex for immediate reversal	If INR < 1.5
Clopidogrel	Irreversible effect on platelets	Proceed with surgery Monitor for blood loss Consider platelet transfusion if concerns regarding bleeding	If anti-platelet monotherapy. GA if dual therapy
Unfractionated iv heparin	1–2 h	Stop iv heparin 2–4 h pre-op	4 h
Low-molecular weight heparin sub-cutaneous prophylactic dose	3–7 h	Last dose 12 h pre-op	12 h
Low-molecular weight heparin sub-cutaneous Treatment dose	3–7 h	Last dose 12–24 h pre-op. Monitor for blood loss	24 h
Ticagrelor	8–12 h	Proceed with surgery with general anaesthetic Monitor for blood loss Consider platelet transfusion if concerns regarding bleeding	5 days or post platelet transfusion at least 6 h post last dose
Aspirin	Irreversible effect on platelets	Proceed with surgery	Continue
Rivaroxiban	7–10 h	Surgery and anaesthesia 24 h after last dose if renal function normal	2 half-lives/24 h after last dose if renal function normal
Dabigatran	12–24 h	Surgery and anaesthesia if thrombin time normal or idarucizumab for immediate reversal if thrombin time prolonged	If thrombin time normal or 30 min following idarucizumab infusion
Apixiban	12 h	Surgery and anaesthesia 24 h after last dose if renal function normal	2 half-lives/24 h after last dose if renal function normal

Understanding the reason for anti-platelet/anticoagulant medication is essential in managing peri-operative risk of thromboembolic events. Patients with cardiac stents are at high risk of thrombosis and cardiac events and anti-platelet medication should either continue or be stopped for the shortest possible time.

Patients with mechanical heart valves (particularly mitral valves), known AF with recent stroke and recent DVT or PE are at high risk of peri-operative thromboembolic complications and bridging strategies should be considered. Treatment-dose subcutaneous low-molecular-weight heparin can be given until 24 h before surgery or intravenous unfractionated heparin until 2–4 h before surgery. The latter requires careful monitoring with 4–6 hourly APTT levels to ensure correct dosing.

Temporary insertion of an inferior vena cava filter should be considered for those with recent proximal DVT or PE.

Tranexamic acid has been shown to reduce the need for transfusion in a small study of patients with hip fracture with no difference in 3-month mortality [20], but in a similar small study, there appeared to be a significant increased risk of thromboembolic events [21]. A meta-analysis involving almost 600 patients suggested that Tranexamic acid administration reduces blood loss and transfusion rates with no significant difference in thrombotic events. The authors recommended a large, high-quality randomised control study to ensure safety and to establish clarity regarding the optimal regimen, dosage and timing before wide recommendation for use in hip fracture surgery [22].

7.5 Anaemia

Anaemia on admission is an independent predictor of poor outcome and is present in about 10–12% of those presenting with hip fracture [23]. It often reflects underlying disease such as malignancy, chronic kidney disease or poor nutrition. It is important to send blood for haematinics pre-transfusion to aid diagnosis and subsequent management. Macrocytic anaemia should not be transfused without an understanding of the cause and in liaison with haematologists. Although the evidence is controversial, most clinicians would aim for a pre-operative haemoglobin of at least 100 g/dL.

It is possible to predict blood loss depending upon the type of fracture with intracapsular fractures losing about 1000 mL, extracapsular about 1200 mL and intertrochanteric or subtrochanteric up to 1600 mL [24]. This may be greater in those on anti-platelet therapy or anti-coagulants.

The FOCUS study was a large randomised controlled trial comparing liberal transfusion with restrictive transfusion in patients following hip fracture which showed no difference in mortality, ability to walk across a room at 60 days or length of hospital stay [25]. However, a decision about transfusion trigger should be made on an individual basis pre-operatively, taking into account frailty, cardiorespiratory reserve and levels of function. Usual practice is to keep haemoglobin above 80 g/dL for those who are well and to aim for a haemoglobin of above 100 g/dL for those with poor cardiorespiratory reserve.

Intravenous iron pre-operatively has been evaluated but its effects are not sufficient or quick enough to reduce the need for blood transfusion in the first week after surgery [26].

7.6 Diabetes

Poor glycaemic control in the peri-operative period can lead to dehydration and poor wound healing with prolonged hyperglycaemia. Hypoglycaemia can also have serious consequences contributing to delirium, falls and seizures.

In the pre-operative period, patients with fragility fracture are often reluctant to eat due to pain, immobility and side effects of analgesia. Immobility may lead to reduced calorie requirements but pain and stress result in hyperglycaemia.

It is important to review diabetes medication pre-operatively and to monitor the blood sugar levels regularly. The AAGBI have produced comprehensive guidelines for peri-operative management of diabetes [27]. Patients who have taken long-acting oral hypoglycaemics or long-acting insulin need close monitoring and may need slow 5% glucose infusion if being kept nil by mouth for surgery.

Pre-operative carbohydrate loading or high-sugar dietary supplements should be withheld in patients with diabetes as these may lead to poorly controlled blood sugar levels.

Most patients on oral hypoglycaemics can be managed by simply omitting usual medication on the day of surgery (NB: there is no need to stop pioglitazone). Metformin should be withheld for 48 h in anyone at risk of renal impairment, as there is an association with lactic acidosis. If pre-operative blood sugars rise above 12 mmol/L, consider variable-rate intravenous insulin infusion (VRIII). Oral medication should restart as soon as the patient is able to eat and drink.

Those usually on short-acting or combined insulin preparations should omit their usual insulin dose and start on VRIII pre-operatively with intravenous fluid. This should be 5% glucose if the blood sugars are low. For patients with type I diabetes, insulin should never be stopped completely.

Long-acting insulin analogues (Glargine, Lantus, Detemir or Levimir) can be continued in the peri-operative period, with some people advocating reducing the dose by one-third.

It is important to make a post-operative plan and to withdraw the VRIII as soon as the patient is eating and drinking, to avoid fluid overload and electrolyte disturbance. Normal insulin doses may need adjusting until the patient is eating, drinking and mobilising normally.

7.7 Chronic Kidney Disease (CKD)

CKD is common in older people and can be associated with excess surgical morbidity [28]. It is important to establish the duration of CKD and baseline renal function. CKD may reflect impaired excretory function with raised urea, creatinine and metabolic products. In addition, there may be impaired synthetic function resulting in acidosis, hyperkalaemia, hypertension and oedema. CKD also results in reduced erythropoietin with anaemia and reduced hydroxylation of vitamin D causing hypocalcaemia and hyperphosphatemia. Platelet dysfunction is common in CKD, increasing the risk of bleeding.

Anaemia and metabolic abnormalities should be corrected to acceptable limits pre-operatively. Fluid overload is difficult to correct pre-operatively but those with end stage renal disease who are dialysis dependent should be dialysed within 24 h pre-operatively to reduce fluid overload.

Many drugs are excreted by the kidneys and can accumulate in patients with CKD. These may require dose adjustment or administration interval adjustment and, in some cases, avoided completely.

Anaesthesia often results in hypotension and a significant reduction in renal blood flow with worsening of renal function in the post-operative period. It is essential that anaesthetists are aware of patients with CKD who have poor renal reserve so that they can make every effort to prevent hypotension.

Patients with CKD often have concomitant ischaemic heart disease and continuation of beta blockers and correction of anaemia may help to reduce the incidence of cardiovascular events.

7.8   Respiratory Disease

Predicting those who are at highest risk of post-operative complications enables pre-operative intervention and optimisation. All patients with hip fracture are at risk of atelectasis and of chest infection which is one of the reasons for early operation and mobilisation. Those with underlying lung disease or smokers with undiagnosed lung disease have a higher risk. Low serum albumin, recent weight loss and dependency are also associated with increased risk [29].

Opiate analgesics and anaesthetic agents can reduce respiratory drive resulting in hypoxia, hypercapnia and atelectasis and should be used with caution.

Obesity also contributes to reduced gas exchange through reduced lung volume and in severe cases can lead to hypercapnic respiratory failure, but there is no evidence that patients with hip fracture and a high BMI have an increased rate of postoperative complications [30].

Cor pulmonale and pulmonary hypertension carry significant morbidity and mortality.

Pre-operative clinical assessment, chest X-ray and arterial blood gases give important baseline information.

Exacerbations of chronic obstructive airways disease may need treatment and optimisation pre-operatively, but most respiratory infections should not delay operation unless accompanied by sepsis, cardiovascular compromise or very high oxygen requirements.

The choice of anaesthetic is discussed in Chap. 8.

7.9   Medication Review

In some countries, medicine reconciliation soon after admission is undertaken by a pharmacist. Understanding how a patient manages a complex regime is important, giving insight into cognition and compliance. Specific medication may suggest certain diagnoses, but care should be taken in making assumptions.

All regular medication should be written up on the drug chart with the indication for each drug and clear documentation of which should be continued or withheld pre-operatively. Most older patients with frailty admitted with fragility fracture will be volume depleted, and it is important to withhold medications which could contribute to renal hypoperfusion and acute kidney failure in the peri-operative period (e.g. diuretics, ACE inhibitors, anti-hypertensives).

Long-term sedatives (e.g. benzodiazepines, antipsychotics) should be reviewed and possibly reduced in the immediate peri-operative period, as many of the anaesthetic drugs will also cause sedation. However, they should not be stopped abruptly or withheld for prolonged periods of time.

Other medications must be given on the morning of surgery with a small sip of water (e.g. beta blockers for angina or rate control, anticonvulsants and medication for Parkinson's disease).

Some medications need reviewing and adjusting during the peri-operative period (see anticoagulants and anti-platelets and management of diabetes). Patients on hydrocortisone for pituitary failure or long-term low-dose steroid with possible adrenal failure should be given an increased dose usually 50 mg of hydrocortisone on induction via intramuscular or intravenous route and three times a day for the first 24 h). Inhalers may be changed to nebulisers for better delivery while a patient is immobile in bed.

Every prescribed medication should have a clear ongoing indication and benefits of the medication should outweigh the risks. Hospital admission with multidisciplinary input is an opportunity to review this. It is an important aspect of comprehensive geriatric assessment and takes considerable time. It should start pre-operatively but will need to continue to be reviewed and adjusted in the postoperative period.

Considerable thought should be given to medication that may contribute to falls (see Chap. 16).

7.10   Preventing Complications: Thromboembolic Events

Patients with fragility fracture are considered at particularly high risk of thromboembolic events, due to the effects of trauma, surgery and immobility. Older patients with frailty may have other co-morbidities such as heart failure or a history of thromboembolic events that increase this risk further. UK NICE guidelines recommend daily prophylactic-dose low-molecular-weight heparin (LMWH) for all hospitalised patients unless there are specific contraindications [31]. LMWH should be prescribed on admission but omitted if the patient is going to surgery within 12 h. If there is likely to be a delay to surgery, pre-operative dosing should be considered taking into account risks of bleeding further into the fracture site.

The incidence of symptomatic venous thromboembolic events (VTE) is between 1% and 9% and symptomatic pulmonary emboli (PE) 0.2–1.7% following hip fracture surgery. However, the risk of significant bleeding with LMWH is 0.8–4.7% [32].

There is no good evidence for compression stockings in patients following hip fracture, and the potential harm in patients with poor skin and circulation should not be underestimated. Local policies should be followed, but with a review of risks and benefits in each individual patient.

7.11   Antibiotic Prophylaxis

Antibiotic prophylaxis is strongly recommended for surgical management of fractures to help to prevent deep wound infection. Each hospital will have its own policy to reflect likely pathogens and local patterns of resistance. This usually involves a single dose pre-operatively and 24-h cover post-operatively. Antibiotic choice may vary for patients who have fallen and fractured while in hospital or from a nursing home environment where the incidence of drug resistance is higher.

7.12   Appropriate Ceilings of Care

Many patients with fragility fracture have significant frailty and a quarter are in their last year of life. It is important that they and their next of kin have a realistic understanding of which treatments may result in benefit and which are likely to cause harm or distress. Organ failure as a result of end-stage chronic disease is usually irreversible, and under these circumstances organ support in an intensive care unit setting is likely to be ineffective and therefore inappropriate. Where there is a reversible element to organ failure, decisions regarding invasive treatments should be discussed in anticipation pre-operatively where possible.

Cardiopulmonary resuscitation in the event of cardiac arrest is unlikely to be effective in those with poor physiological reserve and an anticipatory form (Do Not Attempt Cardiopulmonary Resuscitation or DNACPR form) is required in some countries.

Many older people do not wish to receive life-prolonging treatments and may have discussed this with relatives or completed an advanced care plan. It is important to discuss this with the patient and their next of kin during the pre-operative assessment to ensure that all are aware of the patient's priorities. A DNACPR order may be reversed in the immediate peri-operative period, in theatre and in recovery area to ensure that recovery from anaesthesia is complete and does not contribute to cardiac or respiratory compromise. The use of drugs and techniques often used as part of CPR may be indicated in the short-term [33].

Table 7.3 Reasons for delaying surgery for hip fracture that the AAGBI working party considers unacceptable and acceptable [33]

Acceptable	Unacceptable
Haemoglobin concentration <8 g dL^{-1}	Lack of facilities or theatre space
Plasma sodium concentration <120 or >150 mmol L^{-1}	Awaiting echocardiography
Potassium concentration <2.8 or >6.0 mmol L^{-1}	Unavailable surgical expertise
Uncontrolled diabetes	Minor electrolyte abnormalities
Uncontrolled or acute onset left ventricular failure	
Correctable cardiac arrhythmia with a ventricular rate >120 min^{-1}	
Chest infection with sepsis	
Reversible coagulopathy	

7.13   Conclusion

Pre-operative assessment of patients with fragility fracture requires skill, time and effort. It is best achieved through multi-disciplinary review and information gathering to provide a clear and accurate understanding of a patient's background. Many patients require adjustments to medications in peri-operative period and for some urgent optimisation is necessary. For the majority of patients, proceeding with surgery without delay is in their best interests, as most intercurrent conditions are not rapidly reversible and medical instability will progress with poorly controlled pain from the fracture and an inability to sit upright. The AAGBI have produced guidelines on acceptable reasons to delay surgery [34]—see Table 7.3. Good pre-operative assessment includes shared decision-making with regard to the best form of management for that individual, taking into account the risks and benefits in addition to the patient's priorities. Evidence-based protocols and guidelines are important, but ultimately this process requires clinical judgement and should involve a senior and experienced team.

References

1. Welsh T, Gordon A, Gladman J (2014) Comprehensive geriatric assessment—a guide for the non specialist. Int J Clin Pract 68(3):290–293
2. Marcantonio E, Flacker J, Wright R et al (2001) Reducing delirium after hip fracture: a randomized trial. J Am Geriatr Soc 49(5):516–522
3. Kalisvaart K et al (2005) Haloperidol prophylaxis for elderly hip surgery patients at risk for delirium: a randomised placebo controlled trial. J Am Geriatr Soc 53(10):1658–1666
4. www.the4AT.com
5. Bellelli G et al (2014) Validation of the 4AT; a new instrument for rapid delirium screening: a study in 234 hospitalised older people. Age Ageing 43:496–502. https://doi.org/10.1093/ageing/afu021
6. Jette M et al (1990) Metabolic equivalents (METS) in exercise testing, exercise prescription, and evaluation of functional capacity. Clin Cardiol 13:555–565

7. Goldman L, Caldera DL, Nussbaum SR et al (1977) Multifactorial index of cardiac risk in noncardiac surgical procedures. N Engl J Med 297(9):845–850
8. Lee T, Marcantonio E, Mangione C et al (1999) Derivation and prospective validation of a simple index for prediction of cardiac risk of major noncardiac surgery. Circulation 100:1043–1049
9. Spurrier E, Wordsworth D, Martin S et al (2011) Troponin T in hip fracture patients: prognostic significance for mortality at one year. Hip Int 16:757
10. McBrien M, Heyburn G, Stevenson M et al (2009) Previously undiagnosed aortic stenosis revealed by auscultation in the hip fracture population- echocardiographic findings, management and outcome. Anaesthesia 64:863–870
11. MRHA (2006) Perioperative management pacemakers/ICDs March 2006
12. Scotttish Intercollegiate Guidelines Network (2009) Management of hip fracture in older people
13. Dolman B, Moppett I (2015) Is early hip fracture surgery safe for patients on clopidogrel? Systematic review, meta-analysis and met-regression. Injury 46:954–962
14. Schermann H et al (2019) Safety of urgent hip fracture surgery protocol under the influence of direct oral anticoagulation medications. Injury 50(2):398–402
15. Mullins B, Akehurst H, Slattery D et al (2018) Should surgery be delayed in patients taking direct oral anticoagulants who suffer a hip fracture? A retrospective, case-controlled observational study at a UK major trauma centre. BMJ Open 8(4):e020625
16. Benzon H, Avram M, Green D et al (2013) New oral anticoagulants and regional anaesthesia. BJA 111(S1):i96–i113
17. AAGBI Safety Guideline (2011) Management of proximal femoral fractures
18. Connolly S, Milling T, Eikleboom J et al (2016) Andexanet alfa for acute major bleeding associated with factor Xa inhibitors. N Engl J Med 375:1131–1141
19. White SM et al (2016) Secondary analysis of outcomes after 11,085 hip fracture operations from the prospective UK Anaesthesia Sprint Audit of Practice (ASAP-2). Anaesthesia 71(5):506–514
20. Lee C et al (2015) The efficacy of tranexamic acid in hip hemiarthroplasty surgery: an observational cohort study. Injury 46(10):1978–1982
21. Zufferey P et al (2010) Tranexamic acid in hip fracture surgery: a randomized controlled trial. Br J Anaesth 104:23–30
22. Zhang P, He J, Fang Y et al (2017) Efficacy and safety of intravenous tranexamic acid administration in patients undergoing hip fracture surgery for hemostasis: a meta-analysis. Medicine 96(21):e6940
23. White S et al (2014) Outcome by mode of anaesthesia for hip fracture surgery. An observational audit of 65,535 patients in a national dataset. Anaesthesia 69:224–230. https://doi.org/10.1111/anae.12542
24. Foss N, Kehlet H (2006) Hidden blood loss after surgery for hip fracture. J Bone Joint Surg 88-B:1053–1059
25. Carson J, Michael M, Terrin L, et al for the FOCUS investigators (2011) Liberal or restrictive transfusion in high-risk patients after hip surgery. N Engl J Med 365:2453–2462
26. Moppett I, Rowlands M, Mannings A et al (2019) The effect of intravenous iron on erythropoiesis in older people with hip fracture. Age Ageing 48(5):751–755. https://doi.org/10.1093/ageing/afz049
27. Dhatariya1 K, Levy N, Kilvert A et al, for the Joint British Diabetes Societies (2010) Diabetes UK position statements and care recommendations NHS diabetes guideline for the perioperative management of the adult patient with diabetes. Diabet Med 29:420–433
28. Salifu M et al (2016) Peri-operative management of the patient with chronic renal failure. Medscape. http://emedicine.medscape.com/article/284555-overview#showall. Accessed 6 Apr 2016
29. Arozullah A, Conde M, Lawrence V (2003) Preoperative evaluation for postoperative pulmonary complications. Med Clin North Am 87(1):153–173

30. Batsis J et al (2009) Body mass index and risk of non-cardiac postoperative medical complications in elderly hip fracture patients: a population based study. J Hosp Med 4(8):E1–E9
31. NICE Clinical Guideline 92 (2010) Venous thromboembolism: reducing the risk. www.nice.org.uk/nicemedia/pdf/CG92NICEGuidelinePDF.pdf
32. Rosencher N, Vielpeau C, Emmerich J et al (2005) Venous thromboembolism and mortality after hip fracture surgery: the ESCORTE study. J Thromb Haemost 3(9):2006–2014
33. The Association of Anaesthetists of Great Britain and Ireland (2009) Do not attempt resuscitation decisions in the peri-operative period. www.aagbi.org/sites/default/files/dnar
34. Griffiths R, Alper J, Beckingsale A et al (2012) Management of proximal femoral fractures 2011 Association of Anaesthetists of Great Britain and Ireland. Anaesthesia 67(1):85–98

Orthogeriatric Anaesthesia

8

Stuart M. White

8.1 Introduction

Traditionally, perioperative care of elderly patients requiring surgical hip fracture fixation was less than exemplary. Patients were administered relatively large amounts of opioid analgesia before surgery, which itself was often delayed for more than 48 h for 'organisational' or 'anaesthetic' reasons. A significant proportion of patients were not operated on, because the perioperative risk of death was perceived to be too high, and so received conservative management (bedrest). Patients undergoing surgery would be anaesthetised and operated on by junior clinicians, who administered heavy-handed general anaesthesia with opioid analgesia and used a wide variety of surgical techniques and implants. Postoperative care was coordinated by orthopaedic surgeons, and generally delivered in a passive and intermittent manner. Mortality and morbidity were high, and length of postoperative inpatient stay was long.

This approach to care, however, was economically unsustainable given the rapidly changing demographics of developed (and, increasingly, developing) countries. Although the prevalence of hip fracture has remained stable or has fallen slightly, increased longevity has led to an increase in the number of elderly patients presenting with hip fracture. As a result, several European countries began to develop orthogeriatric services, to streamline and coordinate hip fracture care pathways.

This chapter is a component of Part 2: Pillar I.
For an explanation of the grouping of chapters in this book, please see Chapter 1: 'The Multidisciplinary Approach to Fragility Fractures Around the World—An Overview'.

S. M. White (✉)
Brighton and Sussex University Hospitals NHS Trust, Brighton, UK

© The Author(s) 2021
P. Falaschi, D. Marsh (eds.), *Orthogeriatrics*, Practical Issues in Geriatrics,
https://doi.org/10.1007/978-3-030-48126-1_8

8.2   The Relationship Between Anaesthetist and Orthogeriatrician

Reconfiguration towards multidisciplinary, orthogeriatrician-led care has probably delivered the greatest improvement in hip fracture outcomes in the last two decades. The main benefit of this model is that it allows for continuous, specialised medical care throughout the perioperative period, delivered by anaesthetists and orthogeriatricians.

There are three phases to perioperative care, the preoperative, intraoperative and postoperative phases (Fig. 8.1).

The preoperative phase describes the period from fracture to the patient's arrival in theatres for surgery. Hip fracture is painful, if not always at rest, then usually on movement. Surgical fixation is the only method of providing analgesia and remobilisation in the long term, for which reason it should always be considered an option in preference to non-operative management. Conservative treatment carries the additional risks of immobility—thromboembolism, pressure ulceration and loss of independence. The aim of the preoperative phase, therefore, is to facilitate prompt preparation for surgery. Coordinated orthogeriatric/anaesthetic care enables standardised preoperative assessment (e.g., delivered according to an agreed proforma, detailing history, examination, preoperative investigations and blood cross-matching), risk assessment using scoring systems, analgesia provision according to agreed protocols, fluid resuscitation and organisational and patient-centred preparation for surgery.

Intraoperatively, the aim of anaesthesia is to mitigate the pathophysiological effects of surgery without destabilising the patient's physiology. These patients are at comparatively high risk of perioperative morbidity and mortality, because they

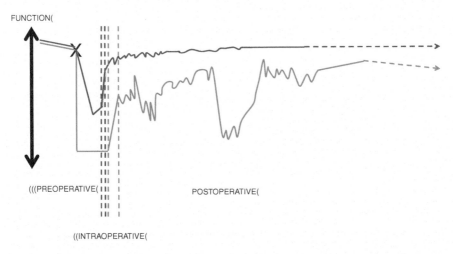

Fig. 8.1 Changes in functional capacity after hip fracture in the three phases of the inpatient episode, with traditional anaesthetic and perioperative care (blue line), compared to proactive multidisciplinary care (red line). See text

are usually frail and elderly (and have limited physiological reserve), and have one or more comorbidities for which they take one or more drugs; cognitive dysfunction is also common. Conceptually, anaesthesia is less about getting high-risk patients through 0.5–2 h of major, emergency surgery, but more about normalising the patient's (patho)physiology so that they are able to return to their normal function within hours following the surgery.

National audits have shown that a wide variety of anaesthesia techniques are used because of a result of personal preference and the lack of conclusive evidence for superiority of one technique over another [1, 2]. However, observational studies and meta-analysis indicate certain anaesthesia techniques probably improve the outcome [3, 4]. Of potentially greater relevance is the idea that hospitals should adopt standardised anaesthesia protocols, so that postoperative care and the management of inevitable complications of anaesthesia and surgery become predictable for orthogeriatricians.

Postoperatively, orthogeriatric care aims to remobilise, re-enable and remotivate patients in preparation for hospital discharge, ideally back to their place of residence before fracture. The early postoperative phase is critical, as delayed remobilisation is associated with a prolonged duration of inpatient stay. Good anaesthesia care facilitates early recovery, by providing non-opioid analgesia, and avoiding delirium, hypotension and anaemia.

Figure 8.1 shows a reconceptualised timeline of what joint anaesthesia/orthogeriatric care should aim to achieve. The blue line represents traditional anaesthesia care. The patient's functional condition has been declining for some time, until they fall and break their hip ('X'), at which point they become entirely dependent. They are taken to hospital but receive minimal care until surgery, and so experience no functional improvement.

Intraoperatively, the fracture is fixed, analgesia, fluids/blood are given, the blood pressure monitored, and the patient's functional status improves, which continues into the immediate postoperative period. However, perhaps the patient develops delirium or feels too nauseous to remobilise for several days in the early postoperative period, as a result of reliance on postoperative opioid analgesia. They recover function in the following few days, but then develop pressure sores or suffer a pulmonary embolism related to their prolonged bedrest, and their functional recovery is delayed again. Eventually, they recover, not quite to their pre-fracture level of function but enough to be discharged from hospital. However, their relatives report that the patient 'was never quite the same' after this episode, with a slow ongoing decline in function after discharge (dotted lines).

In contrast, proactive multidisciplinary care (red line) aims to return patients quickly to their pre-fracture functional status. Simple resuscitation (analgesia, fluids, food) decreases the relative decline in function after fracture, and may indeed begin to improve function preoperatively. The patient undergoes surgery sooner and for a shorter period, during which resuscitation and normalisation of function continues using standardised anaesthesia. The patient's functional status rapidly returns to pre-fracture levels, there are no immobilising complications, the patient is discharged from hospital sooner and remains 'well' after discharge.

8.3   Preoperative Care

International consensus recommendations published by the Fragility Fracture
Network in 2018 detail the organisational and interdisciplinary aspects of anaesthesia
care that hip fracture patients should be expected to receive in any hospital worldwide
[5]. These were endorsed in the 2020 update of the 2012 Association of Anaesthetists
UK guidelines, developed in association with the British Geriatrics Society [6].
Recommendations include the delivery of care by a multidisciplinary team of senior
clinicians, fast-track hospital admission to an acute orthopaedic/hip ward, the provision of daily, and protected trauma lists that prioritise hip fracture surgery.

Several aspects of preoperative care involve coordinated anaesthetic and orthogeriatric input, including analgesia provision, preoperative preparation and ethical/
legal considerations.

8.3.1   Preoperative Analgesia

Hip fractures are usually low impact injuries sustained after a fall from standing
height onto osteoporotic bone. Extracapsular fractures (intertrochanteric, subtrochanteric) are more painful than intracapsular fractures (subcapital, transcervical,
basicervical), due to the greater degree of periosteal disruption.

Approximately a third of the fractures are associated with mild pain, a third with
moderate pain and a third with severe pain. Fractures are usually more painful on
movement, for example when the affected leg is raised passively by 20°.

After admission to the hospital, pain is often poorly assessed. Numerical rating
scales do not adequately describe pain duration or quality. Assessment needs to take
place at rest *and* on movement, before *and* after the administration of analgesia.
Communication difficulties (deafness, blindness, hemiplegia) can make assessment
difficult, as can cognitive impairment related to dementia, or narcotic analgesia
administered in the prehospital phase.

Standardised analgesia protocols ensure that pain is properly assessed and appropriately treated, such that analgesia is provided without opioid-induced cognitive
compromise. In turn, this facilitates other aspects of preoperative care, such as physical assessment, communication, eating and drinking and self-care.

Paracetamol (acetaminophen) is an effective analgesic that is well tolerated by
hip fracture patients, and should be prescribed routinely throughout the perioperative period.

Renal dysfunction is common (~40%) among this patient group, and so non-
steroidal anti-inflammatory drugs (and codeine and tramadol) should be used with
caution, or avoided completely.

Opioid analgesics are effective, but can affect cognition and increasingly so with
older age and/or declining renal function (in such patients the dose should be
reduced and the dosing interval prolonged). Depending on the availability, buprenor-
phine, fentanyl and oxycodone may be preferable to morphine for long-term use.

Preoperative peripheral nerve block has become generally accepted as an analgesic method that minimises the administration of cognition-impairing opioid analgesics [7]. The sensory innervation of the hip involves the femoral, obturator and sciatic nerves, and the skin surrounding the operative incision site, the lateral cutaneous nerve of the thigh. Femoral nerve block and fascia iliaca blocks have been used successfully to reduce pain and limit opioid use preoperatively. Although the efficacy of both blocks is improved by nerve stimulation and (more so by) ultrasound location [8], requiring additional equipment and expertise, both methods have proven to be relatively easy to learn by junior non-anaesthetists, and allied health professionals, such that their protocolised administration by orthogeriatricians should be possible without anaesthetic input. Although additional expertise is required, tunnelled femoral nerve/fascia iliaca catheters can be used to provide prolonged non-opioid analgesia in defined patients for whom surgery is not an option, or where surgery may be delayed for medical reasons.

8.3.2   Preoperative Preparation

Hip fracture patients are often frail and old, with multiple comorbidities demanding polypharmacy. Any of these factors alone or in combination may have contributed to the fall that preceded the fracture, but it is only rarely that the outcome benefits of attempting to improve any of these factors outweigh the risk of delaying surgery. Instead, anaesthetists need reassurance from orthogeriatricians that the patient is appropriately fit for anaesthesia and surgery—'normalised' rather than 'optimised'—and encouragement that risk is best managed by administering an appropriate anaesthetic. Orthogeriatricians should understand what an 'appropriate' anaesthetic involves (see later), and discuss this with anaesthetists who are less familiar with anaesthetising hip fracture patients, and so more likely to cancel patients for medical reasons, delaying surgery.

The Association of Anaesthetists guidelines detail common patient problems that can increase the risk of anaesthesia or its conduct, such as anticoagulation, valvular heart disease, pacemakers and electrolyte abnormalities, and recommend how these should be managed preoperatively [6]. Similarly, generic algorithms are available online that can be modified according to institutional protocols [9]. These are intended as *aides-memoire* for preoperative patient preparation, and are not intended to replace direct communication between anaesthetist and orthogeriatrician.

Most usefully, the Association guidelines identify acceptable and unacceptable reasons for delaying surgery in order to treat certain conditions (Table 8.1). Even so, 'acceptable' is not synonymous with 'obligatory', and surgery may still proceed even if these are present, if the additional risk is managed appropriately. These recommendations serve as a useful starting point when anaesthetists and orthogeriatricians convene to discuss the timing of surgery.

Table 8.1 Acceptable and unacceptable reasons for delaying hip fracture surgery [6]

Acceptable	Unacceptable
• Haemoglobin concentration <8 g dL^{-1} • Plasma sodium concentration <120 or >150 mmol L^{-1} and/or potassium concentration <2.8 or >6.0 mmol L^{-1} • Uncontrolled diabetes • Uncontrolled or acute onset left ventricular failure • Correctable cardiac arrhythmia with a ventricular rate >120 beats min^{-1} • Chest infection with sepsis • Reversible coagulopathy	• Lack of facilities or theatre space • Awaiting echocardiography • Unavailable surgical expertise • Minor electrolyte abnormalities

Table 8.2 The Nottingham hip fracture score

Variable	Points	Total score	Predicted 30-day postoperative mortality (%)
Age 66–85 years	3	0	0.4
Age 86 years or older	4	1	0.6
Male	1	2	1.0
Hb less than or equal to 10 g dL^{-1} on admission to hospital	1	3	1.7
Abbreviated mental test score ≤6/10 at hospital admission	1	4	2.9
Living in an institution	1	5	4.7
More than one co-morbidity*	1	6	7.6
Active malignancy within last 20 years	1	7	12.3
Total score		8	18.2
		9	27.0
		10	38.0

A score out of ten is calculated by summating weighted points for eight criteria (left). The total score is used to predict the risk of a patient dying within 30 days of hip fracture surgery (right). Comorbidities (*) include myocardial infarction, angina, atrial fibrillation, valvular heart disease, hypertension, cerebrovascular accident, transient ischaemic attack, asthma, chronic obstructive pulmonary disease and renal dysfunction

8.3.3 Ethical and Legal Considerations

Hip fracture in elderly patients is associated with significant mortality, morbidity, psychosocial change and reduction in quality of life, although intraoperative mortality is uncommon (<0.5%). Traditionally, discussion between doctors, patients and relatives about the risks and benefits of the various surgical options and recovery approaches has been limited, and hampered by difficulties quantifying risk. National validation of the Nottingham Hip Fracture Score (NHFS) (Table 8.2) supports its use as a risk adjustment for estimating 30-day mortality after hip fracture, in addition to other evidence for its value in predicting 1-year mortality and likelihood of early hospital discharge [10, 11]. The NHFS serves as a useful starting point when discussing risk, but requires patient-specific adjustment. This is best achieved by preoperative communication between the anaesthetist and orthogeriatrician so that discussions with patients and their relatives accurately reflect the possible outcomes of their decisions about treatment.

Similarly, anaesthetists should be involved in discussions about perioperative resuscitation status and/or treatment boundaries, which should be confirmed before every patient undergoes surgery.

Anaesthetic input is also of value when developing patient information literature, for instance, describing what analgesia, antiemesis and anaesthesia interventions the patient can expect to receive.

8.4 Intraoperative Care

In a similar fashion to anaesthetists needing to understand the importance of frailty to orthogeriatric management, orthogeriatricians need to understand how anaesthesia affects postoperative outcome.

Anaesthesia delivered sympathetically to a patient's age, frailty and comorbidity can help re-enable patients after hip fracture surgery by improving analgesia, remobilisation, eating and drinking and cognitive function.

Ideally, in the immediate postoperative period, patients should be sitting up, conversing coherently, drinking and eating, pain free and disconnected from oxygen, intravenous fluids and urinary catheters (all of which impede remobilisation). Although it is not always possible to achieve each of these factors, the aim is to administer anaesthesia in such a way as to facilitate as many as possible.

Evidence for the effect of anaesthetic interventions remains limited. Previously, debate has centred mainly on whether general anaesthesia or spinal anaesthesia (with or without sedation) is preferable in terms of outcome. Randomised controlled trials have proved inconclusive for several reasons: 'general' and 'spinal' anaesthesia can describe a myriad of different techniques, a 2 h period of anaesthesia is probably unrelated to mortality 30 days later, early mortality (within) 5 days is an infrequent outcome for which very large trials would be needed to detect any difference, inclusion and exclusion criteria significantly affect selection bias, equipoise is lacking (most anaesthetists think one or other technique is 'best') and recruitment to follow up is complex [12]. Standardising the outcomes measured in studies should improve comparisons between techniques during meta-analyses [13]. With the advent of 'Big Data', regional and national observational studies have been conducted, but have so far failed to find consistent benefits of one technique over another, at least in terms of mortality [1, 2, 14].

8.4.1 General or Spinal Anaesthesia?

General anaesthesia involves the administration of narcotic and hypnotic anaesthetic agents that render a patient unconscious for the duration of surgery. The patient requires airway support, regardless of whether they are allowed to breathe spontaneously or are paralysed and their lungs ventilated artificially.

Spinal anaesthesia is effectively a reverse dural tap, in which 1–3 mL of local anaesthetic (usually bupivacaine) is injected through a fine bore needle into the subarachnoid cerebrospinal fluid in the lumbar region, providing analgesia, akinesia and anaesthesia below the umbilicus for several hours. Additional sedation is usually administered, either as a bolus or continuously.

Recent meta-analyses, RCTs and large observational studies report conflicting results about whether mortality is lower after general or spinal anaesthesia [2, 3, 14]. However, there is greater consensus in terms of postoperative morbidity and cost, favouring spinal over general anaesthesia. Anecdotally, anaesthetists would prefer to have spinal anaesthesia themselves if they needed hip fracture surgery, orthogeriatricians report better patient recovery after spinal anaesthesia, and physiotherapists report easier patient remobilisation after spinal anaesthesia. Results reported from imminent RCTs (REGAIN, REGARD, iHOPE) should add further information to this determination.

However, of greater relevance than whether spinal or general anaesthesia is better for patients is how well that anaesthesia is delivered. Although there are theoretical and experimental reasons for avoiding general anaesthesia (and sedation) in the elderly, the effect of these is seemingly small compared to numerous other adverse effects of anaesthesia and surgery, including hypotension, pain and analgesia, hypoxia and anaemia. Instead, anaesthetists should focus on careful monitoring of patients during surgery and the provision of appropriate interventions to normalise physiology, for example fluid and vasopressor therapy, depth of anaesthesia/cerebral oxygenation monitoring.

Future research has begun to focus on early postoperative outcomes that are more anaesthesia-specific, such as pain, hypotension and delirium (e.g., ASCRIBED, HIP-HOP and RAGA-delirium RCTs), and clearer definition of the anaesthetic techniques compared (e.g., self-ventilating general anaesthesia + nerve block vs. opioid-free, low-dose spinal anaesthesia + local anaesthetic infiltration without sedation).

8.4.2   Peripheral Nerve Block

Peripheral nerve blockade (fascia iliaca, femoral nerve, lumbar plexus blocks, or local anaesthesia infiltration) should always be administered with either general or spinal anaesthesia, as part of a multimodal analgesia protocol that aims to minimise opioid co-administration [5, 6, 15, 16].

Theoretically, fascia iliaca blocks may provide better analgesia of both the hip and surgical incision site intraoperatively, without dense blockade of the femoral nerve, which can prolong and impair remobilisation. Administered beforehand, a fascia iliaca or femoral nerve block can reduce sedation requirements when positioning patients laterally for spinal anaesthesia administration, and precludes the need to co-administer subarachnoid opioids, which can cause itching, respiratory depression and urinary retention postoperatively.

Co-administration of peripheral nerve blockade beforehand reduces age-adjusted maintenance doses of general anaesthesia.

8.4.3 Spinal Anaesthesia

The aim of spinal anaesthesia is to achieve unilateral blockade on the operative side to a sensory level of ~T_{10-12} for ~2 h maximum operating time, whilst avoiding excessive hypotension related to spinal-induced sympatholysis. This can be achieved using opioid-free 1–1.5 mL subarachnoid 0.5% hyperbaric bupivacaine [17], but these doses are administered to fewer than 20% of patients receiving spinal anaesthesia. Instead, anaesthetists commonly administer in excess of 2 mL 0.5% bupivacaine [14, 18], which is associated with greater relative falls in blood pressure from pre-spinal baseline and a wider range of blood pressure reductions compared to lower doses, changes that can persist into the early postoperative period and prevent patients from sitting out of bed or standing up after surgery. Orthogeriatricians have an important role in encouraging anaesthetists at their institutions to use lower doses of spinal anaesthesia.

8.4.4 Sedation

Similarly, orthogeriatricians have a role in encouraging anaesthetists to consider using less, or no, sedation during spinal anaesthesia.

Commonly, patients co-administered spinal anaesthesia and peripheral nerve block sleep through surgery, because the relative narcotic effect of preoperative opioids increase when pain is alleviated during spinal anaesthesia, and patients are often sleep deprived from the night preceding surgery.

If patients request sedation or sedation is necessary for patient comfort and immobility during surgery, then the minimum amount should be used for the shortest time, to avoid accumulation and sedation in the postoperative period.

Several papers have shown that sedative infusions result in general anaesthesia (without airway support) in a significant proportion of hip fracture patients [19], and so sedation may better be limited to small bolus administration during key periods of surgery (jigsawing, hammering, relocation). Depth of anaesthesia monitors should probably be used to guide sedation if infusions are to be administered.

Theoretically, propofol is the sedative of choice, as it is metabolised rapidly, its metabolites are inert (unlike midazolam) and it does not cause prolonged cognitive impairment (unlike ketamine). There is no evidence supporting the use of combinations of sedatives, although this is common practice.

8.4.5 General Anaesthesia

Older patients are sensitive to the cardiovascular effects of general anaesthesia (negative inochronotropicity and peripheral vasodilation). Hypotension is more common during general anaesthesia compared to spinal anaesthesia, but decreasing the amount of inhalational or intravenous anaesthetic agent administered during surgery can reduce its prevalence. Moreover, compared to younger patients, the elderly require lower doses of drugs to maintain anaesthesia, particularly when a peripheral nerve block is administered preoperatively.

Minimising hypotension while maintaining anaesthesia without awareness can be achieved using depth of anaesthesia monitors (e.g., bispectral index (BIS) and E-Entropy), and it has been recommended that these be used during any type of general anaesthesia in older patients [5, 6]. Alternatively, a Lerou nomogram can be used to adjust inhalational anaesthesia agent dose for age, or age-adjusted doses programmed into a total intravenous anaesthesia syringe pump.

One of the enduring debates among anaesthetists concerns whether the airway of a hip fracture patient administered general anaesthesia should be supported using a laryngeal mask airway, thereby avoiding the pathophysiological effects of mechanical ventilation, or should be intubated, to avoid the risk and consequences of aspiration pneumonia. Respiratory failure is significantly more prevalent after general compared to spinal anaesthesia, and use of paralysing agents is dose-dependently associated within an increased risk of postoperative respiratory complications, but it remains unclear whether hip fracture patients benefit more by avoiding aspiration or by avoiding mechanical ventilation.

8.4.6 Avoiding Ischaemia

Both general and spinal anaesthesia are associated with a high prevalence of hypotension during anaesthesia for hip fracture surgery, general more so than spinal anaesthesia, and postoperative mortality correlates with increased relative fall in blood pressure [14, 18]. Hypotension can be predicted, and ameliorated by administering less anaesthesia, monitoring blood pressure closely, avoiding preoperative dehydration, and administering fluids and vasopressors appropriately.

Hypothetically, avoiding hypotension should reduce the prevalence of postoperative complications related to organ ischaemia, such as confusion/delirium [20], dysrhythmia, acute kidney injury and poor remobilisation. Ischaemic complications may further be attenuated by ensuring adequate postoperative oxygen saturations (e.g., by providing (nasal) oxygen if $SpO_2 \leq 95\%$), avoiding excessive anaemia (e.g., by measuring blood haemoglobin concentration immediately after surgery and on day 1, and considering transfusion) and providing adequate pain relief (to reduce oxygen uptake). Note that simply by reducing anaesthetic dose reduces the prevalence of hypotension, requiring reduced fluid administration, in turn causing less dilutional anaemia, and so, in combination with additional peripheral nerve blockade, less ischaemia.

8.4.7 Bone Cement Implantation Syndrome (BCIS)

BCIS describes a complication occurring during surgical instrumentation and/or cementing of the femoral canal, and is characterised by cardiorespiratory compromise/arrest. It occurs in about 20% of hip fracture operations in which cement is used, and results in cardiopulmonary arrest in about 0.5% [19, 21].

The AAGBI, British Geriatric Society and British Orthopaedic Association have published multidisciplinary guidelines highlighting the need for joint decision-making, team working and attention to detail during the peri-operative period [22].

Of particular importance is the need to identify patients who are at higher risk of BCIS, including those who are very elderly, male, taking diuretic medication and have comorbid cardiorespiratory disease (particularly acute lung pathology).

Compared to uncemented prostheses, the use of cemented prostheses for hip fracture repair increases the likelihood of pain-free mobility after surgery and reduces the risk of re-operation. However, the guidelines recommend that surgeons, anaesthetists and orthogeriatricians discuss preoperatively whether the benefits of using a cemented prosthesis outweigh the risk of BCIS.

8.4.8   Standardisation of Anaesthesia

Clinical outcomes and other measures of care quality have gradually improved in the United Kingdom after hip fracture repair over the last decade. This has resulted from the general standardisation of care, with payments to hospitals for care supplemented by a bonus if they are sure that the defined care targets were met ('payment by results'). Conspicuously absent are targets related to anaesthesia, which combined with an ongoing lack of research evidence and lack of formal professional training in how to anaesthetise hip fracture patients, has meant that there continues to be a wide national variation in anaesthesia practice for hip fracture [1, 2, 12, 15].

Of course, a lack of standardisation may not matter—anaesthesia may have little effect on outcome after hip fracture—but this is unlikely to be the case, given that anaesthesia is administered at the most critical phase of a patient's recovery after hip fracture and has an immediate effect on the trajectory of recovery postoperatively. Until better evidence becomes available, it seems prudent, however, to reject the tacit acceptance of poor, outlying care in support of current evidence-based standardised care as a method for improving safety, in a similar fashion to providing standardised anaesthesia care as part of Enhanced Recovery Protocols.

Although there is some evidence supporting the use of protocolised rather than physician-individualised, there is no evidence supporting physician-individualised care over protocolised care.

In healthcare, standardisation is particularly beneficial when implementing evidence-based care for large numbers of patients with a similar disease process, for whom current treatment is costly, has poor outcomes and is recognised professionally as being of sub-optimal quality—all of which apply in hip fracture.

Standardisation ensures high reliability, consistent, cheaper, higher quality care for the majority of patients, and—most importantly—that the basics of care are not overlooked. Furthermore, standardisation enables monitoring and continuous improvement by amending standards in an evidence-based fashion, reductions in artificial variations in care (caused by slips, lapses or lack of knowledge) whilst improving focus on natural variation in care (caused by differences between patients) and identification of consistently poor performance, areas for future research and educational needs.

Standards for anaesthesia are currently available online (www.hipfractureanaesthesia.com), based on best available current evidence and consensus opinion, describing the rationale behind their formulation and identifying areas for further research. As developed, these standards also provide a method of understanding why individual anaesthetists have deviated from standard practice.

Orthogeriatricians are encouraged to engage anaesthetic colleagues in following these standards, undertaking research in improving them further and engaging in continuous quality improvement cycles, with the aim of optimising care in the critical early postoperative period. This is a mutually cooperative process, as anaesthetists and orthogeriatricians should work together to measure and monitor preoperative care, with the aim of optimising the patient pathway from fracture to early surgical fixation.

8.5   Postoperative Care

Much of anaesthetic involvement in the postoperative phase has been described earlier. Irrespective of whether the patient has been administered general or spinal anaesthetic (with/without sedation), the orthogeriatrician should expect to receive a patient back on the acute orthopaedic ward/hip fracture unit who is immediately ready for re-enablement (resuming activities of daily living) and suitable for rehabilitation to their former place of residence.

The 2012/20 AAGBI guidelines detail the management of common early postoperative complications, including pain, oxygenation, fluid balance and delirium [6]. These are essentially continuations of the primary aims of anaesthesia in the hip fracture population, namely the avoidance of 'ischaemia' through appropriate pain, blood pressure, oxygen, fluid and blood management, so that the consequences of 'ischaemia'—delirium [23], heart pump or rhythm disturbance, acute kidney injury, delay in remobilisation—are avoided.

Gut disturbances are common after hip fracture surgery and often overlooked. Nausea and vomiting delay resumption of oral feeding. Constipation occurs in the majority of patients, particularly those who are dehydrated, not eating or dehydrated. Malnutrition is common especially in frail patients and the cognitively impaired, and close attention to dietary intake is essential to patients' re-enablement.

The role of high dependency or intensive care remains uncertain after hip fracture. Certainly, it is never ethically justified to deny access to these facilities based on a hip fracture patient's age, and in any other group of patients with a similar 30-day postoperative mortality (or indeed mortality >1%, e.g., patients requiring emergency laparotomy), critical care facilities are much more routinely accessed. Indeed, planned admission is important in patients with a pre-operatively identifiable need for single/dual system support postoperatively, when this cannot be achieved to the same degree on an acute orthopaedic ward; for example patients with COPD, acute lung injuries (infection, embolism) and acute left ventricular failure will benefit from critical care. Patients for whom critical care admission is planned have good outcomes compared to patients for whom critical care admission is unplanned, but this reflects the likelihood of intraoperative complications such as bone cement implantation syndrome, on table cardiac arrest or cerebrovascular accident, or massive haemorrhage.

However, adopting systems of orthogeriatric care allows a greater number of elderly patients with comorbidities to receive 'acute' medical care on acute ortho-paedic wards after hip fracture surgery, rather than taxing precious critical care resources. Furthermore, orthogeriatric services are able to coordinate step-down care, reducing the duration of critical care admission. Having managed the patient preoperatively, orthogeriatricians may have a more pragmatic approach to *normalising* patients back to their previous physiological condition, in comparison to the more critical care approach of *optimising* organ function, although this assertion requires further research.

References

1. National Hip Fracture Database (2019) Annual Report 2018. http://www.nhfd.co.uk/files/2018ReportFiles/NHFD-2018-Annual-Report-v101.pdf. Accessed 1 Oct 2019
2. White SM, Moppett IK, Griffiths R (2014) Outcome by mode of anaesthesia for hip fracture surgery. An observational audit of 65 535 patients in a national dataset. Anaesthesia 69:224–230
3. Parker M, Handoll HHG, Griffiths R (2016) Anaesthesia for hip fracture surgery in adults. Cochrane Database Syst Rev 4:CD000521
4. Luger TJ, Kammerlander C, Gosch M et al (2010) Neuroaxial versus general anaesthesia in geriatric patients for hip fracture surgery: does it matter? Osteoporos Int 21:S555–S572
5. White SM, Altermatt F, Barry J et al (2018) International Fragility Fracture Network consensus statement on the principles of anaesthesia for patients with hip fracture. Anaesthesia 73:863–874
6. Association of Anaesthetists (2020) Management of hip fractures 2020. Currently under review
7. Guay J, Parker MJ, Griffiths R, Kopp SL (2017) Peripheral nerve blocks for hip fractures: a Cochrane review. Cochrane Database Syst Rev 1:CD001159
8. Dolan J, Williams A, Murney E, Smith M, Kenny GN (2008) Ultrasound guided fascia iliaca block: a comparison with the loss of resistance technique. Reg Anesth Pain Med 33:526–531
9. White SM (2019) Hip fracture anaesthesia. www.hipfracture.anaesthesia.co.uk. Accessed 25 Oct 2019
10. Moppett IK, Parker M, Griffiths R, Bowers T, White SM, Moran CG (2012) Nottingham Hip Fracture Score: longitudinal and multi-centre assessment. Br J Anaesth 109:546–550
11. Marufu TC, White SM, Griffiths R, Moonesinghe SR, Moppett IK (2016) Prediction of 30-day mortality after hip fracture surgery by the Nottingham hip fracture score and the surgical outcome risk tool. Anaesthesia 71:515–521
12. White SM, Griffiths R, Moppett I (2012) Type of anaesthesia for hip fracture surgery—the problems of trial design. Anaesthesia 67:574–578
13. O'Donnell CM, Black N, McCourt KC et al (2019) Development of a Core Outcome Set for studies evaluating the effects of anaesthesia on perioperative morbidity and mortality following hip fracture surgery. Br J Anaesth 122:120–130

14. White SM, Moppett IK, Griffiths R et al (2016) Secondary analysis of outcomes after 11,085 hip fracture operations from the prospective UK Anaesthesia Sprint Audit of Practice (ASAP-2). Anaesthesia 71:506–514

15. The National Institute of Clinical Excellence. Clinical Guideline 124 (2011) The management of hip fracture in adults. http://www.nice.org.uk/nicemedia/live/13489/54918/54918.pdf. Accessed 1 Apr 2016

16. Scottish Intercollegiate Guidelines Network (2009) Management of hip fracture in older people. National clinical guideline 111. www.sign.ac.uk/pdf/sign111.pdf. Accessed 1 Apr 2016

17. Wood RJ, White SM (2011) Anaesthesia for 1131 patients undergoing proximal femoral fracture repair: a retrospective, observational study of effects on blood pressure, fluid administration and perioperative anaemia. Anaesthesia 66:1017–1022

18. Royal College of Physicians and the Association of Anaesthetists of Great Britain and Ireland (2014) National Hip Fracture Database. Anaesthesia Sprint Audit of Practice 2014. http://www.nhfd.co.uk/20/hipfractureR.nsf/4e9601565a8ebbaa802579ea0035b25d/f085c66488 1d370c80257cac00266845/$FILE/onlineASAP.pdf. Accessed 1 Apr 2016

19. Sieber FE, Gottshalk A, akriya KJ, Mears SC, Lee H (2010) General anesthesia occurs frequently in elderly patients during propofol-based sedation and spinal anesthesia. J Clin Anesth 22:179–183

20. Ballard C, Jones E, Gauge N et al (2012) Optimised anaesthesia to reduce post operative cognitive decline (POCD) in older patients undergoing elective surgery, a randomised controlled trial. PLoS One 7:e37410

21. Donaldson AJ, Thomson HE, Harper NJ, Kenny NW (2009) Bone cement implantation syndrome. Br J Anaesth 102:12–22

22. Griffiths R, White SM, Moppett IK et al (2015) Association of Anaesthetists of Great Britain and Ireland; British Orthopaedic Association; British Geriatric Society. Safety guideline: reducing the risk from cemented hemiarthroplasty for hip fracture 2015: Association of Anaesthetists of Great Britain and Ireland British Orthopaedic Association British Geriatric Society. Anaesthesia 70:623–626

23. Chuan A, Zhao L, Tillekeratne N, Alani S, Middleton PM, Harris IA, McEvoy L, Ní Chróinín D (2019) The effect of a multidisciplinary care bundle on the incidence of delirium after hip fracture surgery: a quality improvement study. Anaesthesia. https://doi.org/10.1111/anae.14840

Hip Fracture: The Choice of Surgery

9

Henrik Palm

9.1 Aim of Surgery

The aim of hip fracture surgery is to allow immediate mobilization with full weight-bearing, aiming to achieve the previous level of function, ranging from maintaining normal walking in self-reliant elderly patients to pain relief in chronic bedridden nursing home residents. Three in four patients are expected to live beyond the first post-operative year, so proper surgery is required to alleviate an otherwise long-standing suboptimal functional level. Surgery is technically challenging, with body weight transfer through a broken oblique column, often with reduced bone quality due to osteoporosis—thus the risk of reoperation is high. A poorly operated hip fracture often leads to unequal leg length, pain and irreversible mobility loss, greatly influencing the quality of life.

9.2 Fracture Types

Hip fractures are divided into different types by the use of classification systems. A fracture classification should ideally have a high degree of reliability and reproducibility, be generally accepted, and have a prognostic validity in the clinical situation.

Historically, several classification systems have been proposed, but the following are the most commonly used in the literature. Hip fracture classifications are based

This chapter is a component of Part 2: Pillar I.
For an explanation of the grouping of chapters in this book, please see Chapter 1: 'The Multidisciplinary Approach to Fragility Fractures Around the World—An Overview'.

H. Palm (✉)
Department of Orthopedics, Copenhagen University Hospital Bispebjerg,
Copenhagen, Denmark
e-mail: henrik.palm@regionh.dk

© The Author(s) 2021
P. Falaschi, D. Marsh (eds.), *Orthogeriatrics*, Practical Issues in Geriatrics,
https://doi.org/10.1007/978-3-030-48126-1_9

125

Fig. 9.1 Antero-posterior radiograph of the right side proximal femur showing the anatomy and fracture positions. *FNF* femoral neck fracture, *TF* trochanteric fracture, *Sub-TF* sub-trochanteric fracture, *LFW* lateral femoral wall

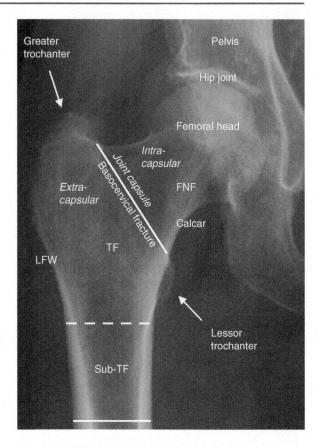

on radiographic fracture patterns, while previous hip surgery, arthritis, cancer, dysplasia, bone quality, soft tissue and pain are normally not taken into account.

Hip fractures cover proximal femoral fractures predominantly located up to 5 cm distal to the lesser trochanter and are classified by fracture anatomy on plain radiographs (Fig. 9.1), if necessary supplemented by CT or MRI [1].

The hip joint capsule divides fractures into two main categories with an almost equal patient distribution: (1) Intra-capsular femoral neck fractures and (2) extracapsular basicervical, trochanteric and sub-trochanteric fractures.

9.2.1   Intra-capsular Fracture Types

In a fragility fracture context, intra-capsular hip fractures are in fact through the femoral neck, as femoral head fractures are uncommon in the elderly.

Femoral neck fractures are at risk of non-union with/without mechanical collapse due to insufficient fixation and/or avascular necrosis of the femoral head. In adults, the femoral head is primarily supplied by the distal recurrent vessels entering the femur on the shaft side of the fracture. Avascular necrosis is caused by ischaemia hypothetically due to either a direct trauma to the arterial supply crossing the

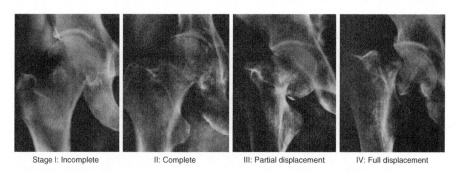

Stage I: Incomplete   II: Complete   III: Partial displacement   IV: Full displacement

Fig. 9.2 Garden's classification. (Reproduced with permission and copyright © of the British Editorial Society of Bone and Joint Surgery)

fracture-line or by a temporary arterial impingement, caused by vessel stretching or intra-capsular hematoma. Preoperative scintigraphy, electrode measurement and arthroscopic visualization of ischaemia have been tested but lack prognostic value. Since ischaemia could be temporary, acute reposition within hours (may be supplemented by hematoma emptying) has been suggested [2, 3].

Femoral neck fracture classification has historically been contentious with several different systems, primarily based on fracture displacement seen in the anterior–posterior radiographs. *Garden's Classification* (Fig. 9.2) has in the last half a century been the most widespread. Fractures are divided into four stages based on fracture displacement [4]. Garden's classification has only fair inter-observer reliability when using all four stages, but moderate to substantial if dichotomized into just undisplaced (Garden I–II) or displaced (Garden III–IV) fractures [5].

In addition, a vertical fracture line in the anterior–posterior radiograph or posterior wall multi-fragmentation, femoral head size and posterior tilt angulation seen in the lateral radiograph are believed to influence outcome [6–9]. However, the dualism of undisplaced versus displaced (with reference to Gardens stages I–II vs. III–IV) remains the most consistent predictor of failure and the most widespread fracture classification, with respectively around one-third and two-third of femoral neck fractures [10, 11].

9.2.2 Extra-capsular Fracture Types

Extra-capsular fractures are at risk of mechanical collapse and non-union due to insufficient fixation. The fracture line is anatomically located laterally to the nutrient vessels to the femoral head, so avascular necrosis is rarely seen, but muscle attachments often dislocate the fragments and bleeding into surrounding muscles can be severe and life-threatening. Classification systems are primarily based on fracture-line location and number of fragments.

Basicervical fractures are a few percent of borderline cases between the intra- and extra-capsular fractures, anatomically positioned on the capsular attachment line. The AO/OTA classification describes them as intra-capsular, but biomechanically they behave like the extra-capsular fractures [12]—except for the risk of rotation of the medial segment due to lack of muscle attachments.

Trochanteric fractures cover the trochanteric area from the capsule until just below the lesser trochanter. The often-used unnecessary prefixes per-, inter- and trans- are undefined, confusing and unhelpful for classification.

The *AO/OTA Classification* (Fig. 9.3) from 1987 is nowadays the most widespread. It divides the 31-A trochanteric area into nine types by severity (1-2-3, each subtyped.1-.2-.3) [13].

Femur, proximal, pertrochanteric simple (only 2 fragments) (31-A1)

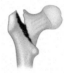 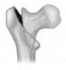 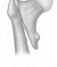

1. Along intertrochanteric line (31-A1.3)

2. Through the greater trochanter (31-A1.1)
(1) nonimpacted
(2) impacted

3. Below lesser trochanter (31-A1.2)

Femur, proximal, trochanteric fracture, pertrochanteric multifragmentary (always have posteromedial fragment with lessor trochanter and adjacent medial cortex (31-A2)

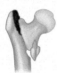 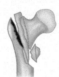 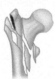

1. With 1 intermediate fragment (31-A2.1)

2. With several intermediate fragments (31-A2.2)

3. Extending more than 1 cm below lessor trochanter (31-A2.3)

Femur, proximal, trochanteric area, intertrochanteric fracture (31-A3)

  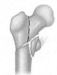

1. Simple oblique (31-A3.1)

2. Simple transverse (31-A3.2)

3. Multifragmentary (31-A3.3)
(1) extending to greater trochanter
(2) extending to neck

Fig. 9.3 AO/OTA Classification for trochanteric fractures (Reproduced with permission from J Orthop Trauma)

Fracture type 31-A1 covers the simple two-part fractures, while 31-A2 demands a detached lesser trochanter, with an intact (31-A2.1) or a detached greater trochanter (31-A2.2-3). 31-A3 covers fracture lines through the lateral femoral wall—defined as the lateral cortex distal to the greater trochanter—in which the subgroup 31-A3.1 represents the reverse fracture and 31-A3.2 the transversal, while the most comminuted 31-A3.3 fracture demands both a fractured lateral femoral wall and a detached lesser trochanter.

The AO/OTA classification covers most fractures within previous classification systems, except the few trochanteric fractures with a detached greater trochanter and an intact lesser trochanter. The reliability when using all nine types is poor, but increases to substantial if only classifying into the three main groups (A1-2-3) [14].

Subtrochanteric fractures are positioned distally to the trochanters, and constitute around 5% of all hip fractures. These have historically been classified by as many as 15 different systems, most often into the 8 types from 0 to 5 cm below the lesser trochanter by Seinsheimer or the 15 types from 0 to 3 cm in the AO/OTA classification for femoral shaft fractures, the type 32ABC(1-3).1 sub-division. A review doubts the value of such division and proposes simplicity into: (1) a stable two-part and unstable, (2) three-part and (3) more comminuted fractures from 0 to 5 cm below the lessor trochanter, without involvement of the trochanters. It however still has to be established whether this easier classification is useful and necessary for decision-making and prognosis [13, 15, 16].

9.3 Implants

There are two major strategies for treating hip fractures, prosthesis or osteosynthesis. A prosthesis involves removing the fracture site, and replacing the femoral head with a hemi-arthroplasty or total hip arthroplasty, the latter also including an acetabular cup. An osteosynthesis involves reducing bone fragments to an acceptable position and retaining them until healing—usually with parallel implants, sliding hip screw or intramedullary nail (Fig. 9.4).

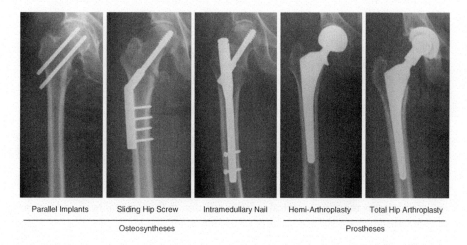

| Parallel Implants | Sliding Hip Screw | Intramedullary Nail | Hemi-Arthroplasty | Total Hip Arthroplasty |
| Osteosyntheses | | | Prostheses | |

Fig. 9.4 The main implant groups for hip fracture surgery

Prostheses are inserted with the patient supine or lateral depending on the surgical approach, while osteosynthesis is always performed through one or more lateral approaches, with the patient supine on a traction table and the use of a radiographic image-intensifier. There are pros and cons for all implants, but all are dependent on proper use, which is why well-defined implant position measurements are needed for optimal evaluation of one implant against another.

Parallel implants are inserted with limited operative bleeding and soft tissue damage through a few lateral stab incisions or a single <5 cm incision. In spite of many clinical and cadaver studies, choice (screws/hookpins) and number (2/3/4) of implants lack consensus [17]. Parallel implants permit fracture compression and they should be inserted as vertically as possible and in different head quadrants. Furthermore, the posterior implant should have posterior cortex contact and the inferior implant calcar contact to achieve three-point fixation that best supports weight transfer from (1) the subchondral bone to (2) a calcar seat and (3) a lateral femoral cortex counterpoint [18]. The main reasons for failure are non-union, with or without mechanical collapse, due to insufficient fixation and/or avascular necrosis. Also, a femoral neck shortened heling position is associated with poor functional outcome [19]. Salvage normally necessitates a hip prosthesis or, depending on the patient's demand, a simple removal of the femoral head. A new fall can result in fractures around the parallel implants, which should be reoperated with a sliding hip screw or an intramedullary nail.

Sliding hip screws have been the Gold Standard for treating trochanteric fractures for several decades—but have recently also gained ground for femoral neck fractures [17]. After reduction, the femoral head fragment is held by a large diameter screw, which can slide inside an approximately 135° angle plate attached laterally to the femoral shaft. The implant is inserted under the lateral vastus muscle through a single lateral approach, around 10 cm long depending on chosen plate length.

To reduce the risk of cut-out of the screw into the hip joint, it should be positioned centrally or central-inferiorly in the femoral neck with the tip attached subchondrally in the femoral head, providing a short so-called tip-apex distance [20]. Beyond cut-out, the common reasons for failure are mechanical collapse, with or without non-union and a distal peri-implant fracture. Depending on femoral head bone status, salvage can be an intramedullary nail or a distally seated hip prosthesis.

Intramedullary nails have, during the last decade, outnumbered sliding hip screws as treatment for trochanteric fractures [21]. After reduction, the femoral head fragment is held by a large diameter screw, which can slide at an angle of approximately 130° through an intramedullary nail with 1–2 distal locking screws. The nail is inserted at the greater trochanter tip, through a 5-cm lateral incision, with the sliding and locking screw(s) inserted by use of a guide through stab incisions in the lateral vastus muscle. A central-inferior position in the femoral head and a short tip–apex distance for the threaded types is important, while the new bladed types might need more distance [22, 23].

Some old nails had a reputation for risking a shaft fracture, but newer nails have moved beyond this, although the many new smaller designs, with different screw, blade, sleeve, locking and anti-rotation mechanisms, lack convincing clinical evidence so far [24, 25].

Reasons for failure are the same as for the sliding hip screws, and salvage can be a distally seated hip prosthesis for bone collapse. In case of a distal peri-implant fracture, a longer nail or a condylar plate can be used, depending on the nail length.

Prostheses involve a metal femoral head replacement attached by a stem seated in the shaft cavity. To fit individual patients' anatomy, implants are modular and assembled during surgery; thus mono-blocks are no longer recommended [26]. Reoperations are primarily caused by repeated dislocations or by a peri-prosthetic fracture (produced during insertion or subsequent to a new fall). For dislocations, closed reduction is the norm, but reposition or modification with a low-range-of-motion constrained liner is necessary in recurrent cases. Peri-prosthetic fractures are treated with circumferential wires and/or a plate, and a loose prosthesis is changed or removed depending on the patient's demands.

Hemi-arthroplasties (HA) traditionally have reduced dislocation rate, shorter operating time and less blood loss than a total hip arthroplasty. Reports of acetabular chondral erosion, following unipolar HA, have encouraged bipolar heads with an additional ball joint—their efficiency is, however, still debated [27–29].

Total Hip Arthroplasties (THA) also replace the acetabular cartilage, theoretically a source of pain and thus reduced functional ability. THAs might provide a better result than HAs in active, independent living, and cognitively intact patients, but more studies are warranted [28, 30–33]. Despite the higher implant price, the total cost of using THA could be lower when taking complications and function into account, in the healthiest patients [34]. THAs, however, have an increased dislocation risk [28, 30, 31, 35], which might be reduced by the technically demanding new dual-mobility type [36–38].

Beyond optimal implant positioning, the dislocation rate following both HA and THA might be reduced to 1–3% of patients if using the antero-lateral approach, compared to 4–14% if using the postero-lateral approach, although the latter can probably be improved by an optimal capsular and muscle repair [39–41]. The only randomized study, however, found no difference in dislocation rate between the two methods [42], and a register study found that the consequences of surgical approach for soft tissue, pain and mobility might be minimal [43]. It may be that dual-mobility cups can justify the continued use of the postero-lateral approach [36–38].

Cementation is associated with more dislocations in some studies but less in others. Cementation seems to improve patient mobility, reduce pain and the rate of peri-prosthetic fractures (1–7% for uncemented prostheses), although only a few studies include the newer hydroxyapatite-coated surfaces. Cementation probably increases risk of air embolism, blood loss and operation time, but registries have shown that a higher acute mortality appears to equilibrate after a couple of months [2, 28, 29, 44–46].

9.4 Surgical Management

Patients should receive their operation as soon as possible, because the negative impact on body functions, while waiting for surgery, appears to be significant. Surgery on the day of, or the day after admission (less than 36 h) is recommended, although studies to prove this are difficult, because stratification by comorbidities is challenging [47–51].

Surgical drains [52], and pre-operative traction is no longer recommended [53]. Conservative treatment should be avoided in modern healthcare systems [54], except in the case of few terminally ill patients who can be kept pain-free by analgesics in their last few days of life.

Patients sustaining a metastatic fracture should be identified, the cancer investigated and the proximal femur fixed in a way that takes into account the growing cancer, normally by use of a long nail or a distally seated THA.

Prophylactic antibiotic treatment should be given. Deep infection is rare (Table 9.1), but potentially devastating, often with several procedures and implant removal. While treating the infection, an external fixator can be used to keep extracapsular fractures reduced. Predictors of infections are primarily the surgeon's experience and the operation duration [55, 56].

9.4.1 Intra-capsular Operations

The overall choice stands between (1) femoral head removal and insertion of a prosthesis, or (2) femoral head preservation by internal fixation, wherein the main overall predictor for failure is initial fracture displacement [3]. However, patient age, co-morbidity, mobility demands and so on should also be taken into account in the choice of implant. Patients should be asked about pre-fracture hip pain and a THA is chosen if hip arthritis coexists.

Table 9.1 Overall rates of surgical complications

	Deep infection (%)	Non-union and cut-out (%)	Avascular necrosis (%)	Distal fracture (%)	Dislocation (%)	Aseptic loosening (%)	Reoperation (%)
Undisplaced FNF, IF	≈1	5–10	4–10	<1	–	–	8–12
Displaced FNF, IF	≈1	20–35	5–20	<1	–	–	15–35
FNF, Prosthesis	1–7	–	–	1–7	1–14	1–3	2–15
Extra-capsular	≈1	1–10	<1	1–4	–	–	2–10

FNF femoral neck fracture, *IF* internal fixation

Undisplaced femoral neck fractures may be complicated by non-union, with or without fracture collapse and, after a minimum of 3–6 months, radiographically evident avascular necrosis of the femoral head (Table 9.1). Around three-quarters of the undisplaced fractures are treated with parallel screws or pins, which appears to be adequate [3, 17]. The sliding hip screw is comparable and enables a more stable fixation due to the fixed angle attachment when three-point fixation is unachievable due to a vertical and/or basal fracture line—but necessitates a larger incision. Also, posterior tilt might increase the reoperation rate [7, 8], suggesting that this may be an indication for prosthesis, rather than osteosynthesis.

Displaced femoral neck fractures are followed by the same complications after internal fixation as the undisplaced—but at a higher rate (Table 9.1).

If using internal fixation, the fracture must be anatomically reduced within a short time and the implants optimally positioned. Prostheses are now the most common treatment for displaced fractures, with improved results (Table 9.1) varying with the approach, cementation and THA/HA [2, 17, 18, 21, 44, 45, 57, 58].

A large number of studies report a significantly lower reoperation rate following a prosthetic replacement. Newer studies also find less pain, better hip function and higher patient satisfaction after a prosthesis. However, this is at the expense of a greater primary operation (operating time, soft tissue damage, blood loss and impact on body functions) resulting in a higher immediate mortality. Fortunately, this appears to equilibrate later [2, 29, 57–59].

Using internal fixation for all displaced fractures, with the insertion of a prosthesis later if required, is not recommended as a salvage prosthesis insertion has a much higher complication risk than a primary. Prostheses, however, have a shorter lifetime in mobile young patients who might outlive their prosthesis once or more. It has therefore been suggested to use an internal fixation in the younger patients, THA in active patients aged around 65–80 years and HA in the oldest. [2, 29, 35, 60].

The subgroup of demented patients might benefit more from internal fixation—their functional scores are generally low—but the literature is so far limited [61, 62]. Osteosynthesis in most fragile patients, who are demented or have a high risk of dying on the operation table, should however be used with caution, as the fixation often turns out to be inadequate and painful in the short term—requiring a reoperation—if the patients live longer than expected. In a few selected bedridden, oldest patients, a simple removal of the femoral head can be chosen as the primary procedure to reduce fracture pain and eliminate complications.

9.4.2 Extra-capsular Operations

Basicervical fractures are treated with a sliding hip screw, attached to a short lateral plate. Parallel implants are insufficient because of the lack of implant support by the calcar bone area [12].

Trochanteric fractures may be complicated by a non-union or mechanical collapse in 1–10% of patients. The pull of muscles often displaces fragments, while a near-anatomical reduction is necessary for the majority of weight to pass through the bone. Use of retractors and/or a posterior-reduction device on the fracture table is recommended to prevent sagging of the fracture.

During the early post-operative months, an inadequate reduction and implant position may lead to femoral shaft medialization and femoral head varus position with risk of a screw cut-out, pain and a shortened femoral neck- and leg-length. The overall rate of reoperation is 2–10%. [25, 63–65]. A salvage prosthesis can be inserted primarily, but this is challenging due to the damaged bone stock.

The choice of implant is between the sliding hip screw and an intramedullary nail but, after many cohort studies and more than 40 RCTs since the past three decades, the comparison remains inconclusive overall. The current status appears to be that, although the sliding hip screw remains the recommended implant, nails might have an advantage on mobility or in the more unstable trochanteric fracture [24, 66, 67]. The Norwegian national registry reported fewer reoperations after sliding hip screws in 7643 stable (AO/OTA type 31A1) and after nails in 2716 unstable trochanteric fractures (AO/OTA type 31A3) [64, 65]. However, a systematic review of the six RCTs on a total of 265 patients with AO/OTA type A3 fractures found comparable fracture healing complication rates for sliding hip screws and intramedullary nails—and more RCTs on fracture subgroups are warranted [68].

Often lateralization and femoral neck shortening are seen following the unstable trochanteric fractures, probably due to a lack of a buttress from the lateral femoral wall. A trochanteric buttress shield might prevent lateralization, but the evidence is not convincing and the method demands a much larger incision than simply inserting the well-known intramedullary femoral nail. The sliding hip screw might be insufficient for fractures with a detached greater trochanter (AO/OTA type A2.2 and A2.3) as the resulting thin lateral femoral wall is at risk of per-operative fracture. The integrity of the lesser trochanter does not seem to influence outcome, and unstable trochanteric fractures should probably thus be defined by a detached greater trochanter or a lateral femoral wall fracture (AO/OTA type 31A.2.2-2.3 + A3) [69, 70].

So far knowledge is limited on whether the use of the longest possible nail can reduce risk of later shaft-fractures, although femoral shaft bending, entry-point and distal locking appears more challenging in long nails [71].

Sub-trochanteric fractures are nowadays most often treated with a long nail, which is probably beneficial with reoperation rates declining by 5–15%. Most literature, however, also included the AO/OTA 31A3 fractures, due to difficulties of differentiation and more knowledge is needed. Circumferential wires can be added for keeping the oblique and comminuted fractures reduced with a low risk of bone-necrosis [15, 72].

9.5   Surgical Algorithms and National Guidelines

As indicated earlier, the published evidence in the last decades has created a degree of consensus for the surgical treatment of hip fractures. In everyday clinical practice, the exact choice of implant however often remains uncertain, and an easily used surgical algorithm for all hip fracture patients might be warranted.

Younger, less experienced surgeons probably feel more confident when guided by a strict algorithm, while older surgeons could feel that their individual right of choice is being restricted. It is, however, important to underline that a treatment algorithm does not negate the individual surgeon's responsibility for the individual patient. A surgeon still has the right and duty, now and then, to defy a guideline due to individual circumstances, but the decision to do so should be justified in the patient record.

Creating an algorithm that embraces the heterogeneous group of hip fracture patients is challenging, and the balance between detail and usability must be considered. Many published articles recommend treatment for some aspects, but only a few authors have published comprehensive decision-tree algorithms for hip fracture surgery—among which the simple, exhaustive and exclusive Copenhagen Algorithm (Fig. 9.5) appears to be the best scientifically evaluated [9, 73].

National guidelines including surgery have emerged in Australia, New Zealand, United States and most European countries during the last decades. Consensus is widespread for some overall recommendations based on the same evidence.

Among the intra-capsular fractures, all recommend internal fixation for undisplaced femoral neck fractures and to some extent prosthetic replacement for the displaced in elderly patients. Among the extra-capsular fractures, the sliding hip screw is recommended for the stable (often defined as AO/OTA type A1) while a nail is recommended for the unstable fractures (often defined as AO/OTA type A3 and further distal). The purpose of national guidelines is to recommend evidence-based surgical treatment for improving outcome. National hip fracture registries have gained ground, especially in the last decades, to enable continued evaluation of treatment quality and the identification of positive and negative outliers. [10, 73, 74].

The multidisciplinary global fragility fracture network has now the strategic focus of facilitating national (or regional) consensus guidelines including quality standards and systematic performance measurement—and offers an easily used minimum data set for hip fracture audit [74]. Hopefully, such knowledge dissemination not only helps to overcome barriers to implementation, but also to globally spread evidence-based national guidelines, standards and registries for improving the surgical quality.

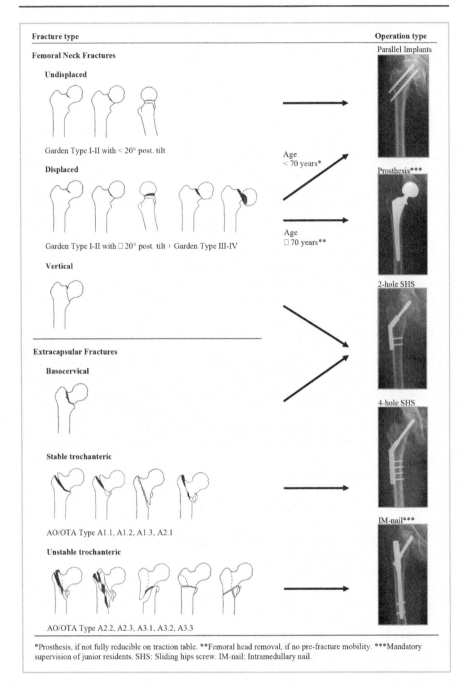

Fig. 9.5 An algorithm for hip fracture surgery (Reproduced with permission from Acta Orthop)

References[1]

1. Cannon J, Silvestri S, Munro M (2009) Imaging choices in occult hip fracture. J Emerg Med 37:144–152
2. Heetveld MJ, Rogmark C, Frihagen F, Keating J (2009) Internal fixation versus arthroplasty for displaced femoral neck fractures: what is the evidence? J Orthop Trauma 23:395–402
3. Loizou CL, Parker MJ (2009) Avascular necrosis after internal fixation of intracapsular hip fractures; a study of the outcome for 1023 patients. Injury 40:1143–1146
4. Garden RS (1961) Low-angle fixation in fractures of the femoral neck. J Bone Joint Surg (Br) 43-B:647–663
5. Gašpar D, Crnković T, Durovic D, Podsednik D, Slišurić F (2012) AO group, AO subgroup, Garden and Pauwels classification systems of femoral neck fractures: are they reliable and reproducible? Med Glas (Zenica) 9:243–247
6. Khan SK, Khanna A, Parker MJ (2009a) Posterior multifragmentation of the femoral neck: does it portend a poor outcome in internally fixed intracapsular hip fractures? Injury 40:280–282
7. Okike K, Udogwu UN, Isaac M, Sprague S, Swiontkowski MF, Bhandari M, Slobogean GP, FAITH Investigators (2019) Not all Garden-I and II femoral neck fractures in the elderly should be fixed: effect of posterior tilt on rates of subsequent arthroplasty. J Bone Joint Surg Am 101(20):1852–1859
8. Palm H, Gosvig K, Krasheninnikoff M, Jacobsen S, Gebuhr P (2009) A new measurement for posterior tilt predicts reoperation in undisplaced femoral neck fractures: 113 consecutive patients treated by internal fixation and followed for 1 year. Acta Orthop 80(3):303–307
9. Palm H, Krasheninnikoff M, Holck K, Lemser T, Foss NB, Jacobsen S, Kehlet H, Gebuhr P (2012) A new algorithm for hip fracture surgery. Acta Orthop 83(1):26–30
10. National Hip Fracture Database (2019) National report. http://www.nhfd.co.uk. Accessed 15 Feb 2020
11. Zlowodzki M, Bhandari M, Keel M, Hanson BP, Schemitsch E (2005) Perception of Garden's classification for femoral neck fractures: an international survey of 298 orthopaedic trauma surgeons. Arch Orthop Trauma Surg 125:503–505
12. Mallick A, Parker MJ (2004) Basal fractures of the femoral neck: intra- or extra-capsular. Injury 35:989–993
13. Marsh JL, Slongo TF, Agel J, Broderick JS, Creevey W, DeCoster TA, Prokuski L, Sirkin MS, Ziran B, Henley B, Audigé L (2007) Fracture and dislocation classification compendium–2007: orthopaedic trauma association classification, database and outcomes committee. J Orthop Trauma 21(Suppl 10):S1–S133
14. Pervez H, Parker MJ, Pryor GA, Lutchman L, Chirodian N (2002) Classification of trochanteric fracture of the proximal femur: a study of the reliability of current systems. Injury 33:713–715
15. Loizou CL, McNamara I, Ahmed K, Pryor GA, Parker MJ (2010) Classification of subtrochanteric femoral fractures. Injury 41:739–745
16. Seinsheimer F (1978) Subtrochanteric fractures of the femur. J Bone Joint Surg 60(3):300–306
17. Parker MJ, Gurusamy KS (2011) Internal fixation implants for intracapsular hip fractures in adults (Review). Cochrane Database Syst Rev. https://doi.org/10.1002/14651858.CD001467
18. Schep NWL, Heintjes RJ, Martens EP, van Dortmont LMC, van Vugt AB (2004) Retrospective analysis of factors influencing the operative result after percutaneous osteosynthesis of intracapsular femoral neck fractures. Injury 35:1003–1009

---

[1] This book chapter is an updated version of: Palm H (2016) An algorithm for hip fracture surgery. Doctor of Medical Science. Dissertation. Copenhagen University. ISBN 978-87-998,922-0-4.

19. Felton J, Slobogean GP, Jackson SS, Della Rocca GJ, Liew S, Haverlag R, Jeray KJ, Sprague SA, O'Hara NN, Swiontkowski M, Bhandari M (2019) Femoral neck shortening after hip fracture fixation is associated with inferior hip function: results from the FAITH trial. J Orthop Trauma 33(10):487–496

20. Baumgaertner MR, Solberg BD (1997) Awareness of tip-apex distance reduces failure of fixation of trochanteric fractures of the hip. J Bone Joint Surg (Br) 79-B:969–971

21. Rogmark C, Spetz C, Garellick G (2010) More intramedullary nails and arthroplasties for treatment of hip fractures in Sweden. Acta Orthop 81:588–592

22. Nikoloski AN, Osbrough AL, Yates PJ (2013) Should the tip-apex distance (TAD) rule be modified for the proximal femoral nail antirotation (PFNA)? A retrospective study. J Orthop Surg Res 8:35

23. Rubio-Avila J, Madden K, Simunovic N, Bhandari M (2013) Tip to apex distance in femoral intertrochanteric fractures: a systematic review. J Orthop Sci 18:592–598

24. Bhandari M, Schemitsch E, Jönsson A, Zlowodzki M, Haidukewych GJ (2009) Gamma nails revisited: gamma nails versus compression hip screws in the management of intertrochanteric fractures of the hip: a meta-analysis. J Orthop Trauma 23:460–464

25. Queally JM, Harris E, Handoll HHG, Parker MJ (2014) Intramedullary nails for extracapsular hip fractures in adults (Review). Cochrane Database Syst Rev. https://doi.org/10.1002/14651858.CD004961.pub4

26. Rogmark C, Leonardsson O, Garellick G, Kärrholm J (2012) Monoblock hemiarthroplasties for femoral neck fractures—a part of orthopaedic history? Analysis of national registration of hemiarthroplasties 2005-2009. Injury 43:946–949

27. Jia Z, Ding F, Wu Y, Li W, Li H, Wang D, He Q, Ruan D (2015) Unipolar versus bipolar hemiarthroplasty for displaced femoral neck fractures: a systematic review and meta-analysis of randomized controlled trials. J Orthop Surg Res 10:8

28. Parker MJ, Gurusamy KS, Azegami S (2010) Arthroplasties (with and without bone cement) for proximal femoral fractures in adults (Review). Cochrane Database Syst Rev. https://doi.org/10.1002/14651858.CD001706.pub4

29. Rogmark C, Leonardsson O (2016) Hip arthroplasty for the treatment of displaced fractures of the femoral neck in elderly patients. Bone Joint J 98-B:291–297

30. Bhandari M, Einhorn TA, Guyatt G, Schemitsch EH, Zura RD, Sprague S, Frihagen F, Guerra-Farfán E, Kleinlugtenbelt YV, Poolman RW, Rangan A, Bzovsky S, Heels-Ansdell D, Thabane L, Walter SD, Devereaux PJ (2019) Total hip arthroplasty or hemiarthroplasty for hip fracture. N Engl J Med 381(23):2199–2208

31. Burgers PT, Van Geene AR, Van den Bekerom MP, Van Lieshout EM, Blom B, Aleem IS, Bhandari M, Poolman RW (2012) Total hip arthroplasty versus hemiarthroplasty for displaced femoral neck fractures in the healthy elderly: a meta-analysis and systematic review of randomized trials. Int Orthop 36:1549–1560

32. Hansson S, Nemes S, Kärrholm J, Rogmark C (2017) Reduced risk of reoperation after treatment of femoral neck fractures with total hip arthroplasty. Acta Orthop 88(5):500–504

33. Parker MJ, Cawley S (2019) Treatment of the displaced intracapsular fracture for the 'fitter' elderly patients: a randomised trial of total hip arthroplasty versus hemiarthroplasty for 105 patients. Injury 50(11):2009–2013

34. Slover J, Hoffman MV, Malchau H, Tosteson ANA, Koval KJ (2009) A cost-effectiveness analysis of the arthroplasty options for displaced femoral neck fractures in the active, healthy, elderly population. J Arthroplast 24:854–860

35. Hansson S, Bülow E, Garland A, Kärrholm J, Rogmark C (2019) More hip complications after total hip arthroplasty than after hemi-arthroplasty as hip fracture treatment: analysis of 5,815 matched pairs in the Swedish Hip Arthroplasty Register. Acta Orthop 18:1–6

36. Adam P, Philippe R, Ehlinger M, Roche O, Bonnomet F, Molé D, Fessy MH, French Society of Orthopaedic Surgery and Traumatology (SoFCOT) (2012) Dual mobility cups hip arthroplasty as a treatment for displaced fracture of the femoral neck in the elderly. A prospective, systematic, multicenter study with specific focus on postoperative dislocation. Orthop Traumatol Surg Res 98:296–300

37. Bensen AS, Jakobsen T, Krarup N (2014) Dual mobility cup reduces dislocation and re-operation when used to treat displaced femoral neck fractures. Int Orthop 38:1241–1245

38. Jobory A, Kärrholm J, Overgaard S, Becic Pedersen A, Hallan G, Gjertsen JE, Mäkelä K, Rogmark C (2019) Reduced revision risk for dual-mobility cup in total hip replacement due to hip fracture: a matched-pair analysis of 9,040 cases from the Nordic Arthroplasty Register Association (NARA). J Bone Joint Surg Am 101(14):1278–1285

39. Enocson A, Tidermark J, Tornkvist H, Lapidus LJ (2008) Dislocation of hemiarthroplasty after femoral neck fracture: better outcome after the anterolateral approach in a prospective cohort study on 739 consecutive hips. Acta Orthop 79:211–217

40. Enocson A, Hedbeck CJ, Tidermark J, Pettersson H, Ponzer S, Lapidus LJ (2009) Dislocation of total hip replacement in patients with fractures of the femoral neck. Acta Orthop 80:184–189

41. Pellicci PM, Bostrom M, Poss R (1998) Posterior approach to total hip replacement using enhanced posterior soft tissue repair. Clin Orthop Relat Res 355:224–228

42. Parker MJ (2015) Lateral versus posterior approach for insertion of hemiarthroplasties for hip fractures: a randomised trial of 216 patients. Injury 46(6):1023–1027

43. Leonardsson O, Rolfson O, Rogmark C (2016) The surgical approach for hemiarthroplasty does not influence patient-reported outcome: a national survey of 2118 patients with one-year follow-up. Bone Joint J 98-B(4):542–547

44. Imam MA, Shehata MSA, Elsehili A, Morsi M, Martin A, Shawqi M, Grubhofer F, Chirodian N, Narvani A, Ernstbrunner L (2019) Contemporary cemented versus uncemented hemiarthroplasty for the treatment of displaced intracapsular hip fractures: a meta-analysis of forty-two thousand forty-six hips. Int Orthop 43(7):1715–1723

45. Kristensen TB, Dybvik E, Kristoffersen M, Dale H, Engesæter LB, Furnes O, Gjertsen JE (2020) Cemented or uncemented hemiarthroplasty for femoral neck fracture? Data from the norwegian hip fracture register. Clin Orthop Relat Res 478(1):90–100

46. Talsnes O, Vinje T, Gjertsen JE, Dahl OE, Engesæter LB, Baste V, Pripp AH, Reikerås O (2013) Perioperative mortality in hip fracture patients treated with cemented and uncemented hemiprosthesis: a register study of 11,210 patients. Int Orthop 37:1135–1140

47. Bretherton CP, Parker MJ (2015) Early surgery for patients with a fracture of the hip decreases 30-day mortality. Bone Joint J 97-B:104–108

48. HIP ATTACK Investigators (2020) Accelerated surgery versus standard care in hip fracture (HIP ATTACK): an international, randomised, controlled trial. Lancet 395:698–708

49. Khan SK, Kalra S, Khanna A, Thiruvengada MM, Parker MJ (2009b) Timing of surgery for hip fractures: a systematic review of 52 published studies involving 291,413 patients. Injury 40:692–697

50. Moja L, Piatti A, Pecoraro V, Ricci C, Virgili G, Salanti G, Germagnoli L, Liberati A, Banfi G (2012) Timing matters in hip fracture surgery: patients operated within 48 hours have better outcomes. A meta-analysis and meta-regression of over 190,000 patients. PLoS One 7:e46175

51. Simunovic N, Devereaux PJ, Sprague S, Guyatt GH, Schemitsch E, Debeer J, Bhandari M (2010) Effect of early surgery after hip fracture on mortality and complications: systematic review and meta-analysis. CMAJ 182:1609–1616

52. Clifton R, Haleem S, Mckee A, Parker MJ (2008) Closed suction surgical wound drainage after hip fracture surgery: a systematic review and meta-analysis of randomised controlled trials. Int Orthop 32:723–727

53. Handoll HHG, Queally JM, Parker MJ (2011) Pre-operative traction for hip fractures in adults (Review). Cochrane Database Syst Rev. https://doi.org/10.1002/14651858.CD000168.pub3

54. Handoll HHG, Parker MJ (2008) Conservative versus operative treatment for hip fractures in adults (Review). Cochrane Database Syst Rev. https://doi.org/10.1002/14651858.CD000337.pub2

55. Harrison T, Robinson P, Cook A, Parker MJ (2012) Factors affecting the incidence of deep wound infection after hip fracture surgery. J Bone Joint Surg (Br) 94-B:237–240

56. Noailles T, Brulefert K, Chalopin A, Longis PM, Gouin F (2016) What are the risk factors for post-operative infection after hip hemiarthroplasty? Systematic review of literature. Int Orthop 40(9):1843–1848

57. Lu-Yao G, Keller R, Littenberg B, Wennberg J (1994) Outcomes after displaced fractures of the femoral neck. A meta-analysis of one hundred and six published reports. J Bone Joint Surg Am 76-A:15–25

58. Parker MJ, Gurusamy KS (2006) Internal fixation versus arthroplasty for intracapsular proximal femoral fractures in adults (Review). Cochrane Database Syst Rev:CD001708

59. Rogmark C, Johnell O (2006) Primary arthroplasty is better than internal fixation of displaced femoral neck fractures: a meta-analysis of 14 randomized studies with 2,289 patients. Acta Orthop 77:359–367

60. Mahmoud SS, Pearse EO, Smith TO, Hing CB (2016) Outcomes of total hip arthroplasty, as a salvage procedure, following failed internal fixation of intracapsular fractures of the femoral neck: a systematic review and meta-analysis. Bone Joint J 98-B(4):452–460

61. Hebert-Davies J, Laflamme G-Y, Rouleau D (2012) Bias towards dementia: are hip fracture trials excluding too many patients? A systematic review. Injury 43:1978–1984

62. Van Dortmont LM, Douw CM, van Breukelen AM, Laurens DR, Mulder PG, Wereldsma JC, van Vugt AB (2000) Outcome after hemi-arthroplasty for displaced intracapsular femoral neck fracture related to mental state. Injury 31:327–331

63. Chirodian N, Arch B, Parker MJ (2005) Sliding hip screw fixation of trochanteric hip fractures: outcome of 1024 procedures. Injury 36:793–800

64. Matre K, Havelin LI, Gjertsen JE, Espehaug B, Fevang JM (2013a) Intramedullary nails result in more reoperations than sliding hip screws in two-part intertrochanteric fractures. Clin Orthop Relat Res 471:1379–1386

65. Matre K, Havelin LI, Gjertsen JE, Vinje T, Espehaug B, Fevang JM (2013b) Sliding hip screw versus IM nail in reverse oblique trochanteric and subtrochanteric fractures. A study of 2716 patients in the Norwegian Hip Fracture Register. Injury 44:735–742

66. Parker MJ, Handoll HHG (2010) Gamma and other cephalocondylic intramedullary nails versus extramedullary implants for extracapsular hip fractures in adults (Review). Cochrane Database Syst Rev. https://doi.org/10.1002/14651858.CD000093.pub5

67. Parker MJ (2017) Sliding hip screw versus intramedullary nail for trochanteric hip fractures; a randomised trial of 1000 patients with presentation of results related to fracture stability. Injury 48(12):2762–2767

68. Parker MJ, Raval P, Gjertsen JE (2018) Nail or plate fixation for A3 trochanteric hip fractures: a systematic review of randomised controlled trials. Injury 49(7):1319–1323

69. Palm H, Jacobsen S, Sonne-Holm S, Gebuhr P (2007) Integrity of the lateral femoral wall in intertrochanteric hip fractures: an important predictor of a reoperation. J Bone Joint Surg Am 89(3):470–475

70. Palm H, Lysén C, Krasheninnikoff M, Holck K, Jacobsen S, Gebuhr P (2011) Intramedullary nailing appears to be superior in pertrochanteric hip fractures with a detached greater trochanter. Acta Orthop 82(2):166–170

71. Norris R, Bhattacharjee D, Parker MJ (2012) Occurrence of secondary fracture around intramedullary nails used for trochanteric hip fractures: a systematic review of 13,568 patients. Injury 43:706–711

72. Ban I, Birkelund L, Palm H, Brix M, Troelsen A (2012) Circumferential wires as a supplement to intramedullary nailing in unstable trochanteric hip fractures: 4 reoperations in 60 patients followed for 1 year. Acta Orthop 83:240–243
73. Palm H, Teixider J (2015) Proxial femoral fractures: can we improve further surgical treatment pathways? Injury Suppl 5:S47–S51
74. Fragility Fracture Network (2020). http://fragilityfracturenetwork.org. Accessed 15 Feb 2020

Proximal Humeral Fractures: The Choice of Treatment

10

Stig Brorson and Henrik Palm

10.1 Aim of Treatment

The overall aim of shoulder fracture treatment is to reduce pain and regain the best possible function. Most patients do not regain previous shoulder function, some patients had an impaired shoulder function prior to the injury, and some patients suffer persistent pain, whether treated surgically or non-surgically.

Generally, pain-free function at shoulder level should be the goal of treatment, allowing daily activities. The achievable treatment result may vary widely and the aim of treatment should be part of the shared decision-making.

Most proximal humeral fractures eventually heal, and non-union is seen in only 1.1% of all fractures [1]. However, malunion is inevitable when displaced fractures are treated non-operatively in adults. This does not entail poor function or pain. Satisfactory patient-reported outcomes can often be obtained without restoring anatomy or replacing the joint with a prosthesis. Radiographic outcomes, range of motion and surgeon-administered outcome measures do not necessarily reflect the needs of the older patient suffering a shoulder fracture.

This chapter is a component of Part 2: Pillar I.
For an explanation of the grouping of chapters in this book, please see Chapter 1: 'The Multidisciplinary Approach to Fragility Fractures Around the World—An Overview'.

S. Brorson (✉)
Zealand University Hospital, Køge, Denmark

Department of Clinical Medicine, University of Copenhagen, Copenhagen, Denmark
e-mail: sbror@regionsjaelland.dk

H. Palm
Bispebjerg University Hospital, Copenhagen, Denmark

Department of Clinical Medicine, University of Copenhagen, Copenhagen, Denmark
e-mail: henrik.palm@regionh.dk

© The Author(s) 2021
P. Falaschi, D. Marsh (eds.), *Orthogeriatrics*, Practical Issues in Geriatrics,
https://doi.org/10.1007/978-3-030-48126-1_10

10.2   Evidence and Literature

The evidence base for the management of proximal humeral fractures has been weak until recently. The increasing amount of literature has so far mostly been unable to inform clinical practice, due to poor methodological quality with only about 3% randomised clinical trials [2]. Consequently, different approaches can be found nationally, regionally and even between care providers at the same institution.

Although the latest Cochrane review [3] reported that surgery was not superior to non-surgical management for most proximal humeral fractures, less than 5% of the scientific literature on proximal humeral fractures deals with non-surgical treatment, while more than 70% deals with surgical treatment modalities [2]. Also, increased surgical activity has been reported [4] and in some parts of the world locking plates remains the gold standard treatment in displaced fractures among the elderly [5]. In recent years, the reverse total shoulder arthroplasty has gained popularity, but strong evidence has still to support this practice.

In the following paragraphs, we outline recent evidence-based principles for the management of these difficult fractures.

10.3   Epidemiology

Proximal humeral fractures are common and account for 4 to 6% of all human fractures [6]. Among the non-vertebral fractures, they are third only to the wrist and hip fractures and, like these, are closely associated with osteoporosis. The lifetime risk is 13% for a woman aged more than 50 years and around half of the patients have sustained a previous fracture [7]. A three-fold increase in incidence has been reported between 1970 and 2002 [8] and the incidence in women aged more than 80 years is as high as 520/100,000 per year [9] but seems to have stabilised in recent years [10].

Previously, it was believed that most proximal humeral fractures were minimally displaced [11]. However, recent epidemiological studies have unequivocally reported that most fractures are displaced [6, 12, 13] and the complexity of the fractures seems to increase with advanced age [14].

10.4   Fracture Classification

Proximal humeral fractures have been classified since the earliest known medical texts [15]. From 1970 the most commonly used classification system for proximal humeral fractures has been the Neer classification [11] followed by the AO classification [16]. Both classification systems describe morphological aspects of the fracture anatomy in an ordinal framework aiming to support diagnostics, treatment and prognostics.

The Neer classification (Fig. 10.1) is based on the description of four anatomical segments of the proximal humerus, as they appear on plain

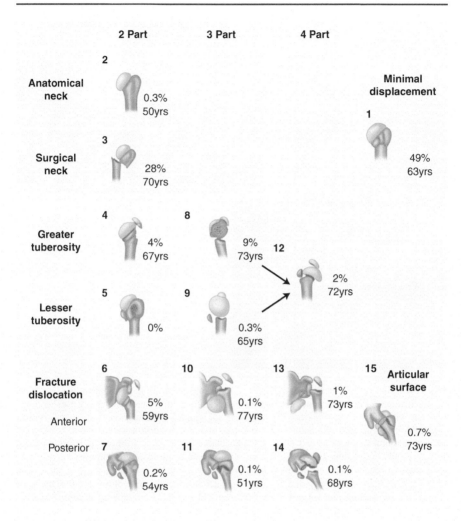

Fig. 10.1 Neer's classification with prevalence and the average age in each category. (Reproduced with permission from Acta Orthop)

anterior–posterior radiographs: (1) the humeral shaft, (2) the articular part of the humeral head, (3) the greater tuberosity and (4) the lesser tuberosity. If any of the four segments are displaced more than 1 cm or angulated more than 45°, the fracture is considered displaced, while all other fractures are categorised as minimally displaced fractures regardless of the number of fracture lines. According to the number of displaced segments, the fractures are termed 2-part, 3-part or 4-part.

This description is further qualified according to the involved segments, for example, 2-part surgical neck fracture (Fig. 10.2a), 3-part greater tuberosity fracture

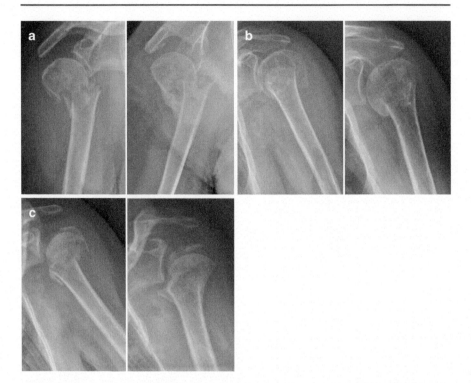

Fig. 10.2 Non-surgical healing of different types of proximal humeral fractures. (**a**) Displaced 2-part fracture of the 'surgical neck' treated non-surgically in an 81-year-old female nursing home resident suffering severe Parkinson's disease. Radiographs at admission (left image) and at 3 months (right image). The patient was pain-free and mobilised in a walker. Good healing but severe malunion was seen after 3 months. (**b**) Displaced 3-part greater tuberosity fracture treated non-surgically in a healthy 75-year old female. Radiographs at admission (left image) and 6 months (right image). The patient was independent living and pain-free. A slight decrease in strength in above shoulder activities was found but the patient achieved a full range of motion. (**c**) Displaced 4-part fracture treated non-surgically in a 66-year old female. Radiographs at admission (left image) and 4 months (right image). The patient was a pain-free function at shoulder level and self-reliant in all daily activities

(Fig. 10.2b) or 4-part fracture involving all segments (Fig. 10.2c). Eighty-six percent of all proximal humeral fractures are either minimally displaced (49%), 2-part surgical neck fractures (28%) or 3-part greater tuberosity fractures (9%) [6].

Additional information about fracture anatomy can be obtained by adding axillary radiographs, CT-scans or 3D-CT scans. Numerous observer studies have demonstrated poor agreement between and within observers using the Neer classification and the AO classification even on very basic observations of displacement and dislocation [17]. Thus, the value of the classification of proximal humeral fractures in clinical decision making and research remains a challenge. The different use of classifications might explain the discrepancies in results and recommendations. Moreover, it has been difficult to establish a translation between the two commonly used classification systems [18].

The integrity of the rotator cuff is rarely assessed in trauma imaging. With advanced age, the incidence of degenerative rotator cuff tears increases. The prognostic importance of concomitant rotator cuff lesions is not known.

10.4.1 Minimally Displaced Fractures

For clinical purposes, proximal humeral fractures are often simply divided into the two main groups explained earlier, the minimally displaced fractures and the displaced fractures.

There is consensus that minimally displaced fractures can be managed non-operatively with short immobilisation in a sling followed by early exercises. Strong evidence is sparse, but randomised trials so far have reported the best results following early mobilisation initiated after 1 week [19–22].

10.4.2 Displaced Fractures

The optimal treatment of displaced proximal humeral fractures has been a matter of controversy for decades. Recommendations have changed over time according to patients' and surgeons' preferences and influenced by the interests of implant providers.

It has proved difficult to demonstrate any beneficial effect of surgery in randomised trials. An increasing number of trials have reported no difference in functional outcome between surgical and non-surgical management and surgery seems to cause an increased risk of subsequent supplemental surgery. A Cochrane review included almost 2000 patients from randomised trials and could not find any benefits of surgery compared to non-surgical management [3]. The studies included displaced 2-part, 3-part and 4-part fractures. No evidence-based recommendations cover fracture-dislocations, articular fractures and isolated tuberosity fractures.

10.5   Treatment

Based on age, comorbidity, functional demand, fracture pattern, bone and soft tissue quality and patient preferences a shared treatment decision can be achieved. Based on the high-quality evidence available [3] non-surgical management should be the treatment of choice in minimally displaced fractures as well as in displaced 2-, 3 and 4-part fractures in older patients. Management of articular surface fractures, fracture-dislocations and isolated tuberosity fractures is not covered by high-quality evidence and these fractures may benefit from surgery (Fig. 10.3).

The use of locking plates in displaced 2-part fractures cannot be recommended, as current high-quality evidence suggests no benefits compared to non-surgical management [23]. Head-preserving osteosynthesis with locking plates in complex fracture patterns and poor bone quality has been accompanied by high complication and reoperation rates [24, 25] and cannot be recommended.

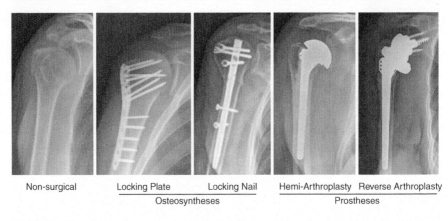

Non-surgical   Locking Plate   Locking Nail   Hemi-Arthroplasty   Reverse Arthroplasty
                       Osteosyntheses   Prostheses

Fig. 10.3 The main treatment groups for proximal humeral fractures

If humeral head replacement with the use of a prosthesis is needed, a reverse total shoulder arthroplasty seems to lead to a better functional outcome than hemiarthroplasty [26]. The superiority of reverse shoulder arthroplasty compared to nonsurgical management has still to be demonstrated in high-quality studies, but results from the first randomised trial indicate that benefits are minimal in 3-, and 4-part fractures if patients are aged more than 80 years [27].

10.5.1 Non-surgical Treatment

Based on the available high-quality evidence [3] and the prevalence of fracture categories reported [6] more than 85% of all proximal humeral fractures can be managed without surgery. As previously mentioned, less than 5% of the scientific literature on proximal humeral fractures deals with non-surgical management [2] and more such studies are warranted, including a focus on pain relief, bandaging methods and systematic training programs.

Several randomised trials have however compared early and late mobilisation in non-surgical cases and reported less pain and better function when initiating training within the first week [20–22]. Early mobilisation can be recommended in most patients except in unstable 3- and 4- part fractures and in tuberosity fractures. In such cases, secondary displacement should be ruled out by outpatient visits, radiographs and controlled loading. The clinical effects of supervised training, home training or no structured training in older patients with proximal humeral fractures have been sparsely studied. Studies on time for the relief of pain are warranted, but our opinion is that most patients experience pain relief after 2 to 3 weeks. Progress in function and pain relief can be expected by 3 to 6 months after surgery.

10.5.2 Surgical Management

Randomised trials and meta-analyses focusing on displaced 2-, 3- and 4-part fractures have been unable to demonstrate superiority of surgery compared to nonsurgical management [3]. There might however be a place for evidence-based surgery in older patients with fracture-dislocations, articular surface fractures and fractures with no contact between the bony fragments.

If surgical management is decided, osteosynthesis with a *locking plate*, or *intramedullary nail* can be an option if the humeral head can be preserved and tuberosity fixation is possible. If head-preserving surgery is not possible a joint prosthesis can be considered. Since the 1950s replacement of the humeral head with a *shoulder hemiarthroplasty* has been preferred, but within the last 20 years, the *reverse total shoulder arthroplasty* has gained increasing popularity as the outcome is less dependent on tuberosity fixation.

10.6   Complications

It is well known that complications can follow surgery. However, complications after non-surgical management are not systematically reported in the scientific literature. Most terms and definitions concern radiographic appearance of the fracture and their relation to functional outcome and patient satisfaction is poorly understood. Consensus-based and validated complication terms are needed [28]. Reported complications include shoulder stiffness, nonunion, malunion, avascular necrosis of the humeral head and persistent pain. Also, the implant itself can be mal-positioned primarily, or subsequently as a result of fracture collapse and/or avascular necrosis of the humeral head.

In cases of failed non-surgical management, as well as in failed osteosynthesis (Fig. 10.4), a reverse total shoulder arthroplasty represents a salvage option. Observational studies thereof have reported good pain relief and reasonable function regardless of tuberosity status.

10.7   Outcome Assessment

Large registry-based studies have reported low revision rates (about 4%) after shoulder arthroplasty for fractures [29]. However, the patient-reported outcome has been less promising, suggesting a possible discrepancy between implant survival and patient satisfaction, as well as between the surgeons' and the patients' perspective on outcome [30].

Most clinical studies report patient outcomes using observer-administered instruments like the Constant-Murley score [31]. These scoring systems are surgeon-derived and tend to emphasise 'objective' measures like the range of motion and strength. It is our impression that patients' focus is more directed towards ADL (independent living) and social and emotional aspects of life (holding

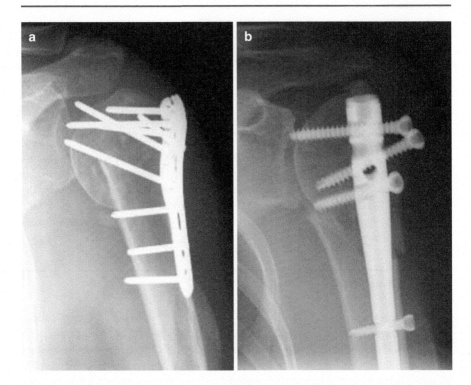

Fig. 10.4 Proximal humeral fracture complications subsequent to osteosynthesis. (**a**) Complications in a displaced 3-part greater tuberosity fracture managed with a locking plate. The humeral head has collapsed due to avascular necrosis. The screws are locked in the plate and subsequently penetrate the glenohumeral joint causing cartilage erosion and pain. (**b**) Complications in a displaced 2-part proximal humeral fracture fixated with a humeral locking nail. The fracture is mal-reduced and a locking screw is protruding into the glenohumeral joint

grandchildren, having dinner with family and friends, caring for disabled relatives). By focusing on 'objective' matters and radiographic appearance of fracture healing healthcare providers may fail to support important preferences of the patients.

Development of patient-related shoulder specific outcome assessment instruments (e.g. OSS, WOOS, ASES) and the use of generic quality of life measures (e.g. EQ-5D, SF-36) for patient evaluation have added to our knowledge of patient preferences. However, the shared decision making on treatment modalities and functional goals for the individual patient remains essential for healthcare providers.

10.8   Conclusions

There are many important aspects when treating an older patient with a proximal humeral fracture (Table 10.1).

Evidence-based management of proximal humeral fractures in the elderly should be based on high-quality clinical studies, as well as well-conducted systematic

Table 10.1   Important points when treating elderly patients with a proximal humeral fracture

Non-surgical management should always be considered, as randomised trials have been unable
to demonstrate benefits from surgery

Immediate surgical treatment is indicated only in patients with fracture-dislocations, articular
fractures (7% of all fractures) and in cases with neurovascular injury

Primary reverse total shoulder prosthesis seems superior to shoulder hemiarthroplasty in such
cases

Shared decision making should include information on patient preferences, comorbidity,
functional level, age and bone quality

A limited goal strategy should be agreed upon regardless of treatment choice. A pain-free and
functional shoulder is a satisfactory outcome for most elderly patients

The radiographic outcome after displaced fractures managed non-surgically correlates poorly to
functional outcome and patient satisfaction

Regaining social and emotional aspects of life is more important than radiographic appearance,
range of motion and strength

Passive exercises should begin within the first week after injury

The evidence base for rehabilitation and different training regimens is poor

Proximal humeral fractures are among the typical osteoporotic fractures and elderly patients
should be examined for osteoporosis

reviews and meta-analyses. Long term follow-up data on benefits and harms should
be provided by national and international registries. The implementation of
evidence-based recommendations should be facilitated by national, regional and
local guidelines and validated algorithms based on the best available evidence.
Resource allocation for patient care and research should be guided by the best evidence and the need for additional knowledge.

Patient preferences should be included at all levels of decision making from the
design of research protocols to the development of patient-derived outcome measures. Not least, the treatment strategy for the individual older patient in the everyday clinic should be decided with the patient and relatives, and based on patient
preferences, comorbidity, functional level, age and bone quality.

References

1. Court-Brown CM, McQueen MM (2008) Nonunions of the proximal humerus: their prevalence and functional outcome. J Trauma 64(6):1517–1521
2. Slobogean GP, Johal H, Lefaivre KA, MacIntyre NJ, Sprague S, Scott T, Guy P, Cripton PA,
   McKee M, Bhandari M (2015) A scoping review of the proximal humerus fracture literature.
   BMC Musculoskelet Disord 16:112
3. Handoll HH, Brorson S (2015) Interventions for treating proximal humeral fractures in adults.
   Cochrane Database Syst Rev (11):CD000434
4. Khatib O, Onyekwelu I, Zuckerman JD (2014) The incidence of proximal humeral fractures
   in New York State from 1990 through 2010 with an emphasis on operative management in
   patients aged 65 years or older. J Shoulder Elb Surg 23(9):1356–1362
5. Klug A, Gramlich Y, Wincheringer D, Schmidt-Horlohé K, Hoffmann R (2019) Trends in surgical management of proximal humeral fractures in adults: a nationwide study of records in
   Germany from 2007 to 2016. Arch Orthop Trauma Surg 139(12):1713–1721

6. Court-Brown CM, Garg A, McQueen MM (2001) The epidemiology of proximal humeral fractures. Acta Orthop Scand 72(4):365–371
7. Johnell O, Kanis J (2005) Epidemiology of osteoporotic fractures. Osteoporos Int 16(Suppl 2):S3–S7
8. Palvanen M, Kannus P, Niemi S, Parkkari J (2006) Update in the epidemiology of proximal humeral fractures. Clin Orthop Relat Res 442:87–92
9. Court-Brown CM, Clement ND, Duckworth AD, Aitken S, Biant LC, McQueen MM (2014) The spectrum of fractures in the elderly. Bone Joint J 96-B(3):366–372
10. Kannus P, Niemi S, Sievänen H, Parkkari J (2017) Stabilized incidence in proximal humeral fractures of elderly women: nationwide statistics from Finland in 1970–2015. J Gerontol A Biol Sci Med Sci 72(10):1390–1393
11. Neer CS 2nd (1970) Displaced proximal humeral fractures. I. Classification and evaluation. J Bone Joint Surg Am 52(6):1077–1089
12. Roux A, Decroocq L, El Batti S, Bonnevialle N, Moineau G, Trojani C, Boileau P, de Peretti F (2012) Epidemiology of proximal humerus fractures managed in a trauma center. Orthop Traumatol Surg Res 98(6):715–719
13. Tamai K, Ishige N, Kuroda S, Ohno W, Itoh H, Hashiguchi H, Iizawa N, Mikasa M (2009) Four-segment classification of proximal humeral fractures revisited: a multicenter study on 509 cases. J Shoulder Elb Surg 18(6):845–850
14. Bahrs C, Stojicevic T, Blumenstock G, Brorson S, Badke A, Stöckle U, Rolauffs B, Freude T (2014) Trends in epidemiology and patho-anatomical pattern of proximal humeral fractures. Int Orthop 38(8):1697–1704
15. Brorson S (2013) Fractures of the proximal humerus. Acta Orthop Suppl 84(351):1–32
16. Marsh JL, Slongo TF, Agel J, Broderick JS, Creevey W, DeCoster TA, Prokuski L, Sirkin MS, Ziran B, Henley B, Audigé L (2007) Fracture and dislocation classification compendium - 2007: Orthopaedic Trauma Association classification, database and outcomes committee. J Orthop Trauma 21(10 Suppl):S1–S133
17. Brorson S, Hróbjartsson A (2008) Training improves agreement among doctors using the Neer system for proximal humeral fractures in a systematic review. J Clin Epidemiol 61(1):7–16
18. Brorson S, Eckardt H, Audigé L, Rolauffs B, Bahrs C (2013) Translation between the Neer- and the AO/OTA-classification for proximal humeral fractures: do we need to be bilingual to interpret the scientific literature? BMC Res Notes 6:69
19. Carbone S, Razzano C, Albino P, Mezzoprete R (2017) Immediate intensive mobilization compared with immediate conventional mobilization for the impacted osteoporotic conservatively treated proximal humeral fracture: a randomized controlled trial. Musculoskelet Surg 101(Suppl 2):137–143
20. Hodgson SA, Mawson SJ, Saxton JM, Stanley D (2007) Rehabilitation of two-part fractures of the neck of the humerus (two-year follow-up). J Shoulder Elb Surg 16(2):143–145
21. Kristiansen B, Angermann P, Larsen TK (1989) Functional results following fractures of the proximal humerus. A controlled clinical study comparing two periods of immobilization. Arch Orthop Trauma Surg 108(6):339–341
22. Lefevre-Colau MM, Babinet A, Fayad F, Fermanian J, Anract P, Roren A, Kansao J, Revel M, Poiraudeau S (2007) Immediate mobilization compared with conventional immobilization for the impacted nonoperatively treated proximal humeral fracture. A randomized controlled trial. J Bone Joint Surg Am 89(12):2582–2590
23. Launonen AP, Sumrein BO, Reito A, Lepola V, Paloneva J, Jonsson KB, Wolf O, Ström P, Berg HE, Felländer-Tsai L, Jansson KÅ, Fell D, Mechlenburg I, Døssing K, Østergaard H, Märtson A, Laitinen MK, Mattila VM, as the NITEP group (2019) Operative versus non-operative treatment for 2-part proximal humerus fracture: a multicenter randomized controlled trial. PLoS Med 16(7):e1002855
24. Brorson S, Rasmussen JV, Frich LH, Olsen BS, Hróbjartsson A (2012) Benefits and harms of locking plate osteosynthesis in intraarticular (OTA Type C) fractures of the proximal humerus: a systematic review. Injury 43(7):999–1005

25. Brorson S, Frich LH, Winther A, Hróbjartsson A (2011) Locking plate osteosynthesis in displaced 4-part fractures of the proximal humerus. Acta Orthop 82(4):475–481
26. Sebastia-Forcada E, Lizaur-Utrilla A, Cebrian-Gomez R, Miralles-Muñoz FA, Lopez-Prats FA (2017) Outcomes of reverse total shoulder arthroplasty for proximal humeral fractures: primary arthroplasty versus secondary arthroplasty after failed proximal humeral locking plate fixation. J Orthop Trauma 31(8):e236–e240
27. Lopiz Y, Alcobía-Díaz B, Galán-Olleros M, García-Fernández C, Picado AL, Marco F (2019) Reverse shoulder arthroplasty versus nonoperative treatment for 3- or 4-part proximal humeral fractures in elderly patients: a prospective randomized controlled trial. J Shoulder Elb Surg 28(12):2259–2271
28. Brorson S, Alispahic N, Bahrs C, Joeris A, Steinitz A, Audigé L (2019) Complications after non-surgical management of proximal humeral fractures: a systematic review of terms and definitions. BMC Musculoskelet Disord 20(1):91
29. Brorson S, Salomonsson B, Jensen SL, Fenstad AM, Demir Y, Rasmussen JV (2017) Revision after shoulder replacement for acute fracture of the proximal humerus. Acta Orthop 88(4):446–450
30. Amundsen A, Rasmussen JV, Olsen BS, Brorson S (2019) Low revision rate despite poor functional outcome after stemmed hemiarthroplasty for acute proximal humeral fractures: 2,750 cases reported to the Danish Shoulder Arthroplasty Registry. Acta Orthop 90(3):196–201
31. Constant CR, Murley AH (1987) A clinical method of functional assessment of the shoulder. Clin Orthop Relat Res 214:160–164

Post-operative Management

11

Giulio Pioli, Chiara Bendini, and Paolo Pignedoli

Older patients with hip fractures are a heterogeneous population [1]. Only 15% are fully independent and with a low level of comorbidity prior to fracture occurrence, while the broad majority presents multiple comorbidities and some frailty-related characteristics. Despite advances in surgical and anaesthetic techniques over time, the risk of complications after hip fracture surgery remains high. The main goal of the post-operative management is to prevent or promptly detect complications in order to reduce morbidity and mortality. A second goal is to mobilise patients as soon as practical in order to avoid the risks of immobilisation and to foster the recovery of pre-fracture walking ability.

11.1 Multidisciplinary Management

The high clinical and functional complexity of hip fracture older patients requires a multidisciplinary approach. Orthogeriatric co-management currently is the standard of care, having been shown to diminish in-hospital stay, time to surgery, in-hospital complications and in-hospital mortality, compared to traditional care [1–5]. Following this model, the orthopaedic surgeon and the orthogeriatrician (a geriatrician skilled in the management of older adults with orthopaedic issues) share

---

This chapter is a component of Part 2: Pillar I.
For an explanation of the grouping of chapters in this book, please see Chapter 1: 'The multidisciplinary approach to fragility fractures around the world—an overview'.

G. Pioli (✉) · C. Bendini
Geriatric Unit, Arcispedale Santa Maria Nuova-IRCCS, Reggio Emilia, Italy
e-mail: giulio.pioli@ausl.re.it; chiara.bendini@ausl.re.it

P. Pignedoli
Orthopaedic Unit, Arcispedale Santa Maria Nuova-IRCCS, Reggio Emilia, Italy
e-mail: paolo.pignedoli@ausl.re.it

© The Author(s) 2021   155
P. Falaschi, D. Marsh (eds.), *Orthogeriatrics*, Practical Issues in Geriatrics,
https://doi.org/10.1007/978-3-030-48126-1_11

responsibility and leadership from admission to discharge. The traditional roles are maintained, with the orthopaedic surgeon assessing the trauma and managing the fracture, and the geriatrician responsible for medical issues and coordinating discharge. Several other healthcare professionals (anaesthesiologist, therapists, specialist nurses, nutritionist and social worker) may be included in the interdisciplinary team during the pathway of care.

In the post-operative period, most needs of older patients with hip fractures are related to medical or geriatric issues; therefore the geriatric team usually contributes to joint preoperative patient assessment, and increasingly takes the lead in postoperative medical care. The orthopaedic surgeon is involved in any issue regarding the surgical site. On the basis of local organisational features, different orthogeriatric models may be implemented, although a dedicated orthogeriatric ward seems to have more consistent results in reducing mortality, compared to other models of orthopaedic/geriatric collaboration [4]. In any case, whatever type of ward the patient is admitted to, it is important that a coordinated multidisciplinary approach ensures continuity of care and responsibility across the clinical pathway from admission to discharge. Former experience, characterised by the use of a geriatric consulting team without continual responsibility for care, demonstrated only small benefits compared to traditional care, and that approach should now be considered outdated [5].

Essential quality standards related to the organisation of orthogeriatric collaboration include senior experience of the members of the team, clinical and service governance responsibility for all stages of the pathway of care, established procedures for communication between different specialists including briefings and meetings, development of shared protocols for the main features of the perioperative phase, continued multidisciplinary reviews, integration with a centre for bone health for secondary prevention and liaison with primary care and social services [6, 7].

11.2   Predicting the Risk of Post-operative Complications

As described in Chap. 7, a key goal of pre-operative orthogeriatric co-management is to identify, and where possible prevent, conditions that predispose to postoperative complications. Several studies have focused on identifying patients at risk after hip fracture surgery [8]. The risk of 30-day mortality has been also explored using scoring systems, some of them very simple, such as the Nottingham Hip Fracture Score [9], which includes relatively few variables.

Specific predictors related to patient risk are not fully consistent, mainly because of a different selection of potential factors across studies. Indeed, patients with the highest pre-fracture comorbidity and disability are those at greater risk of developing clinical complications postoperatively. From an operational point of view, most of the individual preoperative parameters are non-modifiable risk factors. They are useful for identifying patients that require high attention and intensive care. The American College of Surgeons together with the American Geriatrics Society recommends the preoperative evaluation of the older patient for frailty syndrome [10]. This has been defined as a syndrome with multiple reduced physiologic functions that increases an individual's vulnerability for developing increased dependency and/or death. Evidence suggests that frailty, measured with different instruments including those based on Comprehensive Geriatric Assessment, predicts post-operative mortality, complications and prolonged length of stay [11]. Among the hip fracture population, about one-third of patients have significant frailty with a high risk of poor outcomes, one-third with no markers of frailty, and about one-third with an intermediate condition [12].

In clinical practice, a very high risk of complications and short-term mortality is observed in very sick patients with severe organ failure, such as a person with a history of ascites, or end-stage chronic kidney disease on dialysis or dyspnoea at rest [13]. A substantial increase in mortality occurs mainly in severe conditions [14]. Similarly, patients suffering from congestive heart failure or chronic obstructive pulmonary disease are at higher risk of poor outcomes depending on the severity of the underlying disease. Finally, a history of disseminated cancer and full functional dependency increases three to four times the likelihood of death within 30 days [13].

Malnutrition and sarcopenia are other conditions that can increase the occurrence of post-operative complications, but they mainly affect the likelihood of achieving a complete functional recovery. On the other hand, obesity is also associated with negative outcomes. A simple parameter as the BMI shows a U-shaped relationship with respect to the risk of post-operative complications [15], with the highest rates occurring in low-weight (BMI < 20) and morbidly obese (BMI > 40) patients. In particular, the risk of deep surgical site infection increases linearly with increasing BMI.

Among routine admission laboratory testing, several parameters have been found related to negative outcomes including low haemoglobin level, high creatinine value, electrolyte derangements or high Brain Natriuretic Peptide, all of which may be considered an expression of an underlying disease. Probably the most studied laboratory predictor of post-operative outcome is albumin level. There is consistent evidence that albumin lower than 3.5 g/dL is associated with two to three times risk of post-operative complications and mortality [16]. Albumin has commonly been studied as a dichotomous variable, but some data suggest an increasing risk with decreasing values. Serum albumin level is a well-established serum marker of nutritional status, but it is a better predictor of post-operative outcomes than other nutritional indicators, including nutritional assessment [16]. In fact, albumin may have a wider implication, since it is also a negative acute-phase protein, and hypoalbuminemia might represent an increased inflammatory status of the patient—also potentially leading to poor outcomes [17].

Beyond patient-related risk factors, several potentially modifiable process factors may affect the rate of post-operative complications. The most consistently demonstrated across the various studies have been timing of surgery and multidisciplinary management, while inconsistent effects have been found for anaesthetic type and transfusion strategy [8]. A study based on the National Danish Database, analysing post-operative process performance measures, found that mobilisation of patients within 24 h postoperatively was the process with the strongest association with lower 30-day mortality, readmission risk and shorter length of stay [18].

11.3 Early Mobilisation

One of the quality standards developed by NICE for improvement of hip fracture management states that adults with a hip fracture should start mobilisation, at least once a day, no later than the day after surgery [6]. That means assisting patients to quickly re-establish the ability to move between postures, to maintain an upright posture and to ambulate with increasing levels of complexity. Shortening the time of bed rest after hip fracture surgery contributes to a reduction of the length of hospital stay and complications such as thrombosis, pneumonia, respiratory failure, delirium and pressure sores. Early mobilisation impacts especially on the long-term functional status and improves the likelihood of achieving full ambulation recovery [19]. Analyses of data from large databases confirm that patients mobilised on the day of, or the day following surgery have better mobility function 30 days after discharge [20].

Mobilisation involves an early physiotherapist assessment. However, support with mobilisation can be given either by the physiotherapist or by the nursing team, when the physiotherapist is not present [20]. The NICE quality standard recommends that local arrangements (teams) should monitor the accomplishment of early mobilisation by calculating the proportion of hip fracture operations in which the person starts mobilisation within 24 h from surgery [6]. A useful and widespread tool for monitoring basic mobility during acute hospitalisation is the Cumulated Ambulation Score (CAS) that assesses the ability to get in and out of bed, rise from a chair and walk around indoors with a walking aid during the first three post-operative days [21]. With suitable rehabilitation programmes addressing critical issues in the post-operative phase, almost 80% of patients who were able to walk before fracture achieve the ability to walk with aid within the first two post-operative days [22].

Pre-injury functional status and baseline characteristics of patients may clearly affect inpatient rehabilitation as well as final outcomes. Subjects walking with assistive devices before fracture may need more time to be able to transfer postoperatively. Delayed time to mobilisation may be also due to system factors, such as fewer physiotherapists available during the weekends, which may explain why patients undergoing surgery on Friday have a higher risk of delayed mobilisation [22]. Also, surgery performed after 24 h from arrival has been reported to delay the recovery of post-operative ambulatory function, although this finding is not consistent across studies [23, 24].

An essential condition to achieve the goal of early mobilisation is a stable surgical repair, allowing the patient to bear weight as tolerated. When deciding about weight-bearing after surgery, orthopaedic surgeons should take into account that any restriction has the potential to affect recovery and that unrestricted allowance of immediate full weight-bearing should be the standard protocol for the aftercare following fracture fixation in geriatric patients with hip fracture. In addition, it has been proven that older patients treated for hip fractures are not able to adequately follow any weight-bearing restrictions [25], so the patients should be either weight-bearing as tolerated or non-weight-bearing if there is real concern about fixation stability.

In a recent observational study, the most frequent reasons for not completing planned physiotherapy, and not regaining basic mobility independence during the first three post-operative days, were poorly controlled pain and fatigue [26]. The latter is one of the most common limiting symptoms and may occur for multiple reasons such as incomplete volume adequacy, low haemoglobin level or the overall impact of surgery on a patient with frailty. To support early mobilisation, clinicians have to face two main issues: adequate pain control and prevention of post-operative hypotension. Coordinated care pathways addressing both clinical and system issues with the goal to improve functional outcomes after hip fracture surgery should be developed and implemented.

11.4 Pain Management

Standard protocols to manage hip fracture-related pain are currently based on multimodal analgesia that includes a panel of drugs such as IV acetaminophen, pregabalin, oxycodone and—very cautiously—nonsteroidal anti-inflammatory drugs, along with nerve block methods (e.g. femoral nerve or lumbar plexus block or continuous epidural block). Multimodal analgesia offers the advantage of reducing opiate consumption, which has been associated in older patients with nausea, vomiting, sedation, delirium and respiratory depression, particularly in debilitated patients or those with compromised respiratory function [27]. Appropriate parenteral analgesia should start in the Emergency Department and the presence of pain should be regularly checked throughout the peri-operative period in order to ensure that the patient is feeling comfortable. The fascia iliaca compartment block is now quite common, as supplementary pain management in the preoperative phase and seems to have a greater analgesic effect than opioids during movement [28].

Postoperatively, pain is generally higher in patients with trochanteric fractures treated with intramedullary nail than in those with femoral neck fractures who underwent total or partial hip replacements. Nevertheless, patients should continue most of the medications that they received preoperatively. Particularly useful is continuous peripheral nerve block analgesia, through a catheter placed pre- or intra-operatively, connected to a small portable pump, and maintained for some days after surgery. These procedures may offer advantages in early mobilisation since they are more effective than systemic drugs in making the patient feel comfortable enough to ambulate and fully participate in their rehabilitation therapy [27].

11.5 Post-operative Hypotension and Fluid Management

A significant drop in blood pressure can occur early in the post-operative phase, with a further drop when the patient is taking part in rehabilitation, during weight-bearing and in the standing position. In some cases, this may produce symptomatic hypotension, reducing participation in rehabilitation. Several factors may contribute to post-operative hypotension in older adults; these include:

- The effect of ageing, decreasing the ability to compensate and maintain pressure homeostasis when the body is stressed.
- Anaemia due to acute blood loss.
- Dehydration secondary to poor oral intake of fluids.
- The effects of anaesthetic agents.
- The side effects of drugs frequently used in the post-operative phase (e.g. opiates and antiemetics).

Strategies for preventing post-operative hypotension include medication adjustment and fluid management. All antihypertensive drugs should be checked and stopped, starting from the preoperative phase, with the exception of beta-blockers and those with rebound effects like clonidine. Beta-blocker use should be continued during the perioperative phase, while it is no longer recommended for use in naïve patients, as was suggested by earlier studies. Preoperative introduction of beta-blockers can reduce myocardial complications, but may increase the rate of stroke and mortality, possibly due to hypotension [29]. The preoperative pharmaceutical review may also contribute to preventing the intra-operative blood pressure fall that has been found to increase the risk of death within 5 days after surgery [30]. Antihypertensive drugs discontinued before surgical intervention should be resumed in the post-operative period on the basis of the clinical condition and blood pressure values. In some cases, it can be advisable to resume these pharmacological agents only after discharge.

Providing adequate fluid therapy is one of the most important and challenging issues of the management of hip fractures in elderly patients. Fluid administration of 1000 mL is commonly initiated on arrival to compensate for blood loss and maintain basic requirements. During surgery, the anaesthetist usually administers intravenous fluids, on the basis of clinical judgement and according to clinical signs. In the post-operative phase, the administration of about 1.5–2 L of crystalloid is usual practice to attain and maintain intravascular volume [31]. The aim is clearly to optimise cardiac output avoiding cardiovascular overload. In general, this practice is also safe in patients with acknowledged ventricular dysfunction, since the risk of dehydration and hypotension probably exceeds the risks of excessive volume administration. The only exceptions are:

- Patients with severe kidney failure or on dialysis, who require a cautious and controlled fluid administration with control and measurement of fluid balance.
- Patients with severe heart failure or previous episodes of acute pulmonary oedema.

Nevertheless, fluid management should be tailored. In clinical practice, the effect of a standardised fluid protocol should be weighed up by simple available clinical measures such as tissue turgor, heart rate, blood pressure and urine output, in order to decide whether less or extra fluid will provide benefits for the patient. Bedside ultrasound may add further information by measuring inferior vena cava diameter and its collapsibility during one respiratory cycle, while more sensitive methods to assess fluid responsiveness using advanced haemodynamic monitoring techniques to detect cardiovascular changes are not routinely used.

11.6 Management of Postsurgical Anaemia

Anaemia has traditionally been attributed to surgical or post-surgical bleeding, but around 40% of patients with hip fracture have haemoglobin levels below population norms on admission, and values further drop before surgery with an average fall of 0.9 g/dL after 1 day, greater in extracapsular than intracapsular fractures [32]. The maximum post-operative fall is often around 2–3 g/dL and usually occurs 3 days postoperatively.

Current guidelines, based on randomised controlled trials [33], recommend a restrictive transfusion strategy with a safe trigger threshold not greater than 8 g/dL of haemoglobin; as a result, the proportion of patients receiving packed blood cell transfusion has decreased over time. Furthermore, it has been suggested that blood transfusions may be harmful to patients, by reducing the recipient's immune response and thereby increasing the susceptibility to infections [34]. However, blood transfusion should not be dictated by a haemoglobin trigger alone but should be based on an assessment of the patient's clinical status. In particular, the presence of coronary artery diseases or specific signs of haemodynamic instability could suggest a need to transfuse, despite a haemoglobin value greater than 8 g/dL. Some data also suggest that patients with significant frailty, such as nursing home residents, may have some benefit by a more liberal transfusion strategy [35]. On the other hand, in fit and independent patients an even more restrictive transfusion threshold of less than 7 g/dL of haemoglobin might not impair perioperative outcomes [36].

Post-operative anaemia in older subjects is not only related to blood loss during the surgical procedure but also to several other factors which include the effects of intravenous rehydration, inflammation-induced blunted erythropoiesis, pre-existing nutrient deficiency or poor post-operative nutrition that prevents the replenishment of iron stores. The administration of intravenous iron could reduce the need for transfusion but the effect on haemoglobin level in the at-risk days after surgery is small. Benefits have also been seen in post-operative infection and even mortality [37]. Intravenous iron should preferentially be used in post-operative anaemia management, whereas oral iron is of little value because of its even later effect and poor efficacy in functional iron deficiency when iron stores are normal and intestinal absorption suppressed. In some studies, subcutaneous erythropoietin has been administered along with intravenous iron but even, in this case, the effect is too slow to affect significantly the need for transfusion.

Pharmacological reduction of blood loss with tranexamic acid, which is widely implemented in elective orthopaedic surgery and major trauma, is becoming increasingly popular for use in hip fractures too. Some early concerns on the safety in patients with frailty at high risk of thrombotic events seem not to be confirmed by meta-analysis [38]. Either topical or systemic tranexamic acid, or the combined administration of both, have been used in older patients with hip fracture.

11.7 Nutritional Supplementation

Routine nutritional assessment is the standard procedure to draw attention to patients already malnourished on admission. In addition, a huge number of patients may undergo deterioration of their nutritional status during the hospital stay, due to increased energy expenditure related to metabolic stress, and reduced food intake related to lack of appetite, nausea and psychological factors. It has been estimated that in the post-operative days, a quarter of patients ingest less than 25% of meals offered by the hospital, and about half of patients consume between 25 and 50% of meals [39]. The current European and American guidelines recommend at least 1 g protein per kilogram bodyweight per day and around 30 calories per kilogram bodyweight of energy for the majority of sick older patients to maintain nutritional status. In a recent survey on a cohort of geriatric orthopaedic patients, half of them with hip fractures, only 1.5% were able to achieve the energy need and only 21% the resting energy expenditure estimated at 20 calories per kg bodyweight per day [40]. Low dietary intake exposes patients to the risk of infections, pulmonary complications, pressure ulcers and impaired mobility resulting from muscle wasting and reduced muscle power.

Albeit based on low-quality studies, there is evidence that oral supplementation results in fewer complications and also affects mortality [41]. Protein supplementation started before or after surgery, in the form of a commercial protein powder or beverage package is a safe and relatively low-cost means to improve results and promote early rehabilitation. More aggressive nutritional interventions, such as a tube or parenteral feeding, should be reserved for patients with a low level of consciousness, or to malnourished patients unable to eat.

Another part of the nutritional approach is the reduction of preoperative fasting time, in order to improve the comfort of patients and to attenuate the neuroendocrine stress response. Current guidelines have cut the hours of fasting to 6 h for solids and 2 h for clear liquids. An oral carbohydrate preloading beverage is also recommended 3 h prior to surgery to allow the patient to be in a metabolically fed state, which has beneficial effects on reducing insulin resistance and catabolism.

Inconsistent results have been found on the effect of vitamin D supplementation in the perioperative phase. However, vitamin D deficiency is largely prevalent in hip fracture subject and it has been associated with poor functional recovery in frail subjects [42]. The administration of 1000–2000 U per day is, in any case, part of the pharmacological interventions for osteoporosis that should be started before discharge.

To sum up, the nutritional approach includes:

- The reduction of preoperative fasting time to 6 h for solids and 2 h for clear liquids
- Offering an oral carbohydrate preloading beverage 3 h prior to surgery to allow the patient to be in a metabolically fed state

- Implementing a protocol for pharmacologic management of post-operative nausea and vomiting
- Nutrition training for health care staff in order to improve the quality and quantity of feeding assistance
- Involvement of relatives (and volunteers) to help with mealtime assistance
- Providing multiple small meals and snacks throughout the day
- Protein supplementation before or after surgery, in the form of commercial protein powder or beverage package

11.8 Post-operative Medical Complications

Medical complications after hip fracture repair are very common and may significantly influence even long-term outcomes, by increasing length of stay and delaying functional recovery. Major complications affect about 20% of patients with hip fracture but up to 50% of patients may require pharmacological interventions due to clinical issues arising during the first post-operative days. Mortality at 30 days, rather than in-hospital mortality, has been recognised as an important care quality indicator and is used by healthcare systems of several countries in Europe. The data from large national databases show that mortality within 30 days is approximately 6.9–8.2% [43–45]. The most common causes of death are respiratory or cardiac failure and infections, mainly pneumonia or sepsis from other sources [46]. Since pre-existing organ dysfunctions are known risk factors, patients with a history of cardiac or lung diseases should be strictly monitored during the post-operative period, with attention particularly focused on signs and symptoms of organ deterioration or infections. Most of the severe adverse events occur early in the post-operative days. Myocardial infarction, stroke, pneumonia and pulmonary embolism are commonly diagnosed within a week from the surgery, while surgical-site infection and deep vein thrombosis are often diagnosed later [47].

Only a few complications are probably really preventable, but some modifiable features of management may significantly improve outcomes:

- Avoiding surgical delay. Delay to surgery is an established risk factor for mortality and post-operative complications such as pneumonia and pressure ulcers [48]. Patients with significant frailty have likely the greatest advantages in reducing the time of immobilisation and in receiving an intensive approach [49].
- Implementing a standardised approach. In the post-operative phase, several issues should be regularly checked, and all patients should undergo standardised procedures. The best way to face the complex needs of older adults with hip fracture, to improve the quality of the interventions, to minimise errors and omissions, and to reduce post-operative complications is to:
  - Define check-lists individualised for each healthcare professional that should guide healthcare decisions.
  - Standardise and implement specific protocols for the most common issues.

Tailored and individualised interventions based on patients' characteristics, specific needs or clinical instability should be an integral part of daily healthcare, but the overall post-operative management should be as highly standardised as possible. A general principle for each feature of the care should be an intensive approach for a limited time after surgery, followed by recovering of usual function as soon as possible, including removing tubes and catheters and shifting toward oral therapies. In this context, protocols, based on the best available evidence, must be developed, shared, and implemented by the multidisciplinary team, taking into account local resources. A minimum set of standardised protocols that should be implemented in the orthogeriatric setting include the following:

- Prophylaxis of venous thromboembolism
- Antibiotic prophylaxis
- Urinary catheter utilisation
- Pain control
- Skincare and pressure-relieving mattresses
- Constipation and stool impaction prevention
- Delirium prevention
- Post-operative haemoglobin monitoring and management of anaemia
- Malnutrition detection and correction/nutritional support
- Monitoring of vital physiological parameters
- Supplemental oxygen as appropriate
- Early mobilisation

11.9 Prevention and Management of Specific Complications

11.9.1 Delirium

Delirium is a common complication that affects about one-third of older patients with hip fracture in the perioperative period. It has a detrimental effect on functional and clinical outcomes, producing longer length of hospitalisation and slow and incomplete recovery. All the known subtypes may occur after hip fracture. In about two-third of the patients, delirium arises without agitation, as hypoactive or normal psychomotor variants, and therefore is often underdiagnosed [50]. Common symptoms of the hypoactive subtype are decreased levels of activity, speech and alertness as well as apathy, withdrawal and hypersomnolence. In contrast, the hyperactive or mixed variants are characterised by hyperactivity, loudness, and psychomotor agitation, interfering with patients' care and safety and can easily be diagnosed. To avoid missed presentation of delirium all patients must be screened daily and assessed using standardised tools. Both geriatric nurses and physicians should be involved in the early detection of delirium.

11.9.1.1   Prevention of Post-operative Delirium

Patients at risk of developing incident post-operative delirium can already be identified at hospital admission since a number of risk factors have been described [51]. Pre-fracture cognitive impairment is the most weighty risk factor, followed by respiratory failure, low albumin, alcohol consumption and prevalent multiple comorbidities. The type of anaesthesia (particularly neuraxial vs. general anaesthesia) does not appear to affect the incidence of delirium, but deep sedation has been associated with a higher risk of post-operative delirium [52]. Thus, the use of intra-operative monitoring of the depth of anaesthesia and the choice of lighter sedation seems to be effective in reducing post-operative delirium.

Although prevention of delirium in hip fracture patients is possible with preoperative screening and simple interventions, nevertheless early consideration of all risk factors and prompt correction of clinical and laboratory abnormalities is mandatory. This approach requires a multi-component intervention, with good adherence by suitably-trained members of staff, physicians and nurses. When carefully applied, the multi-component intervention has been demonstrated to decrease the incidence of delirium by 40%, compared to traditional care, as well as reducing its duration and severity [53]. Taking into account that for delirium prevention, multiple small interventions can provide substantial benefit, multi-component interventions include:

- Monitoring of vital physiological parameters.
- Reduction of immobilisation and bed rest, mobilising by nursing staff as tolerated to the bathroom, taking meals at the table.
- Improved fluid and nutritional intake, dentures used properly, extra drinks.
- Supplemental oxygen to keep saturation >90%.
- Urinary catheters removed by post-operative day 2, unless otherwise ordered, post-void residual assessment.
- Improved sensory stimulation, appropriate use of glasses and hearing aids.
- Attention to bowel movements by scheduling laxatives.
- Promoting sleep by non-pharmacological measures, if needed trazodone should be used for night-time sedation while benzodiazepines should not be initiated (nor abruptly withdrawn).
- Cognitive activation with environmental aids (calendar, clock) or individual interventions.
- Involvement of relatives to support the patient.
- Post-operative blood tests to detect metabolic/laboratory abnormalities.
- Effective control of pain obtained with acetaminophen, non-opioid medication and nerve blocks rather than opiates, which may increase the risk of delirium.

Pharmacological prevention of delirium through the administration of a low dose of neuroleptic drugs is still a matter of debate [64]. Current evidence does not support the routine use of antipsychotics, albeit, in some trials, they demonstrated a reduced incidence of post-operative delirium, particularly in orthopaedic patients at higher risk.

11.9.1.2 Management of Post-operative Delirium

If delirium occurs, it should be borne in mind that it can represent the first symptom of an underlying/undercurrent complication, such as an infection, coronary syndrome, urinary retention, constipation or dehydration. Therefore, when a patient presents with a new episode of delirium, it is mandatory to undertake a comprehensive clinical assessment, accompanied, as appropriate, by a complete laboratory diagnostic work-up and other specific diagnostic tests. Electrocardiogram and chest radiography may be part of the assessment, while neuroimaging is typically limited to patients with new focal neurologic signs.

The treatment includes addressing all modifiable contributors to delirium that are identified in the evaluation along with a full review of medications, stopping when possible those known to be associated with delirium. Moreover, non-pharmacological measures, listed in the prevention paragraph earlier, should be carefully pursued to help the patient recover from their brain dysfunction.

In case of agitation that can hamper the healthcare or rehabilitation, or even be dangerous for patient and caregiver, pharmacological treatment with antipsychotics is usually employed, but note that antipsychotics do not treat delirium, they simply reduce the symptoms. Antipsychotics should never be used in the hypoactive variant. These pharmacological agents should be used at the lowest effective dose, dosing regimens should be individualised for each patient, and the treatment effects should be monitored daily to correct the dose or discontinue the therapy when appropriate. The antipsychotics commonly used are haloperidol (0.25–2 mg oral or intramuscular), risperidone (0.5–2 mg oral), quetiapine (12.5–50 mg oral), olanzapine (2.5–10 mg oral). QT prolongation contraindicates all these drugs. Benzodiazepines should be avoided in patients with delirium, except for subjects with severe agitation and violent inclination, in which a short-acting formulation (e.g. midazolam 1–5 mg intravenous or intramuscular) may produce rapid tranquillisation. In patients with sleep deprivation, the drug of choice is trazodone (25–100 mg oral).

11.9.1.3 Post-operative Cognitive Dysfunction

Some patients experience a more subtle cognitive disorder, affecting a wide range of cognitive domains, particularly memory and executive function. This condition, dissimilar from delirium, is generally designated as post-operative cognitive dysfunction (POCD) and it may not be evident during the first post-operative days. Compared to delirium, POCD shows a less acute onset, is characterised by normal consciousness and may last weeks to months.

For an accurate diagnosis, neuropsychological testing is required, but, usually, a pre-fracture evaluation for comparison is lacking in patients with hip fractures. The incidence after hip fracture surgery is consequently not known while in older patients undergoing elective arthroplasty, a prevalence of approximately 10% has been found 3 months postoperatively [54]. There are many risk factors for POCD: advanced age, pre-existing cardiovascular disease and mild cognitive impairment. Patients with a level of education more than high school have a lower incidence of POCD compared to those with lower educational levels. In orthopaedic elective interventions, a fast-track approach seems to reduce the incidence of POCD, at least early after surgery [55].

POCD is generally reversible, albeit, in some patients with persistent dysfunction, the apolipoprotein E4 genotype has been found, suggesting a link with the development of dementia [56]. Preventing strategies against POCD include reducing the preoperative stress response, monitoring of anaesthetic depth intraoperatively, maintaining of perioperative hemodynamic stability, a multimodal analgesic approach with cautious use of opioids, early post-operative mobilisation, and all nursing measures described for preventing post-operative delirium [55].

11.9.2 Cardiovascular Complications

Ischemic heart disease and cardiac failure account for more than one-third of early deaths after hip fracture [46] although the incidence of cardiac complications after hip fracture is quite variable in epidemiological studies, depending on the diagnostic criteria considered.

11.9.2.1 Myocardial Infarction

Risk factors for the occurrence of myocardial infarction after hip fracture are all atherosclerotic conditions, not only a history of cardiac disease but also stroke or peripheral vascular disease [57]. Most patients do not experience typical chest pain, while they may present with delirium or congestive heart failure, or even be asymptomatic. Therefore, high-risk subjects or those with suspicious symptoms although atypical should be assessed by recording an electrocardiogram (ECG) and measuring troponin level. Patients with clear myocardial infarction should be considered for coronary angiography and cardiology review.

However, after hip fracture, a considerable number of patients show a subtle and isolated increase of troponin without meeting the full criteria of myocardial infarction that include significant ECG changes and/or new wall motion anomalies and/or typical clinical symptoms. In some studies, up to one-third of patients show an increase of troponin just before or early after surgery, most of them without ECG ischaemic changes [58]. Other clinical conditions associated with isolated troponin increase, such as sepsis, pulmonary embolism, renal failure or acute respiratory failure, explain only a small proportion of such increases in this perioperative biomarker. The prognostic significance of an isolated small troponin increase in older patients with hip fractures is still uncertain, given the inconsistent relationship with short- and long-term mortality [58, 59]. In one study a subgroup of patients with a post-operative isolated increase of troponin >0.5 μg/L, considered a cut-off for more definite myocardial damage, were studied with coronary angiography [60]. All patients were found to have severe coronary disease and underwent percutaneous or surgical revascularisation with a significant improvement in 1-year survival.

11.9.2.2   Heart Failure

Congestive heart failure is another important post-operative complication, related to surgical stress, blood loss, transfusion, or inappropriate fluid administration. The onset may be either typical with dyspnoea, or insidious with a change in functional status, reduction of food intake or delirium.

Diuretic agents are frequently discontinued, as part of the pre-operative drug revision, in order to reduce the risk of dehydration and hypotension. It is important to bear in mind that in patients with ventricular dysfunction, diuresis may be loop diuretic dependent. Therefore, it may be advisable, in patients with pre-fracture congestive heart failure, to continue these pharmacological agents, or discontinue them only for a short period of time. Urinary output measurement is critical for hemodynamic assessment in the early post-operative days. Oliguria could be related either to inadequate volume restoration (most frequent in the first 24–48 h after surgery) or heart and renal failure. Thus, contrasting interventions, such as extra fluid or diuretics administration, require patient-specific decision making. Measurement of the N-terminal fragment of brain natriuretic peptide (NT-proBNP) has been proposed to evaluate post-operative cardiac dysfunction [61], but it has a decreased specificity in older patients.

11.9.2.3   Supraventricular Arrhythmias

New onset atrial fibrillation is particularly frequent after hip fracture surgery occurring in 3–6% of patients [62, 63]. A previous history of atrial fibrillation is the most consistent risk factor. The rapid ventricular rate in atrial fibrillation results in inadequate diastolic filling and a reduced cardiac output leading to hemodynamic instability. Atrial fibrillation may cause exacerbation of heart failure, poor exercise tolerance and thromboembolic events including stroke. The occurrence of atrial fibrillation in the early post-operative days has been consistently associated with a higher risk of mortality within 1 year after fracture [62, 63]. It could be a marker of greater vulnerability, rather than a complication increasing mortality directly. Moreover, evidence links atrial fibrillation after surgery as a risk factor for POCD [55].

Current treatment modalities include anti-arrhythmic medications, radiofrequency ablation, and anticoagulation. Beta-blockers can reduce the risk of this arrhythmia, but their beneficial effects should be balanced against the risk of drug-induced hypotension.

11.9.3   Infections

11.9.3.1   Post-operative Fever

Fever occurs frequently during the post-operative phase; it can either indicate the presence of an infection or be produced by a non-infective cause. The challenge is to identify which patients need immediate screening and which can be skilfully managed with a 'wait and see' approach.

Surgery of any type causes significant cellular injury leading to the release of cytokines into the bloodstream and then fever, as a normal physiologic response. The more tissue is damaged, the greater is the cytokine release. Febrile events occurring within 2 post-operative days in the absence of localising symptoms should be closely monitored, but not acted upon, while they are more suggestive of infection when they occur later than the third post-operative day or if the temperature is greater than 38.5 °C and multiple fever spikes are observed [64].

Studies agree that investigations, particularly chest X-rays or blood and urine cultures, performed to study early post-operative febrile episodes without clinical symptoms or signs of infections are rarely positive and are therefore an inappropriate use of hospital resources [65]. On the other hand, patients with hip fracture with a high degree of frailty, malnutrition, multiple comorbidities, polypharmacy, may have a compromised immune response that predisposes to infection. Early detection of pneumonia or urinary tract infections that are the most common post-operative infections is crucial, since a late diagnosis may have severe detrimental consequences.

Clinical judgement, based on the presence of signs and symptoms of infections, is the only guide to decide when diagnostic procedures and possibly antibiotic therapy should be started. It should be also highlighted that infections in frail older adults may occur without fever, presenting with insidious onset symptoms, such as fatigue and delirium. Traditional biomarkers such as white blood cell count or C-reactive protein may be used to aid in the diagnosis but in the early post-operative days, these blood parameters lack sensitivity and specificity in discriminating inflammation due to a bacterial infection from that of surgical injury response. There is increasing evidence supporting the use of procalcitonin as a useful marker to detect bacterial infections in post-operative days [66, 67]. It is true that, following surgical tissue damage, procalcitonin may have a small and transient increase, but higher and persistent values have a high likelihood of being related to infections. However, at present, it is not clear which is the best cut-off with the most correct balance between specificity and sensitivity. When laboratory biomarkers are required for sepsis confirmation in the first days after hip fracture repair it is probably better to set a high procalcitonin threshold, that is, >0.9 ng/mL, as in trauma patients.

11.9.3.2 Pneumonia

Pneumonia and exacerbation of chronic lung disease occur in about 4% of older patients with hip fractures and account for one-third of post-operative deaths [46]. Predisposing factors are spending most of the day sitting or lying in bed, which leads to incomplete lung expansion and resulting atelectasis. Poor inspiratory effort may also be due to sedation or pain leading to difficulty clearing pulmonary secretions. Moreover, dysphagia or an impaired swallowing function, frequent in frail older patients with declining brain function or decreased muscle mass, may worsen after surgery and cause aspiration and, consequently, aspiration pneumonia.

Patients with an admission diagnosis of COPD have about 2.5 times the risk of developing chest infections during a hospital stay and a substantial excess of mortality compared with patients without COPD [68]. Other reported risk factors for post-operative pneumonia include disorders of the central nervous system, anaemia, diabetes and the use of medication that reduces alertness [69].

Measures and interventions to prevent pneumonia should be implemented in clinical practice in order to quickly restore the capacity of expansion of the lung–chest wall and to avoid aspiration:

- Oral hygiene
- Control of gastroesophageal reflux
- Avoidance of excessive sedation
- Early ambulation
- Adequate nutrition
- Respiratory exercises improving the patient's ability to take deep breaths

11.9.3.3   Urinary Tract Infection

Urinary tract infection is the most common complication after hip fracture surgery occurring in almost one-quarter of all patients. It has been associated with an increased incidence of delirium, prolonged length of hospital stay and even lower functional outcomes [70]. A urinary catheter is the single most important risk factor for this type of infection, but other causes are post-operative urinary retention or neurogenic bladder dysfunction.

Measures to prevent urinary tract infection are:

- Avoiding unnecessary placement of indwelling urinary catheters even intraoperatively.
- Removing a urinary catheter as soon as possible, preferably within the first post-operative day.
- Considering the use of intermittent catheterisation to relieve post-operative urinary retention.
- Planning education of all healthcare professionals around a specific protocol on perioperative use of a urinary catheter and the management of post-operative bladder incontinence or retention.
- Early and repeated mobilisation.

Urinary retention is common among patients with hip fracture, and it is related to urinary infection, prostatic enlargement in males, underlying bladder dysfunction (e.g. diabetic neuropathy, Parkinsonism), and opiate use. Although it is uncertain if a premature removal of the indwelling catheter could favour urinary retention, it should be removed as soon as possible to prevent urinary infections and promote early mobilisation if necessary, patients can be managed through voiding methods, including intermittent catheterisation.

11.9.3.4   Surgical Site Infection

Surgical site infection is the third most frequent cause of infections, and it is discussed among surgical complications. It is less frequent compared to other infections, occurring in 2–4% of patients and usually later, often after discharge.

Patient-specific risk factors are older age, poor nutrition, history of diabetes, smoking, obesity, other concomitant infections and previous history of colonisation. Prevention measures include peri-operative antimicrobial prophylaxis using cefazolin or other antimicrobial agents according to local guidelines, a number of hygiene measures minimising microbial inoculums, and clinical optimisation of the patients. Modifiable patient-related risk factors are malnutrition and uncompensated diabetes. Particularly, blood glucose levels greater than 200 mg/dL in the peri-operative period increase the risk of surgical site infection [71]. Furthermore, patients without a history of diabetes but showing stress-induced hyperglycaemia, with glucose levels greater than 220 mg/day, also have a higher risk of surgical site infection [72]. Close monitoring in the peri-operative period is required to detect and manage glucose fluctuations and is advised before meals. To achieve and maintain good control of glycaemia, fast-acting insulin or basal–bolus regime should be preferred in patients using oral diabetic agents before hospital admission, to limit the risk of hypoglycaemia or other metabolic derangements associated with oral diabetic agents.

11.9.4 Other Complications

Truly, this overview may not be comprehensive, describing the overall constellation of clinical complications presenting in older adults with hip fracture, but a number of other complications should be acknowledged (Table 11.1). Patients with frailty are characterised by an age-associated decline in physiological reserve and function

Table 11.1 Standardised procedures and prevention/management protocols to be implemented for selected medical complications in hip fracture in older adults

Complication	Main goal(s)	Strategies prevention/management
Delirium	Prevention	• Identify high-risk patients on admission
		• Check daily risk factors
		• Correct (when possible) modifiable risk factors
		• Remove delirium-causing medications
		• Monitoring of vital physiological parameters
		• Correct clinical/laboratory abnormalities
		• Control pain, limiting opiates usage
		• Reduce immobilisation and encourage time out of bed
		• Improved fluid and nutritional intake
		• Supplemental oxygen to keep saturation >90%
		• Remove any catheters and tubes as soon as possible
		• Attention to bowel movements
		• Promoting sleep by non-pharmacological measure
		• Cognitive activation with environmental aids
		• Involvement of relatives
		• Pharmacological prevention for patients at very high risk
	Early detection and management	• Assess patients daily using a standardised tool
		• Look for underlying causes
		• Remove (when possible) underlying causes
		• Implement prevention strategies (see Prevention)
		• Pharmacological intervention to reduce symptoms

(continued)

Table 11.1 (continued)

Complication	Main goal(s)	Strategies prevention/management
Post-operative hypotension	Prevention	• Discontinue or reduce doses of antihypertensive drugs and diuretics • Limit the use of hypotensive pharmacological agents • Transfuse patient according to established haemoglobin thresholds • Administer isotonic intravenous fluids pre-, intra- and postoperatively • Tailor fluid management through clinical measures/bedside ultrasound or advanced haemodynamic monitoring techniques if necessary and available
Coronary artery disease	Prevention	• Check for risk factors • Identify high-risk patients on admission • Continue antiplatelet drugs in the perioperative period (in high-risk patients)
	Early detection	• Check for atypical signs/symptoms of ischemia • Measure troponin and ECG in patients with typical or atypical signs/symptoms • Monitor troponin regularly in high-risk patients
Heart failure	Prevention	• Continue beta-blockers • Continue loop diuretics if possible (alternatively, discontinue them briefly and resume rapidly) • Manage fluid administration carefully, checking pulmonary status and early signs/symptoms of acute failure • Measure urine output in the early post-operative days in high-risk patients
Pneumonia	Prevention	• Nutritional supplementation • Avoid excessive sedation • Maintain adequate oral hygiene • Control of gastro-oesophageal reflux • Detect swallowing disorders and modify food consistency • Early surgical repair and ambulation • Deep breathing exercises
	Early detection	• Check daily for typical and atypical signs/symptoms • Laboratory tests and/or chest X-rays in patients at high risk or with clinical signs/symptoms • Measure procalcitonin in selected high-risk patients
Urinary tract infection	Prevention	• Avoiding unnecessary placement on indwelling urinary catheters even intraoperatively • Remove the urinary catheter within the first post-operative day • Considering the use of intermittent catheterisation to relieve post-operative urinary retention • Early and repeated mobilisation • Planning education of all healthcare professional on the management of perioperative use of a urinary catheter and post-operative bladder incontinence or retention • Optimise diabetes control
	Early detection	• Check daily for typical and atypical signs/symptoms • Laboratory tests and/or urine culture in patients at high risk or with clinical signs/symptoms • Measure procalcitonin in selected high-risk patients with signs/symptoms of urinary sepsis

Table 11.1 (continued)

Complication	Main goal(s)	Strategies prevention/management
Surgical site infection	Prevention	• Peri-operative antimicrobial prophylaxis according to guidelines • Hygienic measures in the operating room • Hygienic measures in the management of surgical site minimising the risk of microbial inoculums • Improve malnourishment with nutritional supplementation • Optimise diabetic control maintaining glucose level <220 mg/dL
Acute kidney injury	Prevention	• Identify patients with chronic kidney disease on admission • Monitor perioperative glomerular filtration rate • Manage fluid administration, preventing dehydration and volume overload • Avoid nephrotoxic drug use, including NSAID and certain antimicrobial agents • Avoid intraoperative and post-operative hypotension
Urinary retention	Prevention	• Avoid anticholinergic medications • Manage constipation • Early detection and prompt treatment of urinary infection • Promote early mobilisation
Constipation	Prevention	• Promote early mobilisation • Reducing opioids for pain control • Increasing fluid intake to 1.5 L/day • Reducing fasting time and planning a nutritional support postoperatively • Use laxative when appropriate starting on the day of surgery
Pressure ulcers	Prevention	• Use special beds and equipment to relieve pressure in patients at risk • Improve malnourishment and use nutritional supplements • Reduce time to surgery and promote early mobilisation

across multi-organ systems. Thus, almost every organ is vulnerable, and patients with hip fractures are at risk of multiple adverse health outcomes.

11.9.4.1 Acute Kidney Injury (AKI)

Another very common post-operative complication is a transient worsening of renal function, particularly in patients with pre-fracture impairment of glomerular filtration. Interestingly patients with stage 1 and 2 AKI have similar survival curves but worse when compared to those with no AKI [73], suggesting that a post-operative deterioration of renal function is probably a marker of frailty rather than the direct cause of death. Close monitoring of renal function should be undertaken in the early post-operative days, taking into account the fact that creatinine level overestimates glomerular filtration rate due to the age-related loss of skeletal muscle mass. Estimation of the kidney function with the Cockcroft-Gault method may be useful, being more accurate. Electrolyte imbalances, especially hyponatremia and hypokalaemia, are described frequently and should be promptly corrected.

AKI is potentially preventable in some patients and important measures that should be implemented are:

- Avoidance of nephrotoxic drugs including non-steroidal anti-inflammatory drugs and nephrotoxic antibiotics.
- Appropriate management of fluids, avoiding hypovolaemia by reducing fasting times and by intravenous fluid administration before surgery so that the patient does not arrive in theatre with dehydration.
- Prioritising intraoperative blood pressure control avoiding intraoperative hypotension, irrespective of the type of anaesthesia.
- Temporary discontinuation of antihypertensive drugs, particularly angiotensin converting enzyme (ACE) inhibitors and angiotensin receptor blockers (even if not nephrotoxins per se) especially when AKI or hypotension has developed.

Dialysis-dependent patients are a subgroup of patients with significant frailty and with a high risk of post-operative complications, particularly pneumonia and sepsis/septic shock [74]. Intra-hospital and 30-day mortality rates are 2.5-fold higher than non-dialysis patients. A challenging issue in these patients is well-judged fluid administration in the perioperative period, avoiding both hypovolemia and cardiovascular overload. A team approach, involving an expert nephrologist and orthogeriatrician is essential to reduce early complications and early mortality.

11.9.4.2 Gastrointestinal Complications

Common gastrointestinal complications after hip fracture surgery include dyspepsia, constipation, paralytic ileus and haemorrhage.

The reported incidence of perioperative acute upper gastrointestinal bleeding varies widely in the literature but nowadays seems low [75]. Pre-existing peptic ulcer disease and non-steroidal anti-inflammatory drugs are known risk factors while post-operative use of aspirin is not likely to be a strong risk factor. However, it is possible that the combination of an antiplatelet agent and a prophylactic low molecular weight heparin may exacerbate upper gastrointestinal bleeding. A suspicion of gastrointestinal bleeding requires prompt endoscopic evaluation.

Most patients following hip fracture surgery have problems with the evacuation of faeces during the first post-operative days and a normal defecation pattern is re-established only after several days [76]. In orthopaedic surgery, the effects of constipation on patients are often minor, but sometimes prolonged bowel dysfunction can lead to faecal impaction or post-operative ileus.

Although post-operative nausea and vomiting are rarely associated with a life-threatening condition, they are frequent undesirable side effects of surgery and anaesthesia. Several drugs have been studied to prevent such unpleasant symptoms and the most effective seems to be dexamethasone given pre or intraoperatively at the time of anaesthesia [77].

General measures to prevent gastrointestinal complications are:

- Reducing fasting time (i.e. 2 h for clear liquids) and planning nutritional support postoperatively (i.e. oral nutritional supplement drinks) effective in preventing gastrointestinal stress ulceration, post-operative nausea and vomiting and constipation.
- Increasing fluid intake to 1.5 L/day.
- Early and appropriate mobility.
- Introduction of proton pump inhibitors in patients at risk of bleeding or their continuation if previously taken.
- Avoiding NSAIDs in patients at high risk of bleeding; however, aspirin should not be stopped if it was a regular pre-fracture medication.
- Reducing the use of opioids for pain control.
- Introduction of a laxative, starting on the day of surgery.

11.9.4.3 Pressure Ulcers
Even with the widespread dissemination of nursing protocols, based on attentive skincare and on the use of special bed equipment to relieve pressure, the incidence of pressure ulcers is still approximately 10% which doubles when grade 1 is included [78, 79]. Several features of management have been found to negatively affect the occurrence of pressure ulcers, such as the use of traction and foam splints, while frequent manual repositioning has a positive effect. However, the best strategy for reducing pressure ulcers in patients with hip fracture is shortening the time of bed rest by means of early surgery and mobilisation, along with protein-caloric supplementation.

11.10 Final Remarks

The management of older patients with hip fracture in the post-operative phase requires a comprehensive orthogeriatric approach. Frailty and comorbidity in combination with the hip fracture and surgical repair procedures create a degree of vulnerability that cannot be faced using traditional care models. Currently, orthogeriatric management for patients with a fragility fracture is the gold standard of care all over the world, to prevent complications where possible, or manage them appropriately when they occur. For acute conditions, such as hip fracture, the healthcare needs do not cease after the acute phase, as most patients require treatment in the post-acute phase for further clinical stabilisation and rehabilitation. The susceptibility to complications for these patients may last for several weeks after surgical repair. Thus, discharge destination should match the stability and vulnerability of the patient, his/her rehabilitation program and goals, and the pre-existing level of independence, to ensure long-term positive clinical outcomes. Discharge planning based on discharge needs, patient social supports, patient and family desires is a crucial point in acute management. In recent years, the appropriateness of post-acute settings has become a topic for debate. Similar patients with hip fracture discharged to different post-acute settings (i.e., home-based rehabilitation, post-acute care facilities and inpatient rehabilitation) seem to have different outcomes [80, 81]. The quality of care of post-acute and rehabilitation facilities is another variable that may affect long-term outcomes. Outcomes and standards of care should be monitored in the acute care setting as well as in post-acute care.

References

1. Ranhoff AH, Holvik K, Martinsen MI, Domaas K, Solheim LF (2010) Older hip fracture patients: three groups with different needs. BMC Geriatr 10:65
2. Giusti A, Barone A, Razzano M, Pizzonia M, Pioli G (2011) Optimal setting and care organization in the management of older adults with hip fracture. Eur J Phys Rehabil Med 47(2):281–296
3. Patel JN, Klein DS, Sreekumar S, Liporace FA, Yoon RS (2019) Outcomes in multidisciplinary team-based approach in geriatric hip fracture care: a systematic review. J Am Acad Orthop Surg 28:128. https://doi.org/10.5435/JAAOS-D-18-00425
4. Moyet J, Deschasse G, Marquant B, Mertl P, Bloch F (2019) Which is the optimal orthogeriatric care model to prevent mortality of elderly subjects post hip fractures? A systematic review and meta-analysis based on current clinical practice. Int Orthop 43(6):1449–1454
5. Middleton M, Wan B, Da Assunção R (2017) Improving hip fracture outcomes with integrated orthogeriatric care: a comparison between two accepted orthogeriatric models. Age Ageing 43:465–470
6. National Institute for Health and Care Excellence (2016) Hip fracture in adults. NICE quality standard No. 16. NICE, Manchester
7. Pioli G, Barone A, Mussi C, Tafaro L, Bellelli G, Falaschi P, Trabucchi M, Paolisso G, GIOG (2014) The management of hip fracture in the older population. Joint position statement by Gruppo Italiano Ortogeriatria (GIOG). Aging Clin Exp Res 26(5):547–553
8. Sheehan KJ, Guerrero EM, Tainter D, Dial B, Milton-Cole R, Blair JA, Alexander J, Swamy P, Kuramoto L, Guy P, Bettger JP, Sobolev B (2019) Prognostic factors of in-hospital complications after hip fracture surgery: a scoping review. Osteoporos Int 30:1339. https://doi.org/10.1007/s00198-019-04976-x
9. Moppett IK, Parker M, Griffiths R, Bowers T, White SM, Moran CG (2012) Nottingham hip fracture score: longitudinal and multi-assessment. Br J Anaesth 109(4):546–550
10. Chow WB, Rosenthal RA, Merkow RP, Ko CY, Esnaola NF, American College of Surgeons National Surgical Quality Improvement Program; American Geriatrics Society (2012) Optimal preoperative assessment of the geriatric surgical patient: a best practices guideline from the American College of Surgeons National Surgical Quality Improvement Program and the American Geriatrics Society. J Am Coll Surg 215(4):453–466
11. Lin HS, Watts JN, Peel NM, Hubbard RE (2016) Frailty and post-operative outcomes in older surgical patients: a systematic review. BMC Geriatr 16(1):157
12. Krishnan M, Beck S, Havelock W, Eeles E, Hubbard RE, Johansen A (2014) Predicting outcome after hip fracture: using a frailty index to integrate comprehensive geriatric assessment results. Age Ageing 43(1):122–126
13. Dodd AC, Bulka C, Jahangir A, Mir HR, Obremskey WT, Sethi MK (2016) Predictors of 30-day mortality following hip/pelvis fractures. Orthop Traumatol Surg Res 102(6):707–710
14. Cha YH, Ha YC, Park HJ, Lee YK, Jung SY, Kim JY, Koo KH (2019) Relationship of chronic obstructive pulmonary disease severity with early and late mortality in elderly patients with hip fracture. Injury. pii: S0020-1383(19)30300-6. https://doi.org/10.1016/j.injury.2019.05.021
15. Akinleye SD, Garofolo G, Culbertson MD, Homel P, Erez O (2018) The role of BMI in hip fracture surgery. Geriatr Orthop Surg Rehabil 9:2151458517747414

16. Li S, Zhang J, Zheng H, Wang X, Liu Z, Sun T (2019) Prognostic role of serum albumin, total lymphocyte count, and mini nutritional assessment on outcomes after geriatric hip fracture surgery: a meta-analysis and systematic review. J Arthroplast 34(6):1287–1296
17. Kim S, McClave SA, Martindale RG, Miller KR, Hurt RT (2017) Hypoalbuminemia and clinical outcomes: what is the mechanism behind the relationship? Am Surg 83(11):1220–1227
18. Kristensen PK, Thillemann TM, Søballe K, Johnsen SP (2016) Are process performance measures associated with clinical outcomes among patients with hip fractures? A population-based cohort study. Int J Qual Health Care 28(6):698–708
19. Hulsbæk S, Larsen RF, Troelsen A (2015) Predictors of not regaining basic mobility after hip fracture surgery. Disabil Rehabil 37(19):1739–1744
20. Su B, Newson R, Soljak H, Soljak M (2018) Associations between post-operative rehabilitation of hip fracture and outcomes: national database analysis. BMC Musculoskelet Disord 19(1):211. https://doi.org/10.1186/s12891-018-2093-8
21. Foss NB, Kristensen MT, Kehlet H (2006) Prediction of postoperative morbidity, mortality and rehabilitation in hip fracture patients: the cumulated ambulation score. Clin Rehabil 20(8):701–708
22. Barone A, Giusti A, Pizzonia M, Razzano M, Oliveri M, Palummeri E, Pioli G (2009) Factors associated with an immediate weight-bearing and early ambulation program for older adults after hip fracture repair. Arch Phys Med Rehabil 90(9):1495–1498
23. Villa JC, Koressel J, van der List J, Cohn M, Wellman DS, Lorich DG, Lane JM (2019) Predictors of in-hospital ambulatory status following low-energy hip fracture surgery. Geriatr Orthop Surg Rehabil 10:2151459318814825
24. Ogawa T, Aoki T, Shirasawa S (2019) Effect of hip fracture surgery within 24 hours on short-term mobility. J Orthop Sci 24(3):469–473
25. Kammerlander C, Pfeufer D, Lisitano LA, Mehaffey S, Böcker W, Neuerburg C (2018) Inability of older adult patients with hip fracture to maintain postoperative weight-bearing restrictions. J Bone Joint Surg Am 100(11):936–941
26. Münter KH, Clemmesen CG, Foss NB, Palm H, Kristensen MT (2018) Fatigue and pain limit independent mobility and physiotherapy after hip fracture surgery. Disabil Rehabil 40(15):1808–1816
27. Abou-Setta AM, Beaupre LA, Rashiq S, Dryden DM, Hamm MP, Sadowski CA et al (2011) Comparative effectiveness of pain management interventions for hip fracture: a systematic review. Ann Intern Med 155(4):234–245
28. Steenberg J, Møller AM (2018) Systematic review of the effects of fascia iliaca compartment block on hip fracture patients before operation. Br J Anaesth 120(6):1368–1380
29. Wong SS, Irwin MG (2016) Peri-operative cardiac protection for non-cardiac surgery. Anaesthesia 71(Suppl 1):29–39
30. White SM, Moppett IK, Griffiths R, Johansen A, Wakeman R, Boulton C, Plant F, Williams A, Pappenheim K, Majeed A, Currie CT, Grocott MP (2016) Secondary analysis of outcomes after 11,085 hip fracture operations from the prospective UK Anaesthesia Sprint Audit of Practice (ASAP-2). Anaesthesia 71(5):506–514
31. Moppett IK, Rowlands M, Mannings A, Moran CG, Wiles MD, NOTTS Investigators (2015) LiDCO-based fluid management in patients undergoing hip fracture surgery under spinal anaesthesia: a randomized trial and systematic review. Br J Anaesth 114(3):444–459
32. Puckeridge G, Terblanche M, Wallis M, Fung YL (2019) Blood management in hip fractures; are we leaving it too late? A retrospective observational study. BMC Geriatr 19(1):79
33. Carson JL, Terrin ML, Noveck H, Sanders DW, Chaitman BR, Rhoads GG, Nemo G, Dragert K, Beaupre L, Hildebrand K, Macaulay W, Lewis C, Cook DR, Dobbin G, Zakriya KJ, Apple FS, Horney RA, Magaziner J, FOCUS Investigators (2011) Liberal or restrictive transfusion in high-risk patients after hip surgery. N Engl J Med 365(26):2453–2462
34. Marik PE, Corwin HL (2008) Efficacy of red blood cell transfusion in the critically ill: a systematic review of the literature. Crit Care Med 36(9):2667–2674

35. Gregersen M, Damsgaard EM, Borris LC (2015) Blood transfusion and risk of infection in frail elderly after hip fracture surgery: the TRIFE randomized controlled trial. Eur J Orthop Surg Traumatol 25(6):1031–1038

36. Amin RM, DeMario VM, Best MJ, Shafiq B, Hasenboehler EA, Sterling RS, Frank SM, Khanuja HS (2019) A restrictive hemoglobin transfusion threshold of less than 7 g/dL decreases blood utilization without compromising outcomes in patients with hip fractures. J Am Acad Orthop Surg 28:887. https://doi.org/10.5435/JAAOS-D-18-00374

37. Schack A, Berkfors AA, Ekeloef S, Gögenur I, Burcharth J (2019) The effect of perioperative iron therapy in acute major non-cardiac surgery on allogenic blood transfusion and postoperative haemoglobin levels: a systematic review and meta-analysis. World J Surg 43(7):1677–1691

38. Zhang P, He J, Fang Y, Chen P, Liang Y, Wang J (2017 May) Efficacy and safety of intravenous tranexamic acid administration in patients undergoing hip fracture surgery for hemostasis: a meta-analysis. Medicine (Baltimore) 96(21):e6940. https://doi.org/10.1097/MD.0000000000006940

39. Goisser S, Schrader E, Singler K, Bertsch T, Gefeller O, Biber R et al (2015) Low postoperative dietary intake is associated with worse functional course in geriatric patients up to 6 months after hip fracture. Br J Nutr 113(12):1940–1950

40. Rosenberger C, Rechsteiner M, Dietsche R, Breidert M (2019) Energy and protein intake in 330 geriatric orthopaedic patients: are the current nutrition guidelines applicable? Clin Nutr ESPEN 29:86–91. https://doi.org/10.1016/j.clnesp.2018.11.016

41. Avenell A, Smith TO, Curtain JP, Mak JC, Myint PK (2016) Nutritional supplementation for hip fracture aftercare in older people. Cochrane Database Syst Rev 11:CD001880

42. Pioli G, Lauretani F, Pellicciotti F, Pignedoli P, Bendini C, Davoli ML, Martini E, Zagatti A, Giordano A, Nardelli A, Zurlo A, Bianchini D, Sabetta E, Ferrari A, Tedeschi C, Lunardelli ML (2016) Modifiable and non-modifiable risk factors affecting walking recovery after hip fracture. Osteoporos Int 27(6):2009–2016

43. National Hip Fracture Database annual report (2018). https://www.nhfd.co.uk/2018report

44. Asheim A, Nilsen SM, Toch-Marquardt M, Anthun KS, Johnsen LG, Bjørngaard JH (2018) Time of admission and mortality after hip fracture: a detailed look at the weekend effect in a nationwide study of 55,211 hip fracture patients in Norway. Acta Orthop 89(6):610–614

45. Åhman R, Siverhall PF, Snygg J, Fredrikson M, Enlund G, Björnström K, Chew MS (2018) Determinants of mortality after hip fracture surgery in Sweden: a registry-based retrospective cohort study. Sci Rep 8(1):15695. https://doi.org/10.1038/s41598-018-33940-8

46. Sheikh HQ, Hossain FS, Aqil A, Akinbamijo B, Mushtaq V, Kapoor H (2017) A comprehensive analysis of the causes and predictors of 30-day mortality following hip fracture surgery. Clin Orthop Surg 9(1):10–18. https://doi.org/10.4055/cios.2017.9.1.10

47. Bohl DD, Samuel AM, Webb ML, Lukasiewicz AM, Ondeck NT, Basques BA, Anandasivam NS, Grauer JN (2018) Timing of adverse events following geriatric hip fracture surgery: a study of 19,873 patients in the American College of Surgeons National Surgical Quality Improvement Program. Am J Orthop (Belle Mead NJ) 47(9):1–13. https://doi.org/10.12788/ajo.2018.0080

48. Simunovic N, Devereaux PJ, Sprague S, Guyatt GH, Schemitsch E, Debeer J, Bhandari M (2010) Effect of early surgery after hip fracture on mortality and complications: systematic review and meta-analysis. CMAJ 182(15):1609–1616

49. Pioli G, Lauretani F, Davoli ML, Martini E, Frondini C, Pellicciotti F et al (2012) Older people with hip fracture and IADL disability require earlier surgery. J Gerontol Biol Sci Med Sci 67(11):1272–1277

50. Albrecht JS, Marcantonio ER, Roffey DM, Orwig D, Magaziner J, Terrin M, Carson JL, Barr E, Brown JP, Gentry EG, Gruber-Baldini AL (2015) Stability of postoperative delirium psychomotor subtypes in individuals with hip fracture. J Am Geriatr Soc 63(5):970–976

51. Oh ES, Li M, Fafowora TM, Inouye SK, Chen CH, Rosman LM, Lyketsos CG et al (2015) Preoperative risk factors for postoperative delirium following hip fracture repair: a systematic review. Int J Geriatr Psychiatry 30(9):900–910

52. Orena EF, King AB, Hughes CG (2016) The role of anesthesia in the prevention of postoperative delirium: a systematic review. Minerva Anestesiol 82(6):669–683

53. Oberai T, Laver K, Crotty M, Killington M, Jaarsma R (2018) Effectiveness of multicomponent interventions on incidence of delirium in hospitalized older patients with hip fracture: a systematic review. Int Psychogeriatr 30(4):481–492
54. Kotekar N, Shenkar A, Nagaraj R (2018) Postoperative cognitive dysfunction—current preventive strategies. Clin Interv Aging 13:2267–2273. https://doi.org/10.2147/CIA.S133896
55. Krenk L, Kehlet H, Bæk Hansen T, Solgaard S, Soballe K, Rasmussen LS (2014) Cognitive dysfunction after fast-track hip and knee replacement. Anesth Analg 118(5): 1034–1040
56. Shoair OA, Grasso Ii MP, Lahaye LA, Daniel R, Biddle CJ, Slattum PW (2015) Incidence and risk factors for postoperative cognitive dysfunction in older adults undergoing major noncardiac surgery: a prospective study. J Anaesthesiol Clin Pharmacol 31(1):30–36
57. Sathiyakumar V, Avilucea FR, Whiting PS, Jahangir AA, Mir HR, Obremskey WT, Sethi MK (2016) Risk factors for adverse cardiac events in hip fracture patients: an analysis of NSQIP data. Int Orthop 40(3):439–445
58. Hietala P, Strandberg M, Kiviniemi T, Strandberg N, Airaksinen KE (2014) Usefulness of troponin T to predict short-term and long-term mortality in patients after hip fracture. Am J Cardiol 114(2):193–197
59. Vallet H, Breining A, Le Manach Y, Cohen-Bittan J, Mézière A, Raux M, Verny M, Riou B, Khiami F, Boddaert J (2017) Isolated cardiac troponin rise does not modify the prognosis in elderly patients with hip fracture. Medicine (Baltimore) 96(7):e6169
60. Rostagno C, Peris A, Polidori GL, Ranalli C, Cartei A, Civinini R, Boccaccini A, Prisco D, Innocenti M, Di Mario C (2019) Perioperative myocardial infarction in elderly patients with hip fracture. Is there a role for early coronary angiography?Int. J Cardiol 284:1–5. https://doi.org/10.1016/j.ijcard.2018.10.095
61. Ushirozako H, Ohishi T, Fujita T, Suzuki D, Yamamoto K, Banno T, Takase H, Matsuyama Y (2017) Does N-terminal pro-brain type natriuretic peptide predict cardiac complications after hip fracture surgery? Clin Orthop Relat Res 475(6):1730–1736
62. Gupta BP, Steckelberg RC, Gullerud RE, Huddleston PM, Kirkland LL, Wright RS, Huddleston JM (2015) Incidence and 1-year outcomes of perioperative atrial arrhythmia in elderly adults after hip fracture surgery. J Am Geriatr Soc 63(11):2269–2274
63. Leibowitz D, Abitbol C, Alcalai R, Rivkin G, Kandel L (2017) Perioperative atrial fibrillation is associated with increased one-year mortality in elderly patients after repair of hip fracture. Int J Cardiol 227:58–60
64. Yoo JH, Kim KT, Kim TY, Hwang JH, Chang JD (2017) Postoperative fever after hemiarthroplasty in elderly patients over 70 years of age with displaced femoral neck fracture: necessity of routine workup? Injury 48(2):441–446
65. Ashley B, Spiegel DA, Cahill P, Talwar D, Baldwin KD (2017) Post-operative fever in orthopaedic surgery: how effective is the 'fever workup?'. J Orthop Surg (Hong Kong) 25(3):2309499017727953
66. Zhang L, Cai D, Guo H (2018) Value of procalcitonin for diagnosing perioperative pneumonia, urinary infections and superficial surgical site infections in patients undergoing primary hip and knee arthroplasty. Exp Ther Med 15(6):5403–5409. https://doi.org/10.3892/etm.2018.6124
67. Ingber RB, Alhammoud A, Murray DP, Abraham R, Dixit A, Naziri Q, Ahmed G, Paulino CB, Urban WP, Craig C, Maheshwari AV, Diebo BG (2018) A systematic review and meta-analysis of procalcitonin as a marker of postoperative orthopedic infections. Orthopedics 41(3):e303–e309. https://doi.org/10.3928/01477447-20180409-07
68. Buss L, McKeever TM, Nightingale J, Akyea R, Ollivere B, Moppett IK, Bolton CE (2018) Hip fracture outcomes in patients with chronic obstructive pulmonary disease. Br J Anaesth 121(6):1377–1379
69. Lv H, Yin P, Long A, Gao Y, Zhao Z, Li J, Zhang L, Zhang L, Tang P (2016) Clinical characteristics and risk factors of postoperative pneumonia after hip fracture surgery: a prospective cohort study. Osteoporos Int 27(10):3001–3009
70. Bliemel C, Buecking B, Hack J, Aigner R, Eschbach DA, Ruchholtz S, Oberkircher L (2017) Urinary tract infection in patients with hip fracture: an underestimated event? Geriatr Gerontol Int 17(12):2369–2375

71. Richards JE, Kauffmann RM, Zuckerman SL, Obremskey WT, May AK (2012) Relationship of hyperglycemia and surgical-site infection in orthopaedic surgery. J Bone Joint Surg Am 94(13):1181–1186
72. Karunakar MA, Staples KS (2010) Does stress-induced hyperglycemia increase the risk of perioperative infectious complications in orthopaedic trauma patients? J Orthop Trauma 24(12):752–756
73. Porter CJ, Moppett IK, Juurlink I, Nightingale J, Moran CG, Devonald MA (2017) Acute and chronic kidney disease in elderly patients with hip fracture: prevalence, risk factors and outcome with development and validation of a risk prediction model for acute kidney injury. BMC Nephrol 18(1):20
74. Hickson LJ, Farah WH, Johnson RL, Thorsteinsdottir B, Ubl DS, Yuan BJ, Albright R, Rule AD, Habermann EB (2018) Death and postoperative complications after hip fracture repair: dialysis effect. Kidney Int Rep 3(6):1294–1303
75. Liu J, Gupta R, Hay K, Pulle C, Rahman T, Pandy S (2018) Upper gastrointestinal bleeding in neck of femur fracture patients: a single tertiary centre experience. Intern Med J 48(6):731–735. https://doi.org/10.1111/imj.13809
76. Trads M, Pedersen PU (2015) Constipation and defecation pattern the first 30 days after hip fracture. Int J Nurs Pract 21(5):598–604
77. Chen P, Li X, Sang L, Huang J (2017) Perioperative intravenous glucocorticoids can decrease postoperative nausea and vomiting and pain in total joint arthroplasty: a meta-analysis and trial sequence analysis. Medicine (Baltimore) 96(13):e6382. https://doi.org/10.1097/MD.0000000000006382
78. Lindholm C, Sterner E, Romanelli M, Pina E, Torra y Bou J, Hietanen H, Iivanainen A, Gunningberg L, Hommel A, Klang B, Dealey C (2008) Hip fracture and pressure ulcers—the pan-European pressure ulcer study—intrinsic and extrinsic risk factors. Int Wound J 5(2):315–328. https://doi.org/10.1111/j.1742-481X.2008.00452.x
79. Chiari P, Forni C, Guberti M, Gazineo D, Ronzoni S, D'Alessandro F (2017) Predictive factors for pressure ulcers in an older adult population hospitalized for hip fractures: a prognostic cohort study. PLoS One 12(1):e0169909. https://doi.org/10.1371/journal.pone.0169909
80. Pitzul KB, Wodchis WP, Kreder HJ, Carter MW, Jaglal SB (2017) Discharge destination following hip fracture: comparative effectiveness and cost analyses. Arch Osteoporos 12(1):87
81. Leland NE, Gozalo P, Christian TJ, Bynum J, Mor V, Wetle TF, Teno JM (2015) An examination of the first 30 days after patients are discharged to the community from hip fracture postacute care. Med Care 53(10):879–887

Part III

Pillar II: Rehabilitation

Rehabilitation Following Hip Fracture

12

Suzanne M. Dyer, Monica R. Perracini, Toby Smith,
Nicola J. Fairhall, Ian D. Cameron, Catherine Sherrington,
and Maria Crotty

12.1 The Need for Increased Provision of Rehabilitation Worldwide

The World Health Organization has recently highlighted a substantial unmet need for rehabilitation worldwide, with a 2017 Call-to-Action to increase the role of rehabilitation in health care as an essential component of integrated health services [1]. It was acknowledged that there is a profound unmet need for rehabilitation,

---

This chapter is a component of Part 3: Pillar II.
For an explanation of the grouping of chapters in this book, please see Chapter 1: "The multidisciplinary approach to fragility fractures around the world—an overview".

S. M. Dyer · M. Crotty (✉)
Rehabilitation, Aged and Extended Care, College of Medicine and Public Health, Flinders University, Adelaide, SA, Australia
e-mail: sue.dyer@flinders.edu.au; maria.crotty@flinders.edu.au

M. R. Perracini
Universidade Cidade de São Paulo, São Paulo, Brazil
e-mail: monica.perracini@unicid.edu.br

T. Smith
Department of Orthopaedics, Rheumatology and Musculoskeletal Sciences, University of Oxford, Oxford, UK
e-mail: toby.smith@ndorms.ox.ac.uk

N. J. Fairhall · C. Sherrington
Institute for Musculoskeletal Health, The University of Sydney and Sydney Local Health District, Sydney, NSW, Australia
e-mail: nicola.fairhall@sydney.edu.au; cathie.sherrington@sydney.edu.au

I. D. Cameron
John Walsh Centre for Rehabilitation Research, Kolling Institute, Northern Sydney Local Health District, St Leonards, NSW, Australia
e-mail: ian.cameron@sydney.edu.au

© The Author(s) 2021
P. Falaschi, D. Marsh (eds.), *Orthogeriatrics*, Practical Issues in Geriatrics,
https://doi.org/10.1007/978-3-030-48126-1_12

particularly in LMICs. There was a call for greater access to rehabilitation services recognising it as an essential part of the health system rather than an optional extra. Rehabilitation is "an investment in human capital that contributes to health, economic and social development" and there is under-prioritisation by governments with an absence of planning for services at a national and subnational level. The call to action includes "greater awareness and advocacy, increased investment into rehabilitation workforce and infrastructure, and improved leadership and governance structures". This includes increasing networks and partnerships in rehabilitation, particularly between LMICs and high-income countries.

12.2 The Principles of Rehabilitation Programmes after Hip Fracture

After a hip fracture operation, an older person's recovery is enhanced if they are provided with an optimistic, well-coordinated rehabilitation programme. Recovery after hip fracture starts on admission when the patient and family receive realistic information on the likely course and time of discharge. The earlier patient goals and expectations can be explored and information on barriers or supports for recovery of independence identified, the more likely it is that an individual will retain a sense of control and self-efficacy which is likely to be associated with better outcomes [2, 3]. Consistent information on the planned rehabilitation programme is important as most people will have a recovery pathway which extends for several months across hospital and community settings [4].

During the acute hospital stay (ideally on an orthogeriatrics ward), along with secondary prevention treatments for osteoporosis, a rehabilitation pathway should be established and outlined to the patient and family. Rehabilitation involves diagnosing and treating impairments, preventing and treating complications, slowing loss of function and where this is not possible, compensating for lost functions (e.g. prescribing walking aids, bathroom adaptations, additional home help) [5]. Several systematic reviews and meta-analyses have demonstrated that rehabilitation programmes improve outcomes for patients after hip fracture compared to simply letting time take its course [6–8]. However, the components of recovery/rehabilitation programmes vary, including the length of time and the settings where programmes are delivered (home, inpatient units, outpatients). Standard management of hip fracture patients also varies between different countries. An audit in the UK reported that 70% of hip fracture patients receive orthogeriatrician assessment and 92% a falls assessment. These figures were only 27% for orthogeriatrician assessment and 4% for falls assessment in a tertiary hospital in Beijing [9].

In clinical practice, the cornerstone of a rehabilitation approach is a team of various disciplines (physiotherapy, occupational therapy, nutrition, social work, psychology, medicine) who meet regularly, set goals, review progress towards these goals with the patient and assess outcomes. The chance of recovery is maximised if the following elements are incorporated into the clinical approach:

- *Assessment*: identification of problems to be addressed, which involves understanding the premorbid level of functioning and understanding the current comorbidities (e.g. delirium).

- *Goal-setting*: identifying what can be improved and what cannot. In particular, assessing what level of mobility and independence in bathing and dressing is likely to be achieved in the short, medium and long term. Similarly, identifying what informal and formal supports are available to help recovery.
- *Treatment*: intervening to improve medical and functional problems (such as pain, vitamin D deficiency, undernutrition, depression) as well as physical and psychosocial interventions to meet the rehabilitation goals.
- *Evaluation*: reviewing the effectiveness of interventions (i.e. reassessment).
- *Planning*: organising support services; providing self-management strategies for patients and carers.

The World Health Organization (WHO) International Classification of Functioning, Disability and Health (ICF) framework provides a standardised framework for the classification and description of health, functioning and disability [10]. It moves away from the idea that disability is simply the consequence of disease or ageing towards an approach that acknowledges factors created by the social environment and it attempts to explicitly identify barriers and facilitators to social inclusion. Functioning and disability are seen as multidimensional concepts, relating to:

- Body functions (physiological and psychological functions of body systems) and structures (anatomical parts of the body such as organs, limbs and their components);
- Activities people do and the life areas in which they participate;
- Factors in people's environment (physical, social and attitudinal) which can be barriers or facilitators to functioning.

If this approach is applied to a person who suffers a hip fracture, their disability will be assessed and ranked according to the ICF framework components of health domains (e.g. seeing, hearing, walking, memory) and health-related domains (e.g. their ability to access transport, their level of education and social interactions). Figure 12.1 shows an individual's functioning or disability as a dynamic interaction between health conditions and contextual factors, which encompass both environmental and personal factors [10].

12.3 What Is Known about the Pattern of Recovery Following Hip Fracture?

Talking to people with hip fractures and their families and providing realistic information on approximate expected recovery trajectories allows them to plan. However, it is complex for clinicians to apply evidence from cohort studies to individual patients as the cohorts are heterogeneous and patients have received varying amounts and types of rehabilitation.

Cohort studies suggest that following hip fracture, only 40–60% of people who survive are likely to recover their pre-fracture level of mobility [11]. Up to 70% may recover their level of independence for basic activities of daily living, but this is variable and less than half of all people experiencing hip fracture may regain their ability to perform instrumental ADLs. In Western nations, approximately 10–20% of patients move to a residential care facility following hip fracture. The extent to which these outcomes can be improved with greater access to rehabilitation is not clear.

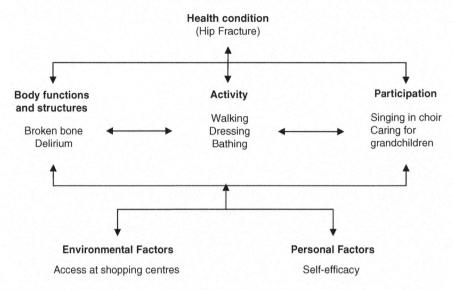

Fig. 12.1 Interactions between the components of the World Health Organization (WHO) International Classification of Functioning, Disability and Health (ICF) framework. *Source*: WHO 2001 [10]

Magaziner et al. described the sequence of recovery across eight different functional abilities following hip fracture [12]. Upper extremity activities of daily living, depression and cognitive function reached maximum recovery within 4 months. Most recovery of gait and balance occurred in the first 6 months, with maximum recovery occurring by 9 months; recovery of instrumental ADLs (such as shopping, preparing meals, house cleaning and handling money) took up to a year. It also took approximately a year for recovery of lower limb function and just over 14 months for walking 3 m without assistance. It seems that the majority of patients who recover their pre-fracture walking and basic activities of daily living do so within the first 6 months after fracture [13], but the role of long-term therapy in recovery pathways is yet to be well investigated.

In LMICs outcomes may be poorer due to reduced rates of optimal management, particularly due to reduced access to rehabilitation services [1]. In many LMICs standard hip fracture management pathways are not established [14]. Barriers to providing rehabilitation services in LMICs are discussed in more detail in Tables 12.10 and 12.11. An audit of practice in China (considered an upper MIC) demonstrated reduced access to surgery and orthogeriatric services at a Beijing hospital in comparison to the United Kingdom [9]. Since that time a retrospective before–after study has demonstrated that improvements in both time to surgery and orthogeriatric management are possible with implementation of a co-management care plan [15].

12.4 Factors Associated with Poor Outcomes After Hip Fracture

Some types of patients with hip fracture appear to be at particular risk of poor outcomes – these include male patients, people living in supported accommodation, those with poorer mobility pre-fracture and those with depression or dementia [13, 16, 17]. People with dementia are also less likely to receive rehabilitation [17, 18]. For people with dementia who receive rehabilitation, improvements comparable to other populations are achievable but this may take longer [19]. Although mortality following hip fracture has been found to be higher in men than women, recovery of mobility is unaffected by gender [17, 20].

Delirium is very common after hip fracture and although it is associated with poorer outcomes, routine assessment by rehabilitation staff remains uncommon [13]. In one prospective study, delirium remained in 39% of people with hip fracture at discharge from hospital and in 32% 1 month after fracture [21]. Even after controlling for pre-fracture physical and cognitive frailty those people who had delirium were twice as likely to have poor functional outcomes (in terms of mobility and recovery of activities of daily living) than those without [21].

Those who are older are more likely to have poorer mobility, need assistance at home, lose their ability to go outside on their own, cook their own dinner and be unable to prepare their own breakfast [17, 20]. Low food intake post-operatively, poor nutrition and malnourishment pre-operatively are associated with worse recovery of mobility and function [22, 23]. A systematic review of nutritional interventions found low-quality evidence to support the effectiveness of multi-nutrient supplements started before or soon after surgery in older people recovering from hip fracture to prevent complications [24]. Amongst nursing home residents, the factors most strongly associated with death or new total mobility dependence are being aged more than 90, having very severe cognitive impairment and receiving non-operative management of the hip fracture [25]. Longer lengths of stay, re-hospitalisation, older age, chronic or acute cognitive deficits and depressive symptoms while in hospital are also predictive of poorer recovery of mobility and activities of daily living [13].

12.5 Key Elements of a Rehabilitation Pathway

After the immediate post-operative period, a rehabilitation pathway should be followed that includes the elements addressed in Table 12.1. In particular, there is a need to assess frailty, establish goals to maximise mobility and other aspects of function, assess the requirement of aids (using occupational therapy services where available) and determine strategies to support and improve independence in activities of daily living [26]. Medication management should ensure all prescribed medications are necessary, minimise the use of antipsychotics and sedatives and ensure adequate pain management. Osteoporosis should be treated as appropriate and falls prevention strategies reinforced with both patients and families.

Table 12.1 Key elements of a typical rehabilitation pathway, based on the Alberta Hip Fracture Restorative Care Pathway [26]

Category of care	
Frailty	Undertake frailty assessment, instigate interventions as appropriate, involve patient in establishing goals to maximise function and achieve safe discharge
Activities of daily living	Ensure progression in recovery of pre-fracture level of independence, aiming for further improvement depending on tolerance
	Assess need for aids and develop strategies to improve independence
	Demonstrate safe transfer using aids and equipment as appropriate
	Ensure there is adequate support in the home environment in terms of assistance from a caregiver or service
	Recommend the family consider a medical alert system if available and appropriate
	Bathing and grooming: Encourage and support independence, bathing and grooming out of bed with assistance if necessary
	Dressing: Support getting out of bed and dressed daily, using dressing aids as necessary
	Toileting: Encourage regular toileting to promote continence, toileting should be in the bathroom, not using bedpans or urinals
	Eating: A high protein/calorie diet should be continued and meals taken in a chair or dining room. An oral nutritional supplement should be considered
	Support for activities of daily living should be provided after discharge. Appropriate home equipment should be provided (mobility aid, raised toilet seat and toilet surround and other items as required)
Mobility	Consider conducting an assessment of mobility/activities of daily living to enable monitoring of recovery of mobility (e.g. the Timed Up and Go test, Barthel Index of Activities of Daily Living)
	Exercise incorporating strengthening, balance and functional components should be continued after discharge
	Walking with or without an aid for at least 50–100 m should be undertaken at least three times daily, or as appropriate depending on pre-fracture mobility
	Capacity to walk the distance required to attend meals in the home setting should be demonstrated
	Ensure ability to manage stairs if necessary and to mobilise safely outside the home in all weather conditions, uneven surfaces, curbs, etc.
	Arrange further mobility training after hospital discharge
Medications	A review of all medications should have been undertaken on admission, polypharmacy should be addressed
	Use of sedatives and antipsychotics should be minimised or ceased and doses should be regularly reviewed
	Medication should be adequate for pain control to enable optimal independence in activities of daily living
Cognitive and mental status	Strategies to prevent and treat delirium should be continued, including ensuring appropriate use of vision and hearing aids, fluid enhancement, orientation, optimising mobility and non-pharmacological sleep supporting strategies. Behaviour monitoring should be undertaken if necessary
	Activity should be encouraged for those with dementia or depression, in terms of ambulation, exercise and social participation
	Caregivers should be provided with support and access to community resources as appropriate
Prevention of further falls/ fractures	Osteoporosis management should be considered if this hasn't already occurred and continued post-discharge
	Fall prevention strategies should be instigated and the use of hip protectors (if available) considered

12.6   What Programmes Should We Recommend to Help with Recovery?

It is widely recognised that a vicious cycle can occur after a hip fracture where pain and hospitalisation result in disuse atrophy of muscles and general deconditioning which increases the risk of immobility and new falls and fractures [27]. While national clinical guidelines recommend providing balance and strengthening exercise [28, 29], it is often unclear how much should be provided, what components of a rehabilitation programme are crucial and how long this programme should be provided for. Analysis of the components of interventions found to be effective in randomised trials can assist in addressing this uncertainty.

The characteristics of all randomised controlled trials of multidisciplinary rehabilitation approaches reporting impact on patient-centred outcomes or mortality (Table 12.2) and exercise and mobility training programmes (Table 12.3), within different settings as identified by systematic review to 2019, are presented below [30, 31]. The quality of the trials is represented with the Physiotherapy Evidence Database (PEDro) score (see https://www.pedro.org.au/), which scores ten items reflecting trial design including randomisation, blinding, balance in baseline characteristics and follow-up. Details of the components of the programmes that have been demonstrated to be effective at improving mobility or function in randomised controlled trials are shown in Table 12.4 (multidisciplinary interventions in hospital or hospital and community setting), Table 12.5 (exercise programmes conducted in hospital settings), Table 12.6 (community-based multidisciplinary interventions) and Table 12.7 (community-based exercise programmes).

12.6.1 In-hospital Rehabilitation

Multidisciplinary programmes have been researched over a long period of time with significant changes to the components of treatment programs. Some trials provide a comparison to a usual care control group while others have a standard rehabilitation programme as the control group. Furthermore, some multidisciplinary programs begin soon after admission (e.g. Prestmo et al. [40]) and others include both in hospital rehabilitation and community components (e.g. Cameron et al. [45]). A 1988 trial demonstrated improvements in function on discharge for provision of multidisciplinary care in comparison to standard orthopaedic care [37].

Table 12.4 shows the characteristics of hospital-based and hospital-plus community-based multidisciplinary rehabilitation interventions in studies with demonstrated effectiveness. Four trials of programmes delivered solely in a hospital setting have demonstrated effectiveness on patient-centred outcomes overall (Table 12.4). One effective in-hospital programme with comprehensive, multidisciplinary geriatric care including early mobilisation, and daily training and a follow-up assessment at 4 months, demonstrated improvements in function at 1 year [42]. Another trial demonstrated improvements in mobility with orthogeriatric care for a subgroup who were living at home [44]. A third trial demonstrated reduced rates of delirium with daily geriatrician visits [38].

Table 12.2 Characteristics of trials of multidisciplinary rehabilitation approaches reporting impact on patient-centred outcomes or mortality

Study	Setting	Sample size	PEDro	Patient-centred outcomes	Characteristics of intervention	Comparator
Hospital-based programmes						
Baroni 2019 [32]	H	430	6[a]	Mortality	Geriatric consultation service	Orthogeriatric comanagement
Chong 2013 [33]	H	162	5[a]	Function, mobility, institutionalisation, mortality, quality of life	Integrated care pathway: Usual care plus structured therapy assessments and checklists	Usual care within multi D team
Fordham 1986 [34]	H	108	5[a]	Poor outcome at discharge,[b] mortality, function, mobility	Joint geriatric and orthopaedic management	Orthopaedic management
Galvard 1995 [35]	H	378	4	Poor outcome at discharge,[b] mortality	Geriatric rehab within geriatric hospital	Usual orthopaedic care
Gilchrist 1988 [36]	H	222	5	Poor outcome at discharge,[b] mortality	Combined geriatric–orthopaedic care in special designated unit	Usual orthopaedic care in orthopaedic ward
Kennie 1988 [37]	H	108	6	Poor outcome at discharge and poor outcome at long-term follow-up,[c] mortality, function	Multi D care in orthopaedic beds at peripheral hospital, plus allied health visits	Usual orthopaedic care in orthopaedic ward, plus allied health
Marcantonio 2001 [38]	H	126	8[a]	Delirium	Proactive geriatrics consultation	Usual care
Naglie 2002 [39]	H	280	7	Poor outcome at long-term follow-up,[d] mortality, function, mobility	Multi D care: Routine post-operative surgical care, daily geriatrician care, allied health, emphasis on prevention, mobilisation, self-care, discharge planning	Usual care on orthopaedic unit
Prestmo 2015 [40]	H	397	6	Mobility, quality of life, function	Comprehensive geriatric care	Usual orthopaedic care
Sanchez Ferrin 1999 [41]	H	206	6[a]	Function, mobility, mortality, institutionalisation	Evaluated by the functional geriatric unit	Usual care

Table 12.2 (continued)

Study	Setting	Sample size	PEDro	Patient-centred outcomes	Characteristics of intervention	Comparator
Stenvall 2007 [42]	H	199	6	Poor outcome at discharge and long-term follow-up,[e] mortality, function, mobility, independent living	Comprehensive geriatric care with assessment at 4-months	Usual care on specialist orthopaedic ward No 4-month assessment
Uy 2008 [43]	H	10	6	Function, mobility	Inpatient multi D rehab programme, using system of accelerated rehab	Usual care (discharge back to NH soon after surgery)
Watne 2014 [44]	H	329	7[a]	Delirium, mortality, mobility	Patients treated in acute geriatric ward: Comprehensive geriatric assessment, daily multi D meetings	Usual care in orthopaedic ward
Hospital- and community-based programmes						
Cameron 1993 [45]	H&C	252	6	Poor outcome at discharge and long-term follow-up,[f] mortality, function	Accelerated rehab and early discharge	Usual care
Crotty 2003 [46]	H&C	66	6	Poor outcome at long-term follow-up,[c] mortality, quality of life, function, mobility	Ambulatory geriatric interdisciplinary rehab programme	Usual care
Huusko 2002 [47]	H&C	260	5	Poor outcome at long-term follow-up,[f] mortality, function	Intensive geriatric rehab in hospital, multi D geriatric team, physio sessions and ongoing treatment at home post-discharge	Discharge to local community hospitals, treatment by GPs, physiotherapists
Jette 1987 [48]	H&C	68	2	Function (ADLs and social function)	Intensive rehab programme: Standard programme plus individualised patient and family education, comprehensive assessment, weekly team meetings, home visit and telephone calls post-discharge	Standard post-surgical rehab programme, including follow-up visits to clinic at 6 weeks, 3, 6, and 12 months post-discharge

(continued)

Table 12.2 (continued)

Study	Setting	Sample size	PEDro	Patient-centred outcomes	Characteristics of intervention	Comparator
Karlson 2016 [49]	H&C	205	8	Mobility, function, delirium, quality of life	Usual care and geriatric multi D home rehab, with aim of early discharge, individually designed, conducted by multi D team, for 10 weeks	Usual care and rehab in geriatric ward with comprehensive geriatric assessment, post-discharge primary HC and outpatient rehab at 3 months as needed
Shyu 2010 [50]	H&C	162	7	Poor outcome at follow-up,[g] function, mortality, mobility, quality of life	Interdisciplinary programme	Usual care on trauma or orthopaedic ward. No follow-up care post-discharge
Shyu 2013 [51]	H&C	299	6[a]	Function	1. Interdisciplinary care 2. Comprehensive care	Usual care: Current routine care of hip fractured elders in Taiwan, no continuation of rehab in home setting
Singh 2012 [52]	H&C	124	5	Function, mortality, residence, mobility, quality of life	Geriatrician supervised, high-intensity resistance exercise and targeted multi D interventions	Standard care: Orthogeriatric care, rehab service and physio
Swanson 1998 [53]	H&C	71	6	Poor outcome at discharge, mortality, mobility, function	Accelerated rehab programme involving multi D team	Standard orthopaedic management. Home visits as needed post-discharge
Vidan 2005 [54]	H&C	321	6	Poor outcome at long-term follow-up,[c] mortality, function, mobility	Multi D care—Geriatric team, assessments, rehab specialist, social worker, comprehensive treatment plan	Usual orthopaedic care. Specialist counselling as required
Ziden 2008 [55]	H&C	102	6	Function, mobility, quality of life	Home Rehab (HR) programme	Conventional Care (CC) and rehab, discharged home or to short-term NH
Community-based programmes						
Crotty 2019 [56]	C	240	7[a]	Mobility, quality of life, function, delirium	Multi D post-op rehab programme within NH	Usual care within NH

Table 12.2   (continued)

Study	Setting	Sample size	PEDro	Patient-centred outcomes	Characteristics of intervention	Comparator
Ryan 2006 [57]	C	71	6	Poor outcome at long-term follow-up,[c] mortality, function	Intensive treatment: ≥6 face-to-face contacts pw from members of a multi D rehab team	Less intensive treatment: ≤3 face-to-face contacts pw with members of multi D rehab team

Note: as identified by systematic review to October 2019. [a]Scored in duplicate by authors

ADLs activities of daily living, *C* community only, *GP* general practitioner, *H* hospital only, *H&C* hospital and community, *HC* health care, *IADLs* instrumental ADLs, *multi D* multidisciplinary, *NA* not available, *NH* nursing home, *physio* physiotherapist/physiotherapy, *post-op* post-operative, *pw* per week, *rehab* rehabilitation

NB Poor outcome = reviewer calculated composite outcome, defined as: [b]mortality at discharge or discharge to more dependent residence/NH, [c]mortality at 12 months or living in more dependent residence/NH, [d]mortality at discharge, discharge to more dependent residence and decline in mobility, [e]mortality at discharge, not discharged to previous residence, not in same residence at 12 months and reduced ADLs, [f]mortality at discharge or discharge to institutional care, mortality at 12 months or institutional care, [g]12-month mortality, admission to institutional care or decline in function

Table 12.3   Characteristics of trials of exercise and mobility training programmes reporting impact on mobility or function outcomes[a]

Study	Setting	Sample size	PEDro	Main mobility outcome	Characteristics of intervention	Comparator
Hospital-based programmes						
Kimmel 2016 [58]	H	92	7	Modified Iowa Level of Assistance (mILOA)	High-intensity functional training	Usual care
Kronborg 2017 [59]	H	90	7	Timed Up and Go	Progressive resistance	Usual care
Mitchell 2001 [30]	H	80	5	Elderly Mobility Scale	High-intensity progressive resistance	Usual care
Monticone 2018 [31]	H	52	7	Western Ontario and McMaster Universities Osteoarthritis Index (WOMAC)	Balance exercises	Usual care/ open kinetic chain exercises in the supine position
Moseley 2009 [60]	H	160	8	PPME	High-intensity weight-bearing	Usual care
Ohoka 2015 [61]	H	27	4	Gait speed	Body weight-supported treadmill training	Usual care
Resnick 2007 [62]	H	208	6	Self-efficacy WES	Exercise plus or exercise only[b]	Usual care
Sherrington 2003 [63]	H	80	7	PPME	Weight-bearing	Non weight-bearing
Van Ooijen 2016 [64]	H	70	5	Elderly Mobility Scale	Treadmill vs. adapted treadmill	Usual care

(continued)

Table 12.3 (continued)

Study	Setting	Sample size	PEDro	Main mobility outcome	Characteristics of intervention	Comparator
Community-based programmes						
Binder 2004 [65]	H&C	90	7	Modified PPT	High-intensity progressive resistance	Low-intensity non-progressive
Hauer 2002 [66]	H&C	28	6	Tinetti's POMA	High-intensity progressive resistance	Placebo motor activity
Langford 2015 [67]	C	30	7	Gait speed	Additional post-discharge physiotherapist telephone support and coaching	Usual care
Latham 2014 [68]	H&C	232	6	SPPB	Home-based exercise	Attention control
Magaziner 2019 [69]	C	210	8[c]	6 min walk distance	Aerobic, strength, balance and functional training	TENS and range-of-motion exercises
Mangione 2005 [70]	C	41	5	6 min walk distance	Resistance or aerobic exercise	Education
Mangione 2010 [71]	C	26	7	6 min walk distance	Home-based resistance	Attention control
Orwig 2011 [72]	C	180	6	Study primary outcome: bone mineral density; mobility: 6 min walk test	Progressive resistance and aerobic	Usual care
Salpakoski 2014 [73]	C	81	8	Short physical performance battery	Progressive resistance, balance and functional	Usual care
Sherrington 1997 [74]	C	42	5	Gait velocity	Weight-bearing	Usual care
Sherrington 2004 [75]	C	120	7	6 m walk time	Weight-bearing or non-weight-bearing	No intervention
Stasi 2019 [76]	C	96	7	Timed Up and Go	Progressive resistance	Usual care
Sylliaas 2011 [77]	C	150	8	6 min walk distance	Progressive resistance	No intervention
Sylliaas 2012 [78]	C	95	8	6 min walk distance	Prolonged resistance	No intervention
Tsauo 2005 [79]	C	54	4	Walking speed	Home-based physiotherapy	Bedside exercise
Williams 2016 [80]	C	61	8	Timed Up and Go	Additional physiotherapy	Usual care

C community only, *H* hospital only, *H&C* hospital and community, *N* no, *PPT* Physical Performance Test, *POMA* Performance Oriented Mobility Assessment, *PPME* Physical Performance Mobility Examination *SPPB* Short Physical Performance Battery, *TENS* transcutaneous electrical nerve stimulation, *WES* Walking Exercise Scale *Y* yes

[a]Based on systematic-review of MEDLINE, EMBASE, CINAHL, CENTRAL and PEDro database search records from inception to April 2019 for randomised controlled trials of exercise-based programmes aiming to improve mobility in older people post-hip fracture reporting data suitable for inclusion in meta-analysis, with a minim PEDro score of 5 or more

[b]Only two out of three comparison groups examined exercise interventions

[c]Scored in duplicate by current authors

Table 12.4 Trials of hospital- and hospital-plus community-based multidisciplinary rehabilitation interventions with demonstrated effectiveness

Study	Participants	Intervention type	Setting	Follow-up times	Outcome effect (95% CI)	Programme length	Control group
Multi D: Hospital only programmes							
Marcantonio 2001 [38]	People aged >65 years	Proactive geriatrics consultation: Daily geriatrician visits, consultation with targeted recommendations based on structured protocol	Acute hospital, USA	During hospital stay	Delirium: RR 0.64 (0.37–0.98) Severe delirium: RR 0.40 (0.18–0.89)	Hospital stay (median LoS 5 days)	Usual care—Management by orthopaedics team, geriatrics consults as needed
Prestmo 2015 [40]	People aged >70 years	Comprehensive geriatric care, structured and systematic interdisciplinary geriatric assessment, focus on physical and mental health, function and social situation, with early discharge planning and early mobilisation and rehab	Central hospital, Norway	1, 4 and 12 months post-surgery	Mean diff (12 months): Mobility (SPPB): 0.69 (0.10–1.28, $p = 0.023$) Function (ADL, Barthel): 1.13 (0.31–1.96, $p = 0.007$) Function IADL: 6.39 (2.59–10.19, $p = 0.001$) QoL (EuroQOL-5D-3L): 0.09 (0.02–0.16, $p = 0.015$)	Hospital stay (mean LoS 12.6 days)	Hospital stay, usual care on orthopaedic ward (mean LoS 11 days)
Stenvall 2007 [42]	People aged ≥70 years 64/N with dementia	Geriatric unit specialising in geriatric orthopaedic care, multi D team providing assessments and rehab, focus on prevention of post-op complications, and early mobilisation, with daily training. Assessment at 4 months for further rehab needs	Teaching hospital, Sweden	On discharge, at 4 and 12 months	Function (12 months): RR 0.65 (0.48, 0.88)	Hospital stay (mean LoS 30 days)	Usual care during hospital stay (mean LoS 40 days)
Watne 2014 [44]	People acutely admitted with hip fracture Subgroup analysis: Participants living in own home at baseline	Acute geriatric ward, key element being use of comprehensive geriatric assessment for treatment planning, plus daily multi D meetings	University hospital, Norway	4 and 12 months	Community-dwelling sub-group[a] (4 months): Mobility (median): CGA 6 vs. con 4 (95% CI for diff 0 to 2; $p = 0.04$)	Hospital stay (median LoS 11 days)	Usual care on orthopaedic ward (median LoS 8 days)

(continued)

Table 12.4 (continued)

Multi D: Hospital and community programmes

Study	Participants	Intervention type	Setting	Follow-up times	Outcome effect (95% CI)	Programme length	Control group
Kennie 1988 [37]	Women aged ≥65 years, surgical repair 51/108 with at least MCI, 35 moderate to severe	Multi D care (GP, geriatrician, orthopaedic specialist) in orthopaedic beds at peripheral hospital. Transferred to rehab ward 0–7 days after trial entry. Patients also received physio, occupational therapy and other services	District hospital, discharged to community, UK	At discharge and 12 months	Poor outcome (12 months): RR 0.48 (0.31, 0.77) Function (more dependent): RR 0.64 (0.46, 0.89)	During hospital stay (mean LoS 37 days), then allied health allied health visits post-discharge similar to usual care	Usual orthopaedic care in orthopaedic ward (a few moved to other short stay wards) (mean LoS 56 days) Patients also received physio, OT and other services
Shyu 2010 [81]	People aged ≥60 years, not severely cognitively impaired One-third with mild cognitive impairment	Interdisciplinary programme— Geriatric consultation, continuous rehab and discharge planning. Early mobilisation. home visits by allied health professionals post-discharge	Teaching hospital, discharged to home, Taiwan	1, 3, 6, 12, 18 and 24 months	Poor function[b] (1 year): RR 0.59 (0.37, 0.95) Mobility (recovery at 2 years): OR 2.72 (11.53–4.84) Function (regression co-eff): $\beta = 9.22$, $p < 0.001$ QoL physical: $\beta = 6.08$, $p < 0.001$	Hospital stay (mean LoS 10.1 days) Usual care + 1 PT session/day (total 4 × ~20 min), 2 × PT assessments, 1 visit rehab physician Post-discharge: one time week 30 min home visits in first month 2 per month in second and third month	Usual care on trauma/orthopaedic ward in Taiwan (mean LoS 9.7 days) Exercises (nurses) in first 2–3 days Sessions varied: 3 sessions ($N = 18$), or 1 session (remainder) Discharge ~7 days from surgery No post-discharge care

Shyu 2013 [51]	People aged ≥60 years, admitted to hospital for fracture from home setting	Comprehensive care model: In addition to interdisciplinary care (geriatric consultation, comprehensive assessment, rehab programme, discharge planning, post-hospital services), also included nutrition consultation, depression management, fall prevention	Hospital and in patients' home, Taiwan	At discharge 1, 3, 6 and 12 months	Function (self-care, 0–12 months): OR 3.19 (1.47–6.89)	Rehab started on first day after surgery, and continued for 1 year in patients' home Mean LoS 8.34 days	Usual care in Taiwan. Average of 1.89 physical therapy sessions in hospital, no continuation of rehab in home setting Mean LoS 8.47 days
Singh 2012 [52]	People aged >55 years with sufficient cognitive ability	HIPFIT intervention: Geriatrician-supervised high-intensity weight-lifting exercise and targeted treatment of balance, osteoporosis, nutrition, vitamin D/calcium, depression, cognition, vision, home safety, polypharmacy, hip protectors, self-efficacy and social support	Public teaching hospital and surrounding geriatric and rehab hospitals, Australia	4 and 12 months	Mobility (assistive devices) relative effect size: −0.45 (−0.86, −0.04) Admission to institution (age-adjusted): OR 0.16 (0.04–0.64) Mortality (age-adjusted): OR 0.19 (0.04–0.91)	In addition to usual care, 80 supervised Exercise training sessions, 10 home visits, and 10 phone calls over 12 months	Standard care in area health service, including orthogeriatric care, rehabilitation service, allied health as required, and physio
Swanson 1998 [53]	People aged ≥55 years, independent and mobile None with dementia	Accelerated rehab programme: Multi D team (orthopaedic surgeon, geriatrician, nurse-coordinator, physio, other allied health). Early surgery, less analgesia, early mobilisation, intense physio, weekly case conference, home assessment before discharge, community services referrals. Follow-up 1 and 6 months post-discharge	Teaching hospital, discharged to home, Australia	At discharge and 6 months	Poor outcome (at discharge): RR 0.50 (0.16, 1.55)	During length of hospital stay (mean LoS 20.8 days), plus 6 months post-discharge	Standard orthopaedic management, daily physio visits, weekly discharge planning during stay. Mean LoS 32.6 days Home visits as needed post-discharge

(continued)

Table 12.4 (continued)

Study	Participants	Intervention type	Setting	Follow-up times	Outcome effect (95% CI)	Programme length	Control group
Ziden 2008 [55]	People aged ≥65 years	Home rehabilitation programme, on admission and after discharge: Early goal-setting, close cooperation with relatives, social home services, focus on early discharge, individual design, physio home visits (focus on self-efficacy and walking outdoors)	University hospital, Sweden	At discharge, at 1, 6, and 12 months	1-year median (range) Function (ADLs and IDLs: Home rehab 85 (46–91) vs. Con 80 (29–91); $P < 0.001$ Function (IADLs): Home rehab 27.0 (0–40) vs. Con 20.0 (0–42); $P = 0.028$	Median home visits 4.5 over 3 weeks post-discharge	Conventional care and rehab, discharged home with no continuing organised rehab or to short-term NH. Participation in standard rehab programme with physio and OT

ADLs activities of daily living, *CI* confidence Interval, *diff* difference, *GP* general practitioner, *IADLs* instrumental ADLs, *LoS* length of stay, *MCI* mild cognitive impairment, *multi D* Multidisciplinary, *NH* nursing home, *OR* odds ratio, *physio* physiotherapist, *OT* occupational therapy, *PT* physical therapy, *rehab* rehabilitation, *QoL* quality of life, *RR* risk ratio, *SPPB* short physical performance battery

[a]Trial effectiveness overall not significant

[b]Non-recovery of function/decline in walking

Table 12.5 Trials of hospital-based exercise and mobility training programmes with demonstrated effectiveness on mobility or function[a]

Study	Participants	Intervention type	Setting Adherence	Outcome effect size SMD (95% CI)	Programme dose	Control group	Control programme dose
Exercise: Hospital only programmes							
Mitchell 2001[b] [30]	People ≥65, mobile ± aid pre-fracture, AMT score ≥ 6	Early post-op, high-intensity bilateral quadriceps muscle strengthening (6 × 12 reps knee extension) progressive from 50% (weeks 1 and 2), 70% (weeks 3 and 4) to 80% (weeks 5 and 6), plus conventional physiotherapy	Rehabilitation unit, supervised, UK Median no. sessions completed (11, range 10–12)	Function: 1.33 (0.67, 1.99)	6 weeks, 2 × pw 30 min[c] Total: 6 h	Conventional physiotherapy	U weeks, 5 × pw, 20 min Total: U
Monticone 2018 [31]	People aged >70 years, MMSE >23, no major recent medical events	Balance task-specific exercises in standing (open and closed eyes, proprioceptive and balance-challenging tasks), 90-min sessions, five times per week for 3 weeks. Walking on a rectilinear trajectory while changing speed and direction, or while performing additional exercises: Gait training (changes in speed and direction, motor-cognitive tasks), sit to stand, stairs and climbing obstacles	Rehabilitation unit, individual sessions supervised by physiatrist/ physiotherapist, Italy	Mobility: 1.91 (1.25, 2.58) Function: 1.31 (0.71, 1.92)	3 weeks, 5 × pw, 90 min Total: 22.5 h	General physiotherapy, including open kinetic chain exercises and walking training. Individual sessions supervised by physiatrist/ physiotherapist	3 weeks, 5 × pw, 90 min Total: 22.5 h

Diff difference, *MMSE* Mini-Mental State Examination, *pw* per week, *SMD* standardised mean difference, *wks* weeks, *U* unclear

[a]Based on analysis at end of intervention period

[b]Weeks, calculated as 1 month = 4 weeks (thus 6 months = 24 weeks)

[c]Estimated

Table 12.6 Characteristics of community-based multidisciplinary rehabilitation interventions in trials with demonstrated effectiveness

Study	Participants	Intervention type	Setting	Follow-up times	Effect: mean difference (95%CI)	Programme length	Control group
Crotty 2019 [56]	People aged ≥70 years, living in long-term care prior to injury, ready for discharge	Ambulatory geriatric interdisciplinary rehabilitation programme. Patients received visits from a hospital outreach team who provided a comprehensive geriatrics assessment, physio (mobility and task specific training), training of care staff and family	Recruitment in hospital, delivered in long-term care, Australia	4 weeks and 12 months	Mobility (NHLSD, 4 weeks): −1.9 (−3.3 to −0.57) QoL DEMQOL (1 year): −7.4 (−12.5 to −2.3) Mortality (4 weeks): Int 8% vs. Con 18% ($p = 0.048$)	4 weeks duration (total 13 h), commencing within 24 h of return to facility	Usual care

DEMQOL Dementia Quality of Life measure, *diff* difference, *h* hour/s, *NHLSD* Nursing Home Life-Space Diameter, *physio* physiotherapist, *QoL* Quality of Life

Table 12.7 Trials of community-based exercise and mobility training programmes with demonstrated effectiveness on mobility or function[a]

Study	Participants	Intervention type	Setting	Effect size SMD (95%CI)	Programme dose[b]	Control group	Control programme dose[b]
Binder 2004 [65]	People ≥65 years, living in community, physically frail	Standard physical therapy, then high-intensity programme of balance, co-ordination and strength exercises with progressive resistance training added after 3 months	Hospital and community rehabilitation, small groups (2–5) led by physical therapist, indoors, USA	Mobility: 0.83 (0.37, 1.29) Function: 0.44 (0, 0.87)	24 weeks, 3 × pw, 45–90 min Total: 81 h	Home-based, low-intensity non-progressive, plus monthly group sessions and weekly 10 min calls	24 weeks, 3 × pw, time NR Total: U
Hauer 2002 [66]	Women aged ≥75 years, recent history of injurious falls	High-intensity progressive resistance training of functionally relevant muscle groups (70–90% max workload), progressive training of functions such as walking, stepping or balancing, started on discharge Additional physio two times week for 25 min	Hospital and community. Small groups (4–6) led by therapeutic recreation specialist, Germany	Mobility (3 months): 1.36 (0.45, 2.26)	12 weeks, 3 × pw, 135 min[c] Total: 81 h	Group-based, placebo motor activity e.g. flexibility exercise, ball games, memory tasks Additional physio two times week for 25 min	12 weeks, 3 × pw, 60 min Total: 36 h
Latham 2014 [68]	≥60 years, functional limitation, able to sit to stand without mobility aid, discharged from rehab ≤20 months of baseline	Home-based exercise, repeating simple functional tasks, using Thera-bands for resistance plus standing exercises using steps of varying height and weighted vests (based on INVEST [84] and Sherrington and Lord [74]). Included cognitive and behavioural strategies addressing exercise, fear of falling and goal setting	Hospital and home-based exercise taught over 3–4 visits of approx. 1 h by physical therapist, with fourth if necessary plus monthly phone calls, USA	Mobility (6 months): 0.33 (0.05, 0.61)	24 weeks, 3 × pw, 60 min Total: 72 h	Attention control, cardiovascular nutrition education by registered dieticians, frequency of contact matched to intervention group	—

(continued)

Table 12.7 (continued)

Study	Participants	Intervention type	Setting	Effect size SMD (95%CI)	Programme dose[b]	Control group	Control programme dose[b]
Stasi 2019 [76]	Community-dwelling, able to walk outdoors for two blocks	Progressive resistance, hip abductor strength training standing and side lying, resistance progressed with cuff weights and loop elastic bands, 2 × 10 reps, progressing to 3 × 15 reps, increasing from 40 to 55 min. Approx. 10 min extra per supervised session commencing week 4, commenced week 6 in control group	Hospital and community, additional intensive resistance programme per supervised session commencing week 4, Greece	Mobility: 3.36 (2.73, 3.99) Function: 1.28 (0.84, 1.72)	12 weeks, 7 × week, 40–55 min Total: 70 h	Standard physiotherapy, daily 1 week in hospital, 11 weeks at home 3 × week supervised, 4 × week independently. Additional resistance from week 6	12 weeks, 7 × pw, 30–45 min Total: 52.5 h
Sylliaas 2011 [77]	People ≥65 years, living at home, ≥23 on MMSE	Progressive resistance (3 × 15 reps at 70% 1-RM weeks 1–3, then 80% with reducing reps maintained at ≥8, increased 3-weekly). 3–6 months after fracture. 10–15 min bike or treadmill warm-up, then standing knee flexion, lunge, sitting knee extension and leg press. Knee flexion and lunge with loading if tolerated Plus advice to walk 30 min per day if tolerated	Two times weekly in outpatient clinic, supervised by physiotherapist, One time weekly home based, Norway	Mobility: 0.51 (0.17, 0.86) Function: 0.37 (0.03, 0.72)	12 weeks, 3 × pw, 45-60 min Total: 32 h[d]	Usual lifestyle, no restrictions on exercise activities	–
Sylliaas 2012 [78]	People ≥65, living at home, ≥23 on MMSE, completed intervention arm of Sylliaas 2011 (12 week programme)	Extended training following from Sylliaas 2011. Prolonged resistance training (at 80% 1-RM, increased 3-weekly). Exercise components as per Sylliaas 2011	One time weekly in outpatient clinic with physiotherapist, One time weekly home based, Norway	Mobility: 1.52 (1.06, 1.97)	24 weeks,[e] 2 × pw, 45–60 min Total: 53 h[d]	Usual lifestyle, no restrictions on exercise activities	–

AMT Abbreviated Mental Test, *h* hour, *equiv* equivalent between both trial arms, *h* hours, *max* maximum, *min* minutes, *MMSE* Mini-Mental State Examination, *pw* per week, *NR* not reported, *1-RM* one-repetition maximum, *SD* standard deviation, *SMD* standardised mean difference, *U* unclear, *wks* weeks

[a] With a minim PEDro score of 5 or more

[b] Calculated as 1 month = 4 weeks (thus 6 months = 24 weeks)

[c] Including breaks

[d] Determined based on average session time of 52.5 min

[e] 12 weeks plus previous 12 week programme of Sylliaas 2011

A more recent hospital-based trial has demonstrated effectiveness on a range of person-centred outcomes including mobility, function and quality of life at 1-year follow-up in comparison to standard orthopaedic care [40]. This programme provided comprehensive interdisciplinary care, early mobilisation and rehabilitation and also addressed psychosocial aspects of care through a focus on social situation and mental health.

Two exercise programmes that have demonstrated effectiveness in terms of improving mobility or function were delivered completely in an in-hospital (rehabilitation) setting (Table 12.5) [30, 31]. One study added progressive resistance training in the form of additional early post-operative, high-intensity bilateral quadriceps muscle strengthening to conventional physiotherapy. A significant improvement in the Elderly Mobility Scale, leg extensor power of the fractured leg and functional reach was reported at 16 weeks, which was 10 weeks after the end of the intervention [30]. The other programme which delivered a high dose of in-patient rehabilitation including supervised balance exercises (five times weekly for 90 min, over 3 weeks), also demonstrated improvements in mobility and function compared to standard rehabilitation on discharge [31].

12.6.2 Rehabilitation in the Community

Six multidisciplinary interventions delivered across both hospital and community settings have demonstrated improvements in patient-centred outcomes in comparison to usual orthopaedic care (Table 12.4) [37, 50–53, 55]. Four of these trials were conducted in high income countries [37, 52, 53, 55] and two were conducted in Taiwan [51, 81]. In general, multidisciplinary programmes that emphasise early assessment through comprehensive geriatric assessment with appropriate early surgery, early mobilisation, higher doses of mobility training and an emphasis on regaining functional independence are more effective. Multidisciplinary rehabilitation programmes (including those with a focus on multidisciplinary factors where specialist teams are not available) should also begin soon after hospital admission and continue for a long period, including after hospital discharge.

It remains unclear what is the best link between orthogeriatric services and hip fracture rehabilitation services to improve coordination for patients, but common governance structures, shared staff, shared information systems or formal arrangements for handovers are all options. These services should treat patients with dementia and delirium and also include patients who are living in, or will live in, residential aged care facilities. High intensity and prolonged multidisciplinary rehabilitation programmes (e.g. Singh et al. [52]) are effective for a selected group of people with hip fracture.

There is an emerging view that hip fracture rehabilitation programmes should also be available to people with significant dementia who live in long-term care, or at home, with severe disabilities. A recent trial of a four-week multidisciplinary programme delivered as a hospital outreach programme within long-term care demonstrated improvements in mobility at the end of the programme, which was not maintained over 12 months, but a small improvement in quality of life was observed at 12 months (Table 12.6) [56]. Whilst the programme was found not to be cost-effective, it demonstrates that improvements in patient-centred outcomes can be made after hospital discharge in a population living in long-term care.

As shown in Table 12.7, the exercise programmes that continued after discharge and were effective were programmes conducted over 12–24 weeks. At least for some individuals, there are benefits from exercise programmes delivered after discharge from hospital. One of the most effective programmes identified in our review of trials of exercise and mobility training programmes was implemented as twice-weekly sessions with a physiotherapist in an outpatient clinic for the first 3 months, then once weekly for a further 3 months (Table 12.7) [77, 78]. This was supplemented with exercises once a week at home. The exercise programme involved prolonged progressive resistance training, fitness warm-up and lower limb strength exercises, compared to a control group of the participant's usual lifestyle, without any restrictions placed on the amount or type of exercise undertaken. This programme significantly improved patient's mobility after 3 months [77], but the magnitude of the effect was even greater after 6 months [78]. While the strength of effect in this study may partly be due to a comparison against patients with no structured exercise programme, two other community-based programmes of progressive resistance training in small groups also demonstrated large effects in comparison to alternative programmes [65, 66]. Another study has demonstrated that extra progressive resistance exercises in addition to a 12-week standard daily physiotherapy programme can provide additional benefits for mobility and function [76].

However, long-term provision of exercise programmes through outpatient clinics for whole populations may not be feasible, even in developed countries, as this would require an enormous expansion of rehabilitation services with associated costs. Greater provision of community exercise options in liaison with health professionals may help to meet this gap, as has been recommended for people with neurological impairments [82].

12.6.3 Rehabilitation in Low Resource Settings

A trial conducted in Taiwan has demonstrated significant improvements in mobility and self-care extending to 2 years post-hip fracture from interdisciplinary rehabilitation programmes in comparison to usual care with no formal rehabilitation programme [81]. A further trial demonstrated additional benefits of a comprehensive care programme addressing nutrition, depression management and falls prevention in addition to interdisciplinary care in the same setting [51]. Whilst the same interdisciplinary care may not be possible in low resource and LMIC settings, rehabilitation programmes that address these principles using professionals with competencies in geriatrics, orthopaedics, physiotherapy, occupational therapy, nutrition, social work and psychology should be the aim.

Supervised exercise programmes may present access difficulties for people in remote locations or in low resource settings so home exercise, wider family involvement or tele-rehabilitation options may be required.

A home-based exercise programme of simple, functionally oriented tasks with minimal supervision had a moderate effect on improving physical function [68]. In this programme, a physical therapist taught the exercises and used cognitive and behavioural strategies to enhance attitudes and beliefs about the benefits of exercise and to overcome fear of falling during three home visits of 1 h (Table 12.7). Monthly telephone calls were also made by the therapists and an additional visit was provided if necessary. The participants were provided with a DVD of the programme to watch and a DVD player if necessary. Participants performed the exercises independently in their own home three times a week for 6 months, supported by a monthly telephone call from the physical therapist. The intervention also included a cognitive-behavioural component in order to improve adherence. A secondary analysis of this trial indicates that self-efficacy may partially mediate the effects of this intervention on longer term functional outcomes [83]. Whilst physical therapists may not be available in all resource settings, this trial demonstrates the potential effectiveness of home-based therapy. Alternative professionals with skills in physical therapy could provide training. Including caregivers in this training, where resources for watching a DVD and follow-up phone calls are not available, appears promising and warrants investigation.

12.7   Rehabilitation and Cognitive Impairment

Rehabilitation for people with dementia after hip fracture is complex. Approximately 40% of patients who sustain a hip fracture have dementia [85, 86]. These patients have more complex care needs, with greater risks of complications, physical disabilities and social care requirements compared to people without dementia [87]. This is due to a number of factors. Firstly, people with dementia are often more disorientated in hospital environments, being more prone to delirium. They often have difficulty expressing problems of pain, nausea and dizziness which impact on physical performance. Many people with dementia have movement limitations, which when combined with hip fracture, makes simple tasks like learning how to use walking aids and equipment very difficult. They often have a critical relationship with informal caregivers (family/friends) which is strained after a hip fracture; greater considerations for supporting the patient–caregiver dyad may be required than for patients without dementia. Daily proactive geriatrician visits starting before or within 24 h of hip fracture surgery, with application of multiple types of treatment, has been demonstrated to reduce delirium occurrence by 36%, and severe delirium by 60% [38]. Similar principles could be followed in LMIC settings with lesser intensity of inputs.

A number of research reports and guidelines recommend intervention with specific strategies including enhanced rehabilitation and care pathways to support recovery from hip fracture for people living with dementia. However, the evidence base for these is sparse. Five trials have investigated enhanced rehabilitation models for this population; evaluating strategies designed specifically for people with dementia following hip fracture surgery. These are larger trials of patients following hip fracture surgery which have presented data specifically for the subgroup of patient with cognitive impairment. These trials have tested two types of interventions: enhanced interdisciplinary inpatient rehabilitation and care models versus conventional

inpatient rehabilitation and care models [43, 88, 89] and secondly, enhanced interdisciplinary inpatient and home-based rehabilitation and care models versus conventional rehabilitation and care models [90, 91]. The characteristics of these trials and
interventions are presented in Table 12.8. The enhanced models generally offer multidisciplinary programmes with greater intensity or length of programmes.

Table 12.8 Characteristics of trials of enhanced rehabilitation for people with dementia following hip fracture

Study	Setting country	Sample size	PEDro	Characteristics of intervention	Comparator
Hospital-based enhanced rehabilitation programmes					
Freter 2017 [88]	Hospital, Canada	283	4	Delirium-friendly care options including: Orientation strategies; night-time sedation, analgesia, and nausea; attention to catheter removal and bowel movements	Standard recovery programme
Stenvall 2012 [89]	Hospital, Sweden	64	6	MultiD team intervention: Individual care planning, monitoring for specific common complications (falls, delirium, bowel and bladder care, sleep, pain, pressure sores, physiological markers and nutrition), early inpatient rehabilitation with increased staffing ratio	Non-formalised and inconsistent provision of team working, individualised care planning, rehabilitation or complication monitoring. Prevention and treatment of decubitus ulcers, pain management and basic care, but no dietitian review
Uy 2008 [43]	Hospital, Australia		8	Early mobility and self-care (nurse delivered). Target of twice-daily physiotherapy with greater multiD team involvement in mobility and enablement	Standard recovery programme
Hospital- and community-based enhanced rehabilitation programmes					
Huusko 2000 [90]	H&C Finland	141	7	Enhanced multi D team rehabilitation including two times daily physiotherapy, multiD team meetings and improved communication across the team and with patients. Plus discharge planning and ten home-based physiotherapy sessions	Standard recovery programme. All participants encouraged to mobilise on the first post-operative day. No further information provided
Shyu 2012 [91]	H&C Taiwan	160	6	Enhanced multiD team, two times daily physio, multiD team meetings, improved communication and individualise care. Plus individualised discharge planning, three home-based physio and eight home-based nurse visits	Standard recovery programme. Inpatient rehabilitation consisted of 3 physiotherapy sessions, and no in-home rehabilitation. No further information provided

C community, *H* hospital, *H&C* hospital and community, *MultiD* multidisciplinary, *physio*
physiotherapy

12.7.1   Enhanced Interdisciplinary Inpatient Rehabilitation and Care

The clinical outcomes of enhanced inpatient rehabilitation care compared to conventional care are summarised in Table 12.9. It appears there was no benefit of enhanced interdisciplinary inpatient rehabilitation over conventional care for outcomes including personal ADL independence at four-month or 12-month follow-up, walking independence without an aid or assistance at four-month or 12-month

Table 12.9 Clinical outcomes of enhanced rehabilitation interventions for people with dementia following hip fracture

Outcome measure	Time-point (months)	Participants	Study	Outcome OR/MD (95% CI)
In-patient enhanced rehabilitation programmes				
Personal activities of daily living independence	4	54	Stenvall 2012 [89]	OR 4.14 (0.40–42.66)
	12	47	Stenvall 2012 [89]	OR 4.62 (0.18–119.63)
Walking independence without an aid or assistance	4	54	Stenvall 2012 [89]	OR 7.63 (0.83–70.53)
	12	47	Stenvall 2012 [89]	OR 7.20 (0.74–70.42)
Mortality	Discharge	151	Freter 2016; Stenvall 2012; Uy 2008 [43, 88, 89]	OR 0.62 (0.22–1.74)
Hospital Length of Stay	Discharge	141	Freter 2016; Stenvall 2012 [88, 89]	MD −3.24 (−8.75 to 2.26)
In-patient and community-based enhanced rehabilitation programmes				
Mortality	3	184	Huusko 2000; Shyu 2012 [90, 91]	OR 1.20 (0.36–3.93)
	12	177	Huusko 2000; Shyu 2012 [90, 91]	OR 1.07 (0.47–2.45)
Requirement of institutional care	3	184	Huusko 2000; Shyu 2012 [90, 91]	OR 0.46 (0.22–0.95)
	12	177	Huusko 2000; Shyu 2012 [90, 91]	OR 0.90 (0.40–2.03)
Regained their pre-fracture walking capability	3	43	Shyu 2012 [91]	OR 5.10 (1.29–20.17)
	12	36	Shyu 2012 [91]	OR 58.33 (3.04–1118.19)
	24	30	Shyu 2012 [91]	OR 3.14 (0.68–14.50)
ADL performance	3	43	Shyu 2012 [91]	MD 18.81 (9.40–28.22)
	12	36	Shyu 2012 [91]	MD 25.40 (10.89–39.91)
	24	30	Shyu 2012 [91]	MD 7.92 (−9.88 to 25.72)
	12	36	Shyu 2012 [91]	OR 0.20 (0.01–4.47)
	24	30	Shyu 2012 [91]	OR 0.77 (0.16–3.74)

CI confidence interval *MD* mean difference *OR* odds ratio

follow-up or the number of drugs prescribed on discharge. Similarly, there were no differences in outcomes for mortality or hospital length of stay for enhanced inpatient rehabilitation models over conventional care.

There was no benefit of an enhanced inpatient rehabilitation programme over conventional rehabilitation for complications including pneumonia, pressure ulcers, postoperative fracture or whether participants were living in care facilities at 4 months or 12 months. However, there was a reduction in the enhanced interdisciplinary rehabilitation care model group for complications including urinary tract infection, nutritional problems, recurrent falls and post-operative delirium. Freter and colleagues also reported greater cognitive function for those who received the enhanced intervention 5 days post-operatively compared to conventional rehabilitation [88].

12.7.2 Enhanced Interdisciplinary Inpatient and Home-Based Rehabilitation

The clinical outcomes of enhanced rehabilitation inpatient and home-based rehabilitation care compared to conventional care are summarised in Table 12.9. Findings suggest that enhanced inpatient and community-based interventions for people with cognitive impairment provide promising early outcomes, but do not differ to conventional rehabilitation models longer term. Whilst people allocated enhanced interdisciplinary rehabilitation were less likely to be living in institutional care at 3 months, this was less certain at 12 months. One trial conducted in Taiwan reported that patients who received enhanced rehabilitation strategies until 3 months post-discharge had improvements in regaining pre-fracture walking levels and better ADL performance at 3 and 12 months, but did not differ from conventional rehabilitation at 24 months [91]. The evidence suggests no benefit of the enhanced inpatient and home-based intervention for outcomes including frequency of hospital admissions, attendance at the emergency room/accident and emergency, incidence of falls or mortality at 4 or 12 months post-operatively.

Whilst the current evidence-base provides a basis, the data remain very low in quality due to the small number of participants and the serious risk of bias in trial designs. The evidence underpinning the rehabilitation of people with dementia following hip fracture is based on subgroup analyses of randomised controlled trials of people with and without cognitive impairment who have a hip fracture. Consequently, the evidence-base is underpowered. No data were provided on behaviour, quality of life, pain or complications. No trials have investigated interventions which have been specifically designed for people with cognitive impairment. It remains unclear whether rehabilitation models are more effective if they include dementia-focused interventions such as provision of cues, reminiscence therapy, the adoption of familiarised routines or the use of assistive technologies. These are areas of research priority. Following this, it is hoped that health professionals will be able to be more evidence-based in addressing the complex care needs for this subgroup of the hip fracture population.

Nevertheless, it is clear that patients with cognitive impairment also benefit from rehabilitation approaches and these patients should not be excluded from rehabilitation following hip fracture.

12.8 Psychosocial Factors and Rehabilitation

Within the WHO ICF framework, psychosocial factors can be environmental or personal "contextual" factors (e.g. social support, self-efficacy, fear of falling) or psychological "body function" factors (e.g. mental health) that interact with health conditions to impact on a person's functioning and recovery. Psychosocial factors are predictors of hip fracture recovery and their role in functional recovery after hip fracture has been acknowledged as important [92]. Depressive symptoms post hip fracture increase the likelihood of poorer mobility, function and psychological outcomes [92–94]. Fear of falling is common in people with hip fracture and is associated with poorer recovery, decreased mobility, anxiety and falls-related self-efficacy [95–97]. Social support and caregiver responses also appear to play a dynamic role in recovery [98, 99]. However, the relationships between psychosocial factors, rehabilitation programmes and outcomes are complex and inadequately understood.

Clinicians need to support patients' adjustment to residual disability when providing rehabilitation to people with fragility fractures. Hip fractures are common and many older people in the community hold the fear that a hip fracture will precipitate a move into a residential aged care facility. In an Australian time–trade-off study, 80% of community-dwelling women at risk of hip fracture said they would rather die rather than suffer a hip fracture requiring relocation into a residential aged care facility [100]. The participants of this study commonly believed that they were living on "borrowed time" having survived beyond usual life expectancy. They perceived any threat to their ability to live independently in the community as potentially catastrophic.

When individuals experience changes in their health states, they often alter their internal standards, their values and concept of quality of life which is sometimes described as a "response shift" [101]. After a hip fracture, many people are left walking with an aid, with restrictions in the use of public transport, hobbies and roles, thus a significant loss of quality of life may occur. Maximising functional recovery is important but providing adequate support for older people to make "response shifts" and adjustments and to identify ways to compensate for changes is equally important e.g. by acknowledging losses in mobility but providing access to alternatives.

A randomised controlled trial of a home-based hip fracture rehabilitation intervention which included psychological strategies improved mobility outcomes for patients [68, 83]. The study found that the intervention protected against the loss of self-efficacy. As self-efficacy appears to play a crucial role in maintaining exercise long-term, a focus on self-efficacy in hip fracture interventions may mean that patients are more likely to continue activity independently [83]. Qualitative studies indicate that hip fracture patients recognise the importance of their own psychological outlook and the need for social support in their recovery. Support from health professionals provides not only information and exercises but also emotional and motivational support and confidence boosting. Support from informal caregivers, family and friends is also seen as invaluable to help with ADLs, emotional support, encouragement and companionship [95, 102, 103]. Thus, inclusion of psychological and social interventions in hip fracture rehabilitation programmes is likely to be beneficial. However, the specifics of how to best design such programmes to improve outcomes are yet unclear [92].

12.9 Delivery of Rehabilitation Following Hip Fracture in LMICs

The prevalence of hip fracture is expected to increase dramatically in middle-income countries in Asia and Latin America, presenting a major challenge to rehabilitation care in coming years. By the year 2050, around 30% of the world's hip fractures will occur in Asia, mostly in China and India. Although the rate of increase in incidence of hip fracture has been attenuated in Hong Kong and Taiwan, it has markedly increased for almost all age groups in both genders in mainland China [104]. India lacks a systematic data registry for fragility hip fractures, but a report in 2004 estimated an annual prevalence of 600,000 hip fractures, which will substantially increase, since the population over 60 years in 2026 will reach nearly 170 million people [105].

Overall hip fractures in the Latin America region will increase by 700% in the population 65 and over with an estimated cost of $13 billion [106]. Based on population ageing estimates in Brazil the increase of hip fracture prevalence is estimated to be nearly 250% between 2015 and 2040 [107]. In Mexico, another highly-populated country, hip fracture rate estimates are sparse, but one study showed similar rates to southern countries in Europe [108].

The impact of hip fractures is unfavourable for patients and their families in LMICs as many do not have health care systems which are able to deliver integrated services including rehabilitation. Barriers exist in terms of human resources capability, infrastructure, cultural and social influences and environmental context.

While research on barriers and facilitators for rehabilitation following hip fracture is still scarce in most LMICs, Tables 12.10 and 12.11 describe known barriers to prompt in-hospital and community rehabilitation following hip fracture surgery in LMICs.

Table 12.10   Barriers to prompt in-hospital rehabilitation following hip fracture surgery in LMICs

Barrier category	Items	Examples
Environmental context and resources	*Delayed surgery* • Long distances to find a proper trauma centre • Lack of ambulance service in rural areas • Overwhelmed public hospitals (scarcity of beds) • Fixed operative days of surgeons • Multiple poorly controlled comorbidities • Bias against admitting frail patients with multiple co-morbidities, pressure sores and those who carry high risks for surgery *Delayed or insufficient mobilisation and functional independence training* • Surgeon's choice of a conservative approach e.g. restricting weight-bearing • Lack of human resources (physiotherapists, occupational therapists, nurses) • Surgery on Fridays with no physiotherapists on weekends • Lack of co-management by orthopaedic and geriatric medicine (geriatric wards or comprehensive geriatric care units or geriatric consulting services) • Lack of in-patient rehabilitation services • Lack of falls prevention programmes *Lack of coordinated discharge plan and referral* • Fragmentation of services and poor transition home programmes. • Lack of caregiving training programmes prior to discharge	Presentation and surgery times: *India:* Patients travelled a mean of 86.4 km to trauma services; 86% patients presented to hospital ≥1 day after fracture (mean 18 days), 10% operated in ≤24 h [109] *Colombia:* 52% patients operated in 1–3 days, 40% 4–6 days, 8% ≥7 days [110] *Beijing:* 8% operated in ≤48 h [9] *Brazil:* Mean 3 days between fracture admission; waiting time for surgery 5.8 days. Nearly 70% operation >48 h [111] *Chile:* Time between admission and surgery 19.3 days, 7% surgery in ≤5 days [112] Assessment: *Colombia:* 64% not evaluated by physiotherapists in hospital [110] *Beijing:* 3.8% falls risk assessment, 22% orthogeriatric assessment [9] *India:* 10% fall-risk assessment, no orthogeriatric care [105] Rehabilitation: WHO: LMICs have scarcity of rehabilitation professionals, many have <10 skilled practitioners per one million population [113] Post-discharge: *Colombia:* Common complaint is lack of interventions to prepare families and patients for discharge to home [110] *China:* Most difficult tasks for family caregivers were providing assistance for stair climbing, emotional problems, management, walking training, rehabilitation and emergency disease management [114, 115]
Cultural and social	*Delayed surgery* • Lack of knowledge or information of family members about the urgency of a fall-injury event • Patients' beliefs in traditional bone healers and aversion to surgical interventions *Burden of family caregivers* • Low socioeconomic background and social vulnerability	*India:* Most patients and relatives had no knowledge of the consequences of hip fracture injury in older people [109] *Internationally:* Family financial overload related to medical appointments, private rehabilitation and transport [115]

(continued)

Table 12.10 (continued)

Barrier category	Items	Examples
Human resources capability	*Delayed surgery* • Untrained health care professionals in primary and secondary care services *Delayed mobilisation and functional independence training* • Evidence-based recommendation of early mobilisation, pain and delirium management, and fall risk assessment is not in routine care yet • Lack of training for nurses, physiotherapists and occupation therapists • Lack of a coordinated multidisciplinary approach • Failure to assess frailty and patients' previous and ongoing cognitive status with consequently limited access to appropriate and timely rehabilitation interventions • Poor attitude or bias against patients who are very old and/or with cognitive decline due to belief that outcomes will be disappointing and rehabilitation ineffective, thereby hopeless	*India and China:* Lack of falls assessment significant gap in care pathway for hip fracture in hospitals [105, 109] *Brazil:* Falls are the main cause of death during the first 30 days after surgery, representing 43.5% of deaths [116]

12.9.1 Key Evidence-Based Recommendations and Their Implementation in LMICs

Implementation of evidence-based recommendations in LMICs is challenging but should not be interpreted as a wasted effort. Table 12.12 lists some key evidence-based recommendations and suggestions for implementation of in-hospital rehabilitation and community rehabilitation following hip fracture surgery in LMICs, based on expert opinion. Suggestions with limited formal evidence but apparent face validity include involving families as partners early and explicitly including them in the care plan and ensuring that ward nurses and therapists jointly commit to delivering the mobility goals.

With limited infrastructure (rehabilitation units and trained therapists) and rapidly growing demand, disruptive approaches to rehabilitation are needed in LMICs. WHO's Integrated Care for Older People (ICOPE) programme for older people is a community-based primary care health ageing approach which focuses on ways of optimising a community dwelling older person's function. However, many of the tools and resources provided in this programme allow community workers to design

Table 12.11 Barriers to rehabilitation in the community in LMICs

Barrier category	Items	Examples
Environmental context and resources	Lack of comprehensive geriatric care services to conduct structured, systematic inter-disciplinary geriatric assessment (including physical and mental health, function and social support condition) Ineffective and under-utilised referral pathways to rehabilitation after hospital discharge No timely and affordable rehabilitation interventions (long waiting times) Lack of adequate service network and rehabilitation facilities to meet different rehabilitation needs (inpatient, outpatient and homecare) Lack of rehabilitation staff, particularly occupational therapists Poor adherence due to lack of transportation, inability of caregiver to take time off work and long distances to rehabilitation facilities Inadequate resources (assistive technologies and devices) Lack of standardised protocols for post-acute care Lack of accessibility and poor neighbourhoods preventing independence in walking outdoors	*Taiwan:* Community-based home care services are designed for people with long-term care needs and are mainly skilled nursing care—doesn't completely fit post-acute care needs [117] *Brazil:* 70% patients had ≤3 months rehabilitation after surgery, mostly one time weekly;[a] 17% had home care rehabilitation [118] *India and Brazil:* Physiotherapy largely delivered in acute care, access difficult in public services. Most families don't have resources to pay for private services *Brazil:* Majority of rehabilitation programmes based on the model of traditional clinic- and hospital-based settings, failing to reach frail older adults at home
Cultural and social influences	Negative social representation of old age Cultural attitudes and beliefs toward disability in old age, older adults have to be convinced that mobility related problems are treatable and falls can be prevented	*Brazil:* Negative connotations of age and a sense of passivity were experienced by older adults after hip fracture surgery, leading to immobility and inactivity (qualitative study) [95]
Human resources capability	Lack of training on systematic inter disciplinary geriatric assessment Lack of training on fragility fractures, frailty, sarcopenia and bone health Lack of training on evidence-based exercise approach (balance and resistance training and falls prevention) Lack of fracture liaison services with a multidisciplinary care approach	

[a]Secondary data from a clinical trial

individualised programmes for older people. Available as an app or on-line some of these practical approaches (e.g. on nutrition, polypharmacy, carer support) could be helpful for primary care workers once a patient with a hip fracture returns home (available from www.who.int/ageing/health-systems/icope/en/).

Table 12.12 Implementation strategies in LMICs, based on expert opinion

In-hospital rehabilitation evidence-based recommendations	Suggested implementation strategies
1. Comprehensive screening and assessment of older adults immediately after admission on trauma or orthopedic ward by a skilled trained nurse	• Make available a short, feasible, reliable and valid tool kit for nurses to screen for frailty and delirium • Identify poor nutritional status and dysphagia as early as possible • Take actions to overcome modifiable risk factors • Where orthogeriatric care is not routine, nurses should request a geriatric consultation for complex cases • Where rehabilitation team members are available (physiatrist, physiotherapist, occupational therapist and speech therapy) a multidisciplinary assessment should be conducted
2. Physiotherapy approach immediately after admission	If surgery is delayed, immediate physiotherapy should begin to prevent muscle strength decline of the non-fractured leg, avoid respiratory problems (such as pneumonia), and pressure ulcers
3. Include caregivers in the care planning from time of ward admission	Caregivers may request to stay with older adults in the ward and should be included in the care plan. Train caregivers to identify signs of complications (such as delirium, swallowing problems, falls, pain) and help with daily basic activities, this can build and strengthen their skills for hospital discharge. Empower caregivers as co-participants in care during hospital stay
4. Surgical planning should target early weight-bearing	Weight-bearing restriction in the post-operative phase should be avoided since it limits what a patient can achieve in terms of mobility and functional independence. Effective surgery allows early weight bearing
5. Early mobilisation after surgery (24 h after surgery)	Unless medically or surgically contraindicated, physiotherapists and/or nurses should sit patients out of bed, and walk as early as possible Care plans delivered co-jointly by nurses and physiotherapists can promote patients' mobility over the entire day
6. Early post-operative goal-directed mobilisation practice with balance and functional exercises	Begin progressive resistance exercises, weight-bearing exercises (unless contra-indicated) and balance exercises during hospital stay, starting as early as possible Some services in LMICs are based on early discharge from hospital to rehabilitation at home ("hospital at home"). Harness informal and formal caregiving training and use technology but be aware how to achieve the best results when relying on families as therapists in LMICs, particularly when education levels are low
7. Fall risk assessment during hospital stay	Provide falls risk assessments to patients/caregivers with educational information and referral to community services after discharge
8. Discharge planning	Nurses should prepare caregivers for the level of care at home. Educational materials and practical carer training should be provided where possible [119]

Access to rehabilitation with the associated opportunity to maximise function and quality of life is increasingly recognised as a human right. Efforts to increase therapist numbers and optimise older patients' access to evidence-based hospital rehabilitation programmes have been strengthened by WHO's recent Rehabilitation 2030: Call to Action [1]. But as the pressure increases for health systems to provide universal coverage with access to rehabilitation it is likely that community-based rehabilitation will become more important as a cost-effective way to deliver services. Globally, community rehabilitation is also likely to become the focus for future research efforts to maximise recovery, partly because of the long trajectories of recovery (particularly of mobility) after hip fracture and partly because older people are increasingly vocal about prioritising returning home as quickly as possible.

12.10 Conclusion

- A rehabilitation pathway includes: (1) early and intensive mobility and self-care retraining with medical minimisation of complications and problems from comorbidities; (2) chronic care interventions (including dementia and frailty assessment and falls prevention) and (3) access to community services, including aged care support services and allied health therapies.
- Patients with cognitive impairment should not be excluded from rehabilitation following hip fracture.
- Recovery time for different functional domains varies from less than 6 months for many activities of daily living and cognitive function to over a year for walking 3 m without assistance.
- Rehabilitation programmes should be multidisciplinary with integration of orthogeriatric and rehabilitation services, or include professionals with multidisciplinary competencies. They should include early comprehensive geriatric assessment, surgery and mobilisation, with higher doses of mobility training and an emphasis on regaining functional independence. Programmes should also begin soon after hospital admission and continue after hospital discharge.
- In-patient rehabilitation programmes should include goal-directed mobilisation practice with balance and functional exercises.
- Structured exercise programmes should continue beyond the hospital setting for at least 12 weeks and may include progressive resistance training.
- Exercise programmes should incorporate components targeting self-efficacy to support patients to build their confidence to undertake exercise programmes post-discharge.
- Where possible a chronic disease self-management approach should be used with patients and families to promote self-efficacy and adherence to falls prevention strategies, osteoporosis treatment and exercise programmes.
- Self-efficacy, social support and caregiver responses play a role in recovery and can assist in rehabilitation in hospital and at home. Caregivers should be included in every phase of the recovery e.g. during care and discharge planning.

216   S. M. Dyer et al.

- Whilst there are many barriers to providing rehabilitation services in lower to middle income countries, implementation of evidence-based recommendations should not be viewed as futile. Health care professionals at all levels should not accept cognitive and physical functioning limitations as a normal age-related pathway for older patients after hip fracture surgery.

References

1. World Health Organisation (2017) Rehabilitation 2030: a call for action. WHO, Geneva
2. Fortinsky RH, Bohannon RW, Litt MD, Tennen H, Maljanian R, Fifield J, Garcia RI, Kenyon L (2002) Rehabilitation therapy self-efficacy and functional recovery after hip fracture. Int J Rehabil Res 25(3):241–246
3. Schwarzer R, Luszczynska A, Ziegelmann JP, Scholz U, Lippke S (2008) Social-cognitive predictors of physical exercise adherence: three longitudinal studies in rehabilitation. Health Psychol 27(Suppl 1):S54–S63
4. National Institute for Health and Care Excellence (2014) Hip fracture: management. NICE Guidelines, vol CG124. National Institute for Health and Care Excellence (NICE), London
5. World Health Organisation (2011) World report on disability. World Health Organisation, Geneva
6. Crotty M, Unroe K, Cameron ID, Miller M, Ramirez G, Couzner L (2010) Rehabilitation interventions for improving physical and psychosocial functioning after hip fracture in older people. Cochrane Database Syst Rev (1):CD007624
7. Diong J, Allen N, Sherrington C (2016) Structured exercise improves mobility after hip fracture: a meta-analysis with meta-regression. Br J Sports Med 50(6):346–355
8. Handoll HH, Sherrington C, Mak JC (2011) Interventions for improving mobility after hip fracture surgery in adults. Cochrane Database Syst Rev (3):CD001704
9. Tian M, Gong X, Rath S, Wei J, Yan LL, Lamb SE, Lindley RI, Sherrington C, Willett K, Norton R (2016) Management of hip fractures in older people in Beijing: a retrospective audit and comparison with evidence-based guidelines and practice in the UK. Osteoporos Int 27(2):677–681
10. World Health Organisation (2002) Towards a common language for functioning, disability and health: ICF. The International Classification of Functioning, Disability and Health. WHO, Geneva
11. Dyer SM, Crotty M, Fairhall N, Magaziner J, Beaupre LA, Cameron ID, Sherrington C (2016) A critical review of the long-term disability outcomes following hip fracture. BMC Geriatr 16(1):158
12. Magaziner J, Hawkes W, Hebel JR, Zimmerman SI, Fox KM, Dolan M, Felsenthal G, Kenzora J (2000) Recovery from hip fracture in eight areas of function. J Gerontol A Biol Sci Med Sci 55(9):M498–M507
13. Magaziner J, Simonsick EM, Kashner TM, Hebel JR, Kenzora JE (1990) Predictors of functional recovery one year following hospital discharge for hip fracture: a prospective study. J Gerontol 45(3):M101
14. Lima CA, Sherrington C, Guaraldo A, SAD M, RDR V, JDA M, Kojima KE, Perracini M (2016) Effectiveness of a physical exercise intervention program in improving functional mobility in older adults after hip fracture in later stage rehabilitation: protocol of a randomized clinical trial (REATIVE Study). BMC Geriatr 16(1):198–198
15. Wu X, Tian M, Zhang J, Yang M, Gong X, Liu Y, Li X, Lindley RI, Anderson M, Peng K, Jagnoor J, Ji J, Wang M, Ivers R, Tian W (2019) The effect of a multidisciplinary co-management program for the older hip fracture patients in Beijing: a "pre- and post-" retrospective study. Arch Osteoporos 14(1):43
16. Beaupre LA, Cinats JG, Jones CA, Scharfenberger AV, Johnston DWC, Senthilselvan A, Saunders LD (2007) Does functional recovery in elderly hip fracture patients differ between patients admitted from long-term care and the community? J Gerontol A Biol Sci Med Sci 62(10):1127–1133

17. Hannan E, Magaziner J, Wang J, Eastwood E (2001) Mortality and locomotion 6 months after hospitalization for hip fracture: risk factors and risk-adjusted hospital outcomes. JAMA 285(21):2736–2742

18. Seitz DP, Gill SS, Gruneir A, Austin PC, Anderson GM, Bell CM, Rochon PA (2014) Effects of dementia on postoperative outcomes of older adults with hip fractures: a population-based study. J Am Med Dir Assoc 15(5):334–341

19. Allen J, Koziak A, Buddingh S, Liang J, Buckingham J, Beaupre LA (2012) Rehabilitation in patients with dementia following hip fracture: a systematic review. Physiother Can 64(2):190–201

20. Osnes E, Lofthus K, Meyer C, Falch M, Nordsletten H, Cappelen E, Kristiansen J, Kristiansen A, Kristiansen L, Kristiansen I, Kristiansen S (2004) Consequences of hip fracture on activities of daily life and residential needs. Osteoporos Int 15(7):567–574

21. Marcantonio ER, Flacker JM, Michaels M, Resnick NM (2000) Delirium is independently associated with poor functional recovery after hip fracture. J Am Geriatr Soc 48(6):618–624

22. Goisser S, Schrader E, Singler K, Bertsch T, Gefeller O, Biber R, Bail HJ, Sieber CC, Volkert D (2015) Malnutrition according to mini nutritional assessment is associated with severe functional impairment in geriatric patients before and up to 6 months after hip fracture. J Am Med Dir Assoc 16(8):661–667

23. Goisser S, Schrader E, Singler K, Bertsch T, Gefeller O, Biber R, Bail HJ, Sieber CC, Volkert D (1940–1950) Low postoperative dietary intake is associated with worse functional course in geriatric patients up to 6 months after hip fracture. Br J Nutr 113(12):2015

24. Avenell A, Smith TO, Curtain JP, Mak JCS, Myint PK (2016) Nutritional supplementation for hip fracture aftercare in older people. Cochrane Database Syst Rev (11):CD001880

25. Neuman MD, Silber JH, Magaziner JS, Passarella MA, Mehta S, Werner RM (2014) Survival and functional outcomes after hip fracture among nursing home residents. JAMA Intern Med 174(8):1273–1280

26. Alberta Health Services. http://www.albertahealthservices.ca/assets/about/scn/ahs-scn-bjh-hf-restorative-care-pathway-hcp.pdf. Accessed 1 May 2019

27. French DD, Bass E, Bradham DD, Campbell RR, Rubenstein LZ (2008) Rehospitalization after hip fracture: predictors and prognosis from a national veterans study. J Am Geriatr Soc 56(4):705–710

28. Australian and New Zealand Hip Fracture Registry (ANZHFR) Steering Group (2014) Australian and New Zealand guideline for hip fracture care: improving outcomes in hip fracture management of adults. Australian and New Zealand Hip Fracture Registry Steering Group, Sydney

29. National Clinical Guideline Centre (2011) The management of hip fracture in adults. London, National Clinical Guideline Centre

30. Mitchell SL, Stott DJ, Martin BJ, Grant SJ (2001) Randomized controlled trial of quadriceps training after proximal femoral fracture. Clin Rehabil 15(3):282–290

31. Monticone M, Ambrosini E, Brunati R, Capone A, Pagliari G, Secci C, Zatti G, Ferrante S (2018) How balance task-specific training contributes to improving physical function in older subjects undergoing rehabilitation following hip fracture: a randomized controlled trial. Clin Rehabil 32(3):340–351

32. Baroni M, Serra R, Boccardi V, Ercolani S, Zengarini E, Casucci P, Valecchi R, Rinonapoli G, Caraffa A, Mecocci P, Ruggiero C (2019) The orthogeriatric comanagement improves clinical outcomes of hip fracture in older adults. Osteoporos Int 30(4):907–916

33. Chong TW, Chan G, Feng L, Goh S, Hew A, Ng TP, Tan BY (2013) Integrated care pathway for hip fractures in a subacute rehabilitation setting. Ann Acad Med Singap 42(11):579–584

34. Fordham R, Thompson R, Holmes J, Hodkinson C (1986) A cost-benefit study of geriatric-orthopaedic management of patients with fractured neck of femur. Working papers 014. CHEDP, Centre for Health Economics, University of York, York

35. Galvard H, Samuelsson SM (1995) Orthopedic or geriatric rehabilitation of hip fracture patients: a prospective, randomized, clinically controlled study in Malmo, Sweden. Aging (Milano) 7(1):11–16

36. Gilchrist WJ, Newman RJ, Hamblen DL, Williams BO (1988) Prospective randomised study of an orthopaedic geriatric inpatient service. BMJ 297(6656):1116–1118
37. Kennie DC, Reid J, Richardson IR, Kiamari AA, Kelt C (1988) Effectiveness of geriatric rehabilitative care after fractures of the proximal femur in elderly women: a randomised clinical trial. BMJ 297(6656):1083–1086
38. Marcantonio ER, Flacker JM, Wright RJ, Resnick NM (2001) Reducing delirium after hip fracture: a randomized trial. J Am Geriatr Soc 49(5):516–522
39. Naglie G, Tansey C, Kirkland JL, Ogilvie-Harris DJ, Detsky AS, Etchells E, Tomlinson G, O'Rourke K, Goldlist B (2002) Interdisciplinary inpatient care for elderly people with hip fracture: a randomized controlled trial. CMAJ 167(1):25–32
40. Prestmo A, Hagen G, Sletvold O, Helbostad JL, Thingstad P, Taraldsen K, Lydersen S, Halsteinli V, Saltnes T, Lamb SE, Johnsen LG, Saltvedt I (2015) Comprehensive geriatric care for patients with hip fractures: a prospective, randomised, controlled trial. Lancet 385(9978):1623–1633
41. Sánchez Ferrín P, Mañas M, Márquez A, Dejoz M, Quintana S, González F (1999) Valoración geriátrica en ancianos con fractura proximal de fémur. Rev Esp Geriatr Gerontol 34(2):65–71
42. Stenvall M, Olofsson B, Nyberg L, Lundstrom M, Gustafson Y (2007) Improved performance in activities of daily living and mobility after a multidisciplinary postoperative rehabilitation in older people with femoral neck fracture: a randomized controlled trial with 1-year follow-up. J Rehabil Med 39(3):232–238
43. Uy C, Kurrle SE, Cameron ID (2008) Inpatient multidisciplinary rehabilitation after hip fracture for residents of nursing homes: a randomised trial. Australas J Ageing 27(1):43–44
44. Watne LO, Torbergsen AC, Conroy S, Engedal K, Frihagen F, Hjorthaug GA, Juliebo V, Raeder J, Saltvedt I, Skovlund E, Wyller TB (2014) The effect of a pre- and postoperative orthogeriatric service on cognitive function in patients with hip fracture: randomized controlled trial (Oslo Orthogeriatric Trial). BMC Med 12:63
45. Cameron ID, Lyle DM, Quine S (1993) Accelerated rehabilitation after proximal femoral fracture: a randomized controlled trial. Disabil Rehabil 15(1):29–34
46. Crotty M, Whitehead C, Miller M, Gray S (2003) Patient and caregiver outcomes 12 months after home-based therapy for hip fracture: a randomized controlled trial. Arch Phys Med Rehabil 84(8):1237–1239
47. Huusko TM, Karppi P, Avikainen V, Kautiainen H, Sulkava R (2002) Intensive geriatric rehabilitation of hip fracture patients: a randomized, controlled trial. Acta Orthop Scand 73(4):425–431
48. Jette AM, Harris BA, Cleary PD, Campion EW (1987) Functional recovery after hip fracture. Arch Phys Med Rehabil 68(10):735–740
49. Karlsson A, Berggren M, Gustafson Y, Olofsson B, Lindelof N, Stenvall M (2016) Effects of geriatric interdisciplinary home rehabilitation on walking ability and length of hospital stay after hip fracture: a randomized controlled trial. J Am Med Dir Assoc 17(5):464. e469–464.e415
50. Shyu YI, Liang J, Wu CC, Su JY, Cheng HS, Chou SW, Chen MC, Yang CT (2008) Interdisciplinary intervention for hip fracture in older Taiwanese: benefits last for 1 year. J Gerontol A Biol Sci Med Sci 63(1):92–97
51. Shyu YI, Liang J, Tseng MY, Li HJ, Wu CC, Cheng HS, Yang CT, Chou SW, Chen CY (2013) Comprehensive care improves health outcomes among elderly Taiwanese patients with hip fracture. J Gerontol A Biol Sci Med Sci 68(2):188–197
52. Singh NA, Quine S, Clemson LM, Williams EJ, Williamson DA, Stavrinos TM, Grady JN, Perry TJ, Lloyd BD, Smith EU, Singh MA (2012) Effects of high-intensity progressive resistance training and targeted multidisciplinary treatment of frailty on mortality and nursing home admissions after hip fracture: a randomized controlled trial. J Am Med Dir Assoc 13(1):24–30
53. Swanson CE, Day GA, Yelland CE, Broome JR, Massey L, Richardson HR, Dimitri K, Marsh A (1998) The management of elderly patients with femoral fractures. A randomised controlled trial of early intervention versus standard care. Med J Aust 169(10):515–518

54. Vidan M, Serra JA, Moreno C, Riquelme G, Ortiz J (2005) Efficacy of a comprehensive geriatric intervention in older patients hospitalized for hip fracture: a randomized, controlled trial. J Am Geriatr Soc 53(9):1476–1482

55. Ziden L, Frandin K, Kreuter M (2008) Home rehabilitation after hip fracture. A randomized controlled study on balance confidence, physical function and everyday activities. Clin Rehabil 22(12):1019–1033

56. Crotty M, Killington M, Liu E, Cameron ID, Kurrle S, Kaambwa B, Davies O, Miller M, Chehade M, Ratcliffe J (2019) Should we provide outreach rehabilitation to very old people living in Nursing Care Facilities after a hip fracture? A randomised controlled trial. Age Ageing 48(3):373–380

57. Ryan T, Enderby P, Rigby AS (2006) A randomized controlled trial to evaluate intensity of community-based rehabilitation provision following stroke or hip fracture in old age. Clin Rehabil 20(2):123–131

58. Kimmel LA, Liew SM, Sayer JM, Holland AE (2016) HIP4Hips (High Intensity Physiotherapy for HIP fractures in the acute hospital setting): a randomised controlled trial. Med J Aust 205(2):73–78

59. Kronborg L, Bandholm T, Palm H, Kehlet H, Kristensen MT (2017) Effectiveness of acute in-hospital physiotherapy with knee-extension strength training in reducing strength deficits in patients with a hip fracture: a randomised controlled trial. PLoS One 12(6):e0179867

60. Moseley AM, Sherrington C, Lord SR, Barraclough E, St George RJ, Cameron ID (2009) Mobility training after hip fracture: a randomised controlled trial. Age Ageing 38(1):74–80

61. Ohoka T, Urabe Y, Shirakawa T (2015) Therapeutic exercises for proximal femoral fracture of super-aged patients: effect of walking assistance using Body Weight-Supported Treadmill Training (BWSTT). Physiotherapy 101:e1124–e1125

62. Resnick B, Magaziner J, Orwig D, Yu-Yahiro J, Hawkes W, Shardell M, Hebel JR, Zimmerman S, Golden J, Werner M (2007) Testing the effectiveness of the exercise plus program in older women post-hip fracture. Ann Behav Med 34(1):67–76

63. Sherrington C, Lord SR, Herbert RD (2003) A randomised trial of weight-bearing versus non-weight-bearing exercise for improving physical ability in inpatients after hip fracture. Aust J Physiother 49(1):15–22

64. Van Ooijen MLW, Roerdink M, Trekop M, Janssen TWJ, Beek PJ (2016) The efficacy of treadmill training with and without projected visual context for improving walking ability and reducing fall incidence and fear of falling in older adults with fall-related hip fracture: a randomized controlled trial. BMC Geriatr 16(1):215

65. Binder EF, Brown M, Sinacore DR, Steger-May K, Yarasheski KE, Schechtman KB (2004) Effects of extended outpatient rehabilitation after hip fracture: a randomized controlled trial. JAMA 292(7):837–846

66. Hauer K, Specht N, Schuler M, Bärtsch P, Oster P (2002) Intensive physical training in geriatric patients after severe falls and hip surgery. Age Ageing 31(1):49–57

67. Langford D, Fleig L, Brown K, Cho N, Frost M, Ledoyen M, Lehn J, Panagiotopoulos K, Sharpe N, Ashe MC (2015) Back to the future—feasibility of recruitment and retention to patient education and telephone follow-up after hip fracture: a pilot randomized controlled trial. Patient Prefer Adherence 2015:1343–1351

68. Latham NK, Harris BA, Bean JF, Heeren T, Goodyear C, Zawacki S, Heislein DM, Mustafa J, Pardasaney P, Giorgetti M, Holt N, Goehring L, Jette AM (2014) Effect of a home-based exercise program on functional recovery following rehabilitation after hip fracture: a randomized clinical trial. JAMA 311(7):700–708

69. Magaziner J, Mangione KK, Orwig D, Baumgarten M, Magder L, Terrin M, Fortinsky RH, Gruber-Baldini AL, Beamer BA, Tosteson ANA, Kenny AM, Shardell M, Binder EF, Koval K, Resnick B, Miller R, Forman S, McBride R, Craik RL (2019) Effect of a multicomponent home-based physical therapy intervention on ambulation after hip fracture in older adults: the CAP randomized clinical trial. JAMA 322(10):946–956

70. Mangione KK, Craik RL, Tomlinson SS, Palombaro KM (2005) Can elderly patients who have had a hip fracture perform moderate- to high-intensity exercise at home? Phys Ther 85(8):727–739

71. Mangione KK, Craik RL, Palombaro KM, Tomlinson SS, Hofmann MT (2010) Home-based leg-strengthening exercise improves function 1 year after hip fracture: a randomized controlled study. J Am Geriatr Soc 58(10):1911–1917

72. Orwig D, Hochberg M, Yu-Yahiro J, Resnick B, Hawkes W, Shardell M, Hebel J, Colvin P, Miller R, Golden J, Zimmerman S, Magaziner J (2011) Delivery and outcomes of a yearlong home exercise program after hip fracture: a randomized controlled trial. Arch Intern Med 171(4):323

73. Salpakoski A, Törmäkangas T, Edgren J, Kallinen M, Sihvonen SE, Pesola M, Vanhatalo J, Arkela M, Rantanen T, Sipilä S (2014) Effects of a multicomponent home-based physical rehabilitation program on mobility recovery after hip fracture: a randomized controlled trial. J Am Med Dir Assoc 15(5):361–368

74. Sherrington C, Lord SR (1997) Home exercise to improve strength and walking velocity after hip fracture: a randomized controlled trial. Arch Phys Med Rehabil 78(2):208–212

75. Sherrington C, Lord SR, Herbert RD (2004) A randomized controlled trial of weight-bearing versus non-weight-bearing exercise for improving physical ability after usual care for hip fracture. Arch Phys Med Rehabil 85(5):710–716

76. Stasi S, Papathanasiou G, Chronopoulos E, Dontas IA, Baltopoulos IP, Papaioannou NA (2019) The effect of intensive abductor strengthening on postoperative muscle efficiency and functional ability of hip-fractured patients: a randomized controlled trial. Indian J Orthop 53(3):407–419

77. Sylliaas H, Brovold T, Wyller TB, Bergland A (2011) Progressive strength training in older patients after hip fracture: a randomised controlled trial. Age Ageing 40(2):221–227

78. Sylliaas H, Brovold T, Wyller TB, Bergland A (2012) Prolonged strength training in older patients after hip fracture: a randomised controlled trial. Age Ageing 41(2):206–212

79. Tsauo JY, Leu WS, Chen YT, Yang RS (2005) Effects on function and quality of life of post-operative home-based physical therapy for patients with hip fracture. Arch Phys Med Rehabil 86(10):1953–1957

80. Williams NH, Roberts JL, Din NU, Totton N, Charles JM, Hawkes CA, Morrison V, Hoare Z, Williams M, Pritchard AW, Alexander S, Lemmey A, Woods RT, Sackley C, Logan P, Edwards RT, Wilkinson C (2016) Fracture in the Elderly Multidisciplinary Rehabilitation (FEMuR): a phase II randomised feasibility study of a multidisciplinary rehabilitation package following hip fracture. BMJ Open 6(10):e012422–e012422

81. Shyu YI, Liang J, Wu CC, Su JY, Cheng HS, Chou SW, Chen MC, Yang CT, Tseng MY (2010) Two-year effects of interdisciplinary intervention for hip fracture in older Taiwanese. J Am Geriatr Soc 58(6):1081–1089

82. Rimmer JH, Henley KY (2013) Building the crossroad between inpatient/outpatient rehabilitation and lifelong community-based fitness for people with neurologic disability. J Neurol Phys Ther 37(2):72–77

83. Chang FH, Latham NK, Ni P, Jette AM (2015) Does self-efficacy mediate functional change in older adults participating in an exercise program after hip fracture? A randomized controlled trial. Arch Phys Med Rehabil 96(6):1014–1020

84. Bean JF, Herman S, Kiely DK, Frey IC, Leveille SG, Fielding RA, Frontera WR (2004) Increased Velocity Exercise Specific to Task (InVEST) training: a pilot study exploring effects on leg power, balance, and mobility in community-dwelling older women. J Am Geriatr Soc 52(5):799–804

85. Seitz DP, Adunuri N, Gill SS, Rochon PA (2011) Prevalence of dementia and cognitive impairment among older adults with hip fractures. J Am Med Dir Assoc 12(8):556–564

86. Royal College of Physicians (2018) National hip fracture database (NHFD). Royal College of Physicians, London

87. National Clinical Guideline Centre (2017) The management of hip fracture in adults. London, National Clinical Guideline Centre

88. Freter S, Koller K, Dunbar M, MacKnight C, Rockwood K (2017) Translating delirium prevention strategies for elderly adults with hip fracture into routine clinical care: a pragmatic clinical trial. J Am Geriatr Soc 65(3):567–573

89. Stenvall M, Berggren M, Lundstrom M, Gustafson Y, Olofsson B (2012) A multidisciplinary intervention program improved the outcome after hip fracture for people with

dementia—subgroup analyses of a randomized controlled trial. Arch Gerontol Geriatr 54(3):e284–e289

90. Huusko TM, Karppi P, Avikainen V, Kautiainen H, Sulkava R (2000) Randomised, clinically controlled trial of intensive geriatric rehabilitation in patients with hip fracture: subgroup analysis of patients with dementia. BMJ 321(7269):1107–1111

91. Shyu YI, Tsai WC, Chen MC, Liang J, Cheng HS, Wu CC, Su JY, Chou SW (2012) Two-year effects of an interdisciplinary intervention on recovery following hip fracture in older Taiwanese with cognitive impairment. Int J Geriatr Psychiatry 27(5):529–538

92. Bischoff-Ferrari HA, Dawson-Hughes B, Platz A, Orav EJ, Stähelin HB, Willett WC, Can U, Egli A, Mueller NJ, Looser S, Bretscher B, Minder E, Vergopoulos A, Theiler R (2010) Effect of high-dosage cholecalciferol and extended physiotherapy on complications after hip fracture: a randomized controlled trial. Arch Intern Med 170(9):813–820

93. Liu H, Yang C, Tseng M, Chen C, Wu C, Cheng H, Lin Y, Shyu Y (2018) Trajectories in post-operative recovery of elderly hip-fracture patients at risk for depression: a follow-up study. Rehabil Psychol 63(3):438–446

94. Cristancho P, Lenze EJ, Avidan MS, Rawson KS (2016) Trajectories of depressive symptoms after hip fracture. Psychol Med 46(7):1413–1425

95. Moraes SA, Furlanetto EC, Ricci NA, Perracini MR (2019) Sedentary behavior: barriers and facilitators among older adults after hip fracture surgery. A qualitative study. Braz J Phys Ther. https://www.sciencedirect.com/science/article/abs/pii/S1413355518310232?via%3Dihub. Accessed 10 July 2019

96. Bower ES, Wetherell JL, Petkus AJ, Rawson KS, Lenze EJ (2016) Fear of falling after hip fracture: prevalence, course, and relationship with one-year functional recovery. Am J Geriatr Psychiatry 24(12):1228–1236

97. Visschedijk J, van Balen R, Hertogh C, Achterberg W (2013) Fear of falling in patients with hip fractures: prevalence and related psychological factors. J Am Med Dir Assoc 14(3):218–220

98. Lim KK, Matchar DB, Chong JL, Yeo W, Howe TS, Koh JSB (2019) Pre-discharge prognostic factors of physical function among older adults with hip fracture surgery: a systematic review. Osteoporos Int 30(5):929–938

99. Shyu YI, Chen MC, Wu CC, Cheng HS (2010) Family caregivers' needs predict functional recovery of older care recipients after hip fracture. J Adv Nurs 66(11):2450–2459

100. Salkeld G, Cameron ID, Cumming RG, Easter S, Seymour J, Kurrle SE, Quine S (2000) Quality of life related to fear of falling and hip fracture in older women: a time trade off study. BMJ 320(7231):341–346

101. Schwartz CE, Bode R, Repucci N, Becker J, Sprangers MA, Fayers PM (2006) The clinical significance of adaptation to changing health: a meta-analysis of response shift. Qual Life Res 15(9):1533–1550

102. Pol M, Peek S, van Nes F, van Hartingsveldt M, Buurman B, Krose B (2019) Everyday life after a hip fracture: what community-living older adults perceive as most beneficial for their recovery. Age Ageing 48(3):440–447

103. Langford D, Edwards N, Gray SM, Fleig L, Ashe MC (2018) "Life goes on" everyday tasks, coping self-efficacy, and independence: exploring older adults' recovery from hip fracture. Qual Health Res 28(8):1255–1266

104. Yu F, Xia W (2019) The epidemiology of osteoporosis, associated fragility fractures, and management gap in China. Arch Osteoporos 14(1):32

105. Rath S, Yadav L, Tewari A, Chantler T, Woodward M, Kotwal P, Jain A, Dey A, Garg B, Malhotra R, Goel A, Farooque K, Sharma V, Webster P, Norton R (2017) Management of older adults with hip fractures in India: a mixed methods study of current practice, barriers and facilitators, with recommendations to improve care pathways. Arch Osteoporos 12(1):55

106. Riera-Espinoza G (2009) Epidemiology of osteoporosis in Latin America 2008. Salud Publica Mex 51(Suppl 1):S52–S55

107. Zerbini CA, Szejnfeld VL, Abergaria BH, McCloskey EV, Johansson H, Kanis JA (2015) Incidence of hip fracture in Brazil and the development of a FRAX model. Arch Osteoporos 10:224

108. Dhanwal DK, Dennison EM, Harvey NC, Cooper C (2011) Epidemiology of hip fracture: worldwide geographic variation. Indian J Orthop 45(1):15–22
109. Dash SK, Panigrahi R, Palo N, Priyadarshi A, Biswal M (2015) Fragility hip fractures in elderly patients in Bhubaneswar, India (2012–2014): a prospective multicenter study of 1031 elderly patients. Geriatr Orthop Surg Rehabil 6(1):11–15
110. González ID, Becerra MC, González J, Campos AT, Barbosa-Santibáñez J, Alvarado R (2016) Fracturas de cadera: satisfacción posquirúrgica al año en adultos mayores atendidos en Méderi-Hospital Universitario Mayor, Bogotá, D.C. Rev Cienc Salud 14(3):409–422
111. Arliani GG, da Costa AD, Linhares GK, Balbachevsky D, Fernandes HJ, Dos Reis FB (2011) Correlation between time until surgical treatment and mortality among elderly patients with fractures at the proximal end of the femur. Rev Bras Ortop 46(2):189–194
112. Dinamarca-Montecinos JL, Amestica-Lazcano G, Rubio-Herrera R, Carrasco-Buvinic A, Vasquez A (2015) [Hip fracture. Experience in 647 Chilean patients aged 60 years or more]. Rev Med Chil 143(12):1552–1559
113. World Health Organisation. https://www.who.int/news-room/fact-sheets/detail/rehabilitation. Accessed 22 Aug 2019
114. Lin PC, Hung SH, Liao MH, Sheen SY, Jong SY (2006) Care needs and level of care difficulty related to hip fractures in geriatric populations during the post-discharge transition period. J Nurs Res 14(4):251–260
115. Rocha SA, Avila MA, Bocchi SC (2016) The influence of informal caregivers on the rehabilitation of the elderly in the postoperative period of proximal femoral fracture. Rev Gaucha Enferm 37(1):e51069
116. Vidal EI, Coeli CM, Pinheiro RS, Camargo KR (2006) Mortality within 1 year after hip fracture surgical repair in the elderly according to postoperative period: a probabilistic record linkage study in Brazil. Osteoporos Int 17(10):1569–1576
117. Chen Y-T, Peng L-N, Liu C-L, Chen L-K (2011) Orthogeriatrics in Taiwan: overview and experiences. J Clin Gerontol Geriatr 2:66e70
118. Lima CA, Sherrington C, Guaraldo A, Moraes SA, Varanda RD, Melo JA, Kojima KE, Perracini M (2016) Effectiveness of a physical exercise intervention program in improving functional mobility in older adults after hip fracture in later stage rehabilitation: protocol of a randomized clinical trial (REATIVE Study). BMC Geriatr 16(1):198
119. Furlan AD, Irvin E, Munhall C, Giraldo-Prieto M, Fullerton L, McMaster R, Danak S, Costante A, Pitzul K, Bhide RP, Marchenko S, Mahood Q, David JA, Flannery JF, Bayley M (2018) Rehabilitation service models for people with physical and/or mental disability living in low- and middle-income countries: a systematic review. J Rehabil Med 50(6):487–498

The Psychological Health of Patients and their Caregivers

13

Stefano Eleuteri, Maria Eduarda Batista de Lima, Paolo Falaschi, and On behalf of the FFN Education Committee

13.1 Why Is Psychological Status Important in the Management of Hip Fracture?

Hip fractures are associated with reduced health-related quality of life (QoL). Buckling and colleagues [1] have found a pre-existing need for care, limited function, cognitive impairment and depression to be independent factors associated with lower QoL during a patient's post-surgical period. To assign a realistic value to osteoporosis and osteoporotic fracture treatment, it is important to understand the full impact that osteoporotic fractures have on QoL. In fact, QoL can predict mortality, as well as physical and psychological functioning [2].

This chapter is a component of Part 3: Pillar II.
For an explanation of the grouping of chapters in this book, please see Chapter 1: 'The multidisciplinary approach to fragility fractures around the world—an overview'.

On behalf of the FFN Education Committee

S. Eleuteri (✉)
Sapienza University of Rome, Rome, Italy

Education Committee Chair of the Fragility Fracture Network, Rome, Italy

M. E. B. de Lima
Fondazione Don Carlo Gnocchi, Rome, Italy

P. Falaschi
Education Committee Chair of the Fragility Fracture Network, Rome, Italy
e-mail: paolo.falaschi@fondazione.uniroma1.it

© The Author(s) 2021
P. Falaschi, D. Marsh (eds.), *Orthogeriatrics*, Practical Issues in Geriatrics,
https://doi.org/10.1007/978-3-030-48126-1_13

13.1.1 Why Is Psychological Status Important in the Outcome of Hip Fracture?

Depression, delirium, and cognitive-impairment rates, at the time of hip fracture, have been estimated at between 9% and 47% (mean 29%), between 43% and 61% (mean 49%), and between 31% and 88% (mean 47%), respectively [3]. Mental health status at the time of surgery has been reported as being an important determinant of the outcome, with mental disorders associated with poorer functional recovery and higher mortality rates [4]. For example, a functional decline can lead to disability and may lead to prolonged hospital stays, institutionalisation and even death [5].

It has also been suggested that pre-fracture dependence in ADL is a stronger predictor of further functional decline—resulting in institutionalisation or death—than pre-fracture dementia [6]. Furthermore, delirium is associated with lower functional outcome in both short and long term and recovery increased length of stay, high risk of dementia and persistent cognitive deficits [7]. Delirium is also associated with other hospital-acquired complications that translate into higher rates of institutionalisation, greater need for rehabilitation and home healthcare services after discharge, increased mortality and healthcare costs, as well as an additional burden on the patient, hospital staff and family caregivers [8].

13.1.2 Why Is Psychological Status Important in Rehabilitation from Hip Fracture?

A study [9] showed that delirium was independently associated with poor functional outcome 1 month after fracture even after adjusting for pre-fracture frailty. Also at the 6-month follow-up, it constitutes an independent risk factor for institutionalisation among hip-fracture patients who live at home before the fracture. In the case of patients who are able to return to their homes, delirium is a strong predictor of functional decline at the 6-month follow-up [10]. Regarding depression, the literature showed that approximately one in five people who are not depressed at the time of their fracture become so after 8 weeks [11]. In a long-term study [12], functional healing was evaluated after 2 years in elderly cases with hip fractures, and depression was reported to have affected healing. A negative effect of depression on daily living activities emerged also at the end of a 6-month period. A patient's active participation in the rehabilitation process has a positive effect on healing. However, the presence of depression disrupts this process because of reluctance, negative cognition and symptoms similar to psychomotor retardation. Depression in elderly hip-fracture cases was found to have affected daily living activity negatively.

The psychological state of the individual who suffers from a hip fracture is highly relevant when determining how well that person may recover [13]. The affective responses to a hip fracture predict both psychological and physical functioning over time, providing a potential target for the enhancement of recovery from this debilitating injury [14]. It is also suggested that the effect of rehabilitation after hip fracture can be less effective if functions are restricted due to fear of falling (FOF) [15]. For all the aspects mentioned earlier, it seems important to take care of the HF patient's psychological status.

13.1.3 Why Is Caregivers' Psychological Status also Important?

Hip-fracture (HF) patients are among the most vulnerable of hospitalised patients. The associated caregiving rehabilitation task often falls to a member of the family. Most caregivers (86%) are family members (predominantly women) also known as 'informal caregivers' [16]. They fulfil their role for between 7 and 11 h per day on average and anything up to 10–15 h when clinical conditions worsen: the more serious the fracture, the more support is needed [17, 18]. Usually, they have no professional assistance-procedure skills. Informal caregivers must cope with physical, psychological and social stressors that affect their health status and quality of life negatively.

The primary stressors experienced by informal caregivers are related to the severity of the patient's disease and the amount of time devoted to assisting him/her. Informal caregivers are an important resource for elderly patients suffering from hip fractures because they play a key role during their recovery. One important task is that of motivating the patients to adhere to their therapy programme. Elderly patients with a hip fracture may present with a complexity of other problems, which may be challenging to both them and their carers.

13.1.4 Consequences of Caregiving

The level of family caregivers' mental health has been shown to be an important predictor of care recipients' institutionalisation [19], and a risk factor for care–recipient mortality. Objective primary stressors can affect various dimensions of burden differently: functional health has been found to be associated with time-dependent, physical and developmental burdens; cognitive status has been found to be associated with a time-dependent burden. Patterns of change in family caregivers' mental health over time have also been explored, as have the relationships between family caregivers' mental health and recovery outcomes of elderly hip-fractured patients. The findings suggest that, during the first year following patient discharge, family caregivers' mental health is associated with patients' post-fracture recovery, including the recovery of physical functionality, reduced pain and better health-related outcomes.

These results also suggest that, when estimating recovery times and health-related outcomes of patients who have suffered from hip fractures, healthcare providers should also consider the mental well-being of family caregivers. An understanding of the relationships between caregiver-related predictors and the recovery of elderly persons after hip-fracture surgery might provide a more holistic view of that recovery [20]. The perspective that tends to dominate much of the literature is that care by family members is provided solely to older adults living at home. When caregivers are monitored over considerably long periods of time, it becomes evident that family caregiving responsibilities do not end with institution-alisation of the disabled relative. Instead, this key transition appears to affect the type and intensity of help provided.

Unlike earlier studies that treated institutionalisation as an 'endpoint' in family caregiving, recent research has emphasised the continued involvement of relatives in care and the effects of nursing-home admission upon the stress and mental health of family members. There is a lack of literature addressing family caregiving for frail elderly people and its consequence on the life quality of family caregivers. The subjective responses of individuals to the environments in which they live play an important role in maintaining the status of their care recipients. High levels of depressive symptoms and low levels of life satisfaction in caregivers may also be associated with the low quality of the care provided to their frail care recipients and even with maltreatment of the elderly [21].

Caregiver burden and its associated stress impact negatively upon the caregivers' perceived general physical and mental health [22] and have been negatively corre-lated with the functional status of elderly family members 1 month after discharge following hip-fracture surgery [23, 24].

13.1.5 The Relationship Between Caregivers' and Patients' Psychological Status

In a recent study, we found a correlation between the patient's psychological well-being and the caregiver's burden. At the 2-month follow-up, the outcome of ADL scores was negatively associated with caregiver burden ($p < 0.01$). Follow-up functional ability was higher in patients whose caregivers reported lower burden during their hospitalisation ($p = 0.03$). Interesting results regard the correlation existing between a patient's psychological well-being and his/her mood; greater psychological well-being corresponds, in fact, to lower likelihood of depression.

A mutual relationship seems, therefore, to exist between the patient's psychologi-cal well-being and the caregiver's burden, so that improvements in the state of health of the one boost that of the other, and vice versa. This datum confirms the importance of using a bio-psycho-social approach when dealing with both patients and caregivers and evaluating the HF patient's and caregiver's psychological status [25, 26].

13.2 How Should the Psychological Status of Patients and Caregivers Be Assessed?

In Table 13.1, we illustrate the different areas we believe it is important to evaluate to obtain a complete assessment of HF patients and relative caregivers during the different stages of the illness and recovery.

Table 13.1 Areas to be evaluated in an integrative assessment in HF patients and caregivers, at different staging (1 = admission; 2 = discharge; 3 = 90 days follow-up; 4 = 1 year follow-up; 5 = 2 years follow-up)

Areas	Staging				
	1	2	3	4	5
Patient					
Quality of life	X		X	X	
Fear of falling			X		
Pain			X	X	
Activities of daily living	X		X	X	
Delirium	X	X			
Depression	X		X	X	X
Cognitive status	X				
Stress		X	X		
Anxiety		X	X		
Caregiver					
Psychological well-being	X		X	X	
Caregiver's burden	X		X	X	

13.2.1   The Psychological Evaluation of the Patient

The recovery process that follows surgery varies based on the patients' comorbidities, cognitive and functional status and their psychosocial state. Well-being in this sense means more than health as such. It is important to evaluate different negative and positive dimensions to assess patients' psychological status when following a bio-psycho-social approach.

13.2.1.1   Quality of Life

Health-related Quality of Life (QoL) is recognised as an important measure of health status that may be used for evaluating disease and health care services [27]. It is a broad, multidimensional construct that includes domains such as physical, psychological and social functionality [28], which permits identification of specific aspects of QoL and targeting of interventions needed.

Some patients suffer from QoL [29] and well-being loss [30] while others move to nursing home facilities [31]. According to Rasmussen and colleagues [32], well-being and self-efficacy are resources for both health and illness to be considered when exploring ways of promoting possibilities of recovery. The importance of patients' perception of the care they receive has been highlighted in the literature over the past few years [33]. Without QoL data, the burden of osteoporotic fractures is likely to be underestimated [34]. The EQ-5D has been recommended for the assessment of QoL in elderly patients [35]. Although this instrument shows good psychometric properties in elderly patients, assessing the QoL of cognitively impaired patients is difficult. In people with mild and moderate dementia, these tests yield good validity and good-to-average test–retest reliability for the descriptive system, but not for the Visual Analogue Scale (VAS), which is a part of this questionnaire.

Proxy assessment is, in some cases, the only way to gather information regarding QoL, when patients are unable to respond. Family caregivers tend to overestimate health limitations concerning less visible items (pain and anxiety/depression). Very frequently, healthcare professionals rate patients at the same level for all five domains (some problems with everything). No consensus has been reached as to the most appropriate proxy to apply, but a proxy assessment of EQ-5D seems, in our opinion, to be the best option when assessing QoL in patients with severe dementia. QoL should be assessed using the EQ-5D method upon admission to determine pre-fracture QoL and in post-admission 90-day and 1-year follow-ups. In patients affected by severe dementia, EQ-5D should be completed by a proxy, if one is available [36].

13.2.1.2 Fear of Falling

Fear of falling is linked to self-efficacy—the belief people have about their capability to perform certain tasks [37].

After a hip fracture, older people have reported that their lives have changed physically, personally and socially [38]. McMillan and colleagues [39] conducted interviews 3 months after discharge from the hospital and found that during hip fracture rehabilitation, older people struggled to take control of their future lives by trying to balance risk-taking and help-seeking. The interviewees were aware that, on the one hand, it might prove risky to move around and that they were afraid of falling but, on the other, they wanted to be active and were trying to do things. They were determined to regain independence. To make progress, some of the interviewees stressed the importance of giving information to patients and to include them in talks regarding their progress. In the patient follow-up, FOF should be assessed 90 days after admission.

13.2.1.3 Pain

In the HF patients, pain should be assessed, initially, during the EQ-5D test; however, as we said before, the VAS used by EQ-5D is not reliable in cognitively impaired patients [35]. Therefore, VAS within EQ-5D rates overall body pain, while we are also interested in the pain at the site of the fracture. The Verbal Rating Scale (VRS) performs well in cases of patients with dementia, and it is more informative regarding fracture-site pain [40]. Liem and colleagues [36] agree that this test should be used on the second day after surgery—or, in cases of conservative treatment, the second day after admission—and at 90 days and 1 year after admission.

13.2.1.4 Activities of Daily Living

Activities of daily living (ADLs) are an important health outcome in the orthogeriatric population. Recovery of pre-fracture health and functional levels is one of the main goals in hip fracture management. Therefore, it is important to assess deterioration in functional level over time. The literature provides a vast selection of ADL measurement tools, but the Katz Activities of Daily Living Scale [41], is the most widely used. In many cases, it may prove difficult to assess pre-injury ADLs accurately at the time of admission. In such cases, we suggest consulting a proxy, who will typically be a family member, friend or caregiver. ADLs should be assessed upon admission to evaluate pre-fracture status. During patient follow-up, ADLs should be assessed after 90 days and 1 year after admission.

13.2.1.5   Delirium

Delirium in hip-fracture patients usually occurs during the 2–5 days following surgery. It is common in elderly hip fracture patients, occurring in 10–61% of cases [42]. It can represent a difficult clinical condition to assess, as a fluctuation of symptoms can lead to failure to recognise its onset [43]. Dementia and cognitive decline, measured by MMSE, were found to be independent risk factors for delirium [44]. The Confusion Assessment Method (CAM) [45] is a reliable and valid measure of delirium in the general medical and surgical population. The CAM focuses on four features: (1) acute change in mental status with a fluctuating course, (2) inattention, (3) disorganised thinking and (4) altered level of consciousness and is a valuable instrument with which to assess delirium. Delirium should be assessed upon admission to evaluate the pre-fracture status and on discharge after acute hospitalisation.

13.2.1.6   Depression

Depression is the most common hip-fracture-related psychological disorder, although it is frequently difficult to assess it [46]. An independent relationship was found to exist between low functional capacity and depression symptoms in the elderly [47]. In elderly people who cannot walk well enough to perform daily living activities, social isolation often occurs, and social isolation is in itself a risk factor for depression [48]. Therefore, we can say that a vicious circle of low ADL is created between pre-existing depression and an increase in depression that feelings of inadequacy when performing daily activities can produce. The Geriatric Depression Scale (GDS) may be a valuable instrument by which to assess depression [49]. Depression was observed more often in females and those who had lost their spouses [11]. Depression should be assessed upon admission to evaluate its pre-fracture status. During patient follow-up, it should be assessed after 90 days, 1 and 2 years from the date of admission.

13.2.1.7   Cognitive Impairment

Some studies suggest that cognitive impairment, found in 31–88% of elderly patients experiencing hip fractures, was a predictor of poor functional recovery after hip-fracture surgery [13]. Furthermore, pre-fracture cognitive impairment is also associated [4] with higher mortality rates. The Mini-Mental State Examination (MMSE) [50] may prove to be a valuable instrument for the assessment of cognitive impairment. Cognitive impairment should be assessed upon admission to evaluate the pre-fracture status.

13.2.1.8   Stress

The importance of the overlapping mechanisms of osteoporosis and psychological stress were documented recently.

These factors can be extended to fragility fractures [51]. The Perceived Stress Scale [52] can prove useful when assessing stress. Stress should be appraised at discharge and 90 days after admission.

13.2.1.9 Anxiety

This emerged as one of the most important aspects regarding patients, especially their evaluation upon admission [26]. The Short Anxiety Screening Test [53] has been shown to be an easy and valuable one for the assessment of anxiety in this type of patient. Anxiety should also be assessed upon discharge and 90 days after admission.

13.2.2 The Psychological Evaluation of Caregivers

The increased risk of burnout identified among informal caregivers is closely related to their perceived level of burden, defined as a multidimensional response to negative appraisals and perceived stress [54]. Joint assessment of the dimensions of burden and well-being, that coexist in caregivers' experience, allows for the identification of personal and relational resources that may be usefully included in interventions addressed to caregivers [16, 17, 54].

13.2.2.1 Psychological Well-Being

The concept of subjective well-being (SWB) is multi-component by nature. It is affected by positive (e.g. happiness), negative (e.g. depressive symptoms) and cognitive components (e.g. life satisfaction). Its multiple components are affected by different sets of social determinants and develop differently at successive life stages [55]. High care-demand levels may affect multiple aspects of caregivers' lives, including free time, social life, emotional and physical health as well as personal development. These subjectively defined stressors are also called caregiver burden. Perceived caregiver burden may adversely affect their self-esteem and their sense of competency as a caregiver [21]. These might cause caregivers to suffer from higher levels of depressive symptoms and become less satisfied with their lives.

In other words, multidimensional caregiver burdens may play a mediatory role in the association between objective primary stressors and caregivers' SWB. The Psychological General Well-Being Index (PGWBI) [56] can prove to be a valuable test for the investigation of patients' and caregivers' psychological well-being. Psychological well-being should be assessed after admission and at 90 days and 1 year after admission.

13.2.2.2 The Caregiver Burden

Informal caregivers have to cope with physical, psychological and social stressors that affect their health conditions and quality of life negatively [57]. Over the last 30 years, researchers have paid special attention to the investigation and assessment of burden [58]. The Caregiver Burden Inventory (CBI) [59] provides information regarding both the Objective Burden (OB)—the time and commitment caregivers devote to caring activities daily—and the Subjective Burden (SB)—perceived lack of everyday opportunities, fatigue, physical problems, issues related to socialisation and participation, and how they feel towards the care–recipient. Caregiver burden is an all-encompassing term used to describe the physical, emotional and financial responses of a caregiver to the changes and demands caused by providing help to another person with a physical or mental disability.

Increasing numbers of studies have examined the caregiver-burden phenomenon, the lack of support given to caregivers and interventions focused on relieving caregiver burden; this increase is probably due in part to greater evidence of caregiver burden being a determining factor in the quality of life (QoL) of caregivers. Several studies have revealed an association between the characteristics of patients and caregivers and caregivers' QoL, with caregiver burden serving as an important predictor of QoL. Caregiver burden has also been used as an outcome variable rather than a predictor [60], suggesting that caregiver burden and QoL are closely related. Thus, caregiver burden seems to be a potential moderator of the associations between patients' and caregivers' characteristics and caregivers' QoL. Some studies have shown that caregivers of elderly people suffering from hip fractures experienced a multidimensional burden, including tiredness, emotional distress and role conflicts [22, 23].

Many caregivers assume the caregiver role with little or no preparation and have to learn to deal with several aspects of care in a very short time. Often caregivers do not know what to expect during hip fracture recovery. They face situations where they have to address various care-related tasks, such as the arrangement of rehabilitation services and assistive devices. These situations become more stressful when caregivers must juggle their work and family lives. The care burden related to hip fracture, an acute injury, may decrease over time; however, it is often prolonged over 12 months or more [61]. Caregivers tend to experience the greatest stress during the first 2 months after fracture, the stress being associated with increased care demands and costs. Family caregivers of hip-fractured patients were reported as experiencing moderate burden [23]. Furthermore, the caregiver's burden was negatively related to the physical function of older patients with hip fracture. On the other hand, social support has been associated with a diminution of the caregiver burden [24]. The caregiver's burden should be assessed after admission as well as at 90 days and 1 year after admission.

13.3   How Can Psychological Status Be Influenced Positively by the Orthogeriatric Team?

We have found that a mutual relationship seems to exist between the patient's psychological well-being and the caregiver's burden, so that improvement in the state of health of the one boost that of the other, and vice versa. The correlation emerging between patients' psychological well-being and their caregivers' burden confirms the importance of using a bio-psycho-social approach towards patients and caregivers [25, 26]. Unfortunately, no specific researches have nowadays studied how the psychological status of the patient and the caregiver can be positively influenced by the orthogeriatric team. Further studies are therefore needed to better understand what can be done to improve psychological health.

In the previous paragraphs, we showed the different negative and positive dimensions that are important to evaluate, the staging we suggest and instruments we believe to be the most appropriate. The orthogeriatric team should address these aspects following a bio-psycho-social approach. The inclusion of a psychologist in the team can help in the assessment of the patients' and the caregivers' psychological well-being, using the tools we have detailed earlier, but also enables psychological counselling. In the course of counselling, the psychologist can also obtain more qualitative data, to tailor the intervention based on the resources and needs emerging and give feedback to the patients and their caregivers on the problems and the strengths that emerged in the assessment. A pilot study suggested, for example, the positive influence that twice-a-week counselling, for about 45 min, had a positive influence on HF patients' depressive and anxious symptoms. Although long-term follow-up studies are necessary to evaluate whether good early results are sustained over a longer period, these data suggest that counselling can be useful in these patients [61].

The literature shows that these patients risk much longer, and more frequent hospital stays than other adults. Comprehensive discharge-planning programmes, including early identification of those at risk, can alter these statistics. Upon admission to care facilities, early multidimensional assessment can provide significant indications of how to address the entire course of patient treatment more efficiently. In our experience, the organisation of formative courses for caregivers and the implementation of a 'caregiver help desk', with the collaboration of case manager nurses, can be additional tools that the orthogeriatric team can use to promote a comprehensive discharge-planning programme enhancing, in this way, the psychological health of HF patients and their caregivers.

Greater psycho-educational support can be provided to patients and caregivers during rehabilitation, given the longer length of stay, compared to admission in other post-surgical settings.

13.4   Cultural Influence and the Anthropology of Care

To support patients and caregivers better, it is important to include cultural and anthropological influence in the dynamics of care.

All over the world women are the predominant providers of informal care to family members with chronic medical conditions or disabilities, including the elderly and adults with mental illnesses. It has been suggested that several societal and cultural demands are made on women obliging them to assume the role of family caregiver.

Stress-coping theories propose that women are more likely to be exposed to caregiving stressors, and are likely to perceive, report and cope with these stressors differently from men [62, 63].

Many studies, which have examined gender differences among family caregivers looking after people with mental illnesses, have concluded that women spend more time in providing care and carrying out personal care tasks than men. These studies have also found that women experience greater mental and physical strain, greater caregiving-burden, and higher levels of psychological distress while providing care [64, 65].

However, an almost equal number of studies have not found any differences between men and women as far as these aspects are concerned. This has led to the view that though there may be certain differences between male and female caregivers, most of these are small and of doubtful clinical significance. Accordingly, caregiver–gender is thought to explain only a negligible proportion of the variance in negative caregiving outcomes [66, 67].

A similar inconsistency characterises the explanations provided for gender differences in caregiving such as role expectations, differences in stress, coping and social support, and response biases involved in reporting distress. Apart from the equivocal and inconsistent evidence provided, there are other problems in the literature on gender differences regarding the issue of caregiving. Most of the evidence has been derived from studies on caregivers dealing with elderly people suffering either from dementia or a variety of physical conditions [68, 69].

With changing demographics and social norms men are increasingly assuming the role of caregiver. However, the experience of care-providing men has not been adequately explored. The impact of gender on the outcome of caregiving may be mediated by several other variables including patient-related factors, socio-demographic variables, and the effects of kinship, culture and ethnicity, but these have seldom been considered in research into gender differences [70, 71].

Beyond the gender aspect, each culture and nation have its own way of establishing the care relationship between the patient and the caregiver. A study conducted in different European countries, for example, found that in countries where cross-generational support is more strongly established (Italy, Spain), the impact of fragility fractures on caregivers is generally higher than in the other countries (i.e. France) [72]. Contemporary literature reveals that global economic shifts, migration, and chronic disease are enlarging the demand for care of the elderly while, at the same time, altering intergenerational expectations; the critical roles older persons play in familial care systems as global care chains are becoming increasingly clear [73]. Migrant care workers frequently look after elderly people with significantly different bodily and historical experiences, drawing creatively upon their models of care to define cultural and gender-based identities and make claims concerning their contribution to the nation [74].

These aspects need to be considered, for example, during training courses for caregivers.

References

1. Bueckling B, Struewer J, Waldermann A, Horstmann K, Schubert N, Balzer-Geldsetzer M et al (2014) What determines health-related quality of life in hip fracture patients at the end of acute care? A prospective observational study. Osteoporos Int 25:475–484

2. Kao S, Lai KL, Lin HC, Lee HS, Wen HC (2005) WHOQOL-BREF as predictors of mortality: a two-year follow-up study at veteran homes. Qual Life Res 14:1443–1454
3. Fenton FR, Cole MG, Engelsmann F, Mansouri I (1997) Depression in older medical inpatients. Int J Geriatr Psychiatry 12:389–394
4. Holmes JD, House AO (2000) Psychiatric illness predicts poor outcome after surgery for hip fracture: a prospective cohort study. Psychol Med 30:921–929
5. Miller EA, Weissert WG (2000) Predicting elderly people's risk for nursing home placement, hospitalization, functional impairment, and mortality: a synthesis. Med Care Res Rev 57:259–297
6. Krogseth M, Wyller TB, Engedal K, Juliebø V (2014) Delirium is a risk factor for institutionalization and functional decline in older hip fracture patients. J Psychosom Res 76:68–74
7. Marcantonio ER, Flacker JM, Michaels M, Resnick NM (2000) Delirium is independently associated with poor functional recovery after hip fracture. J Am Geriatr Assoc 48:618–624
8. Saczynski JS, Marcantonio ER, Quach L, Fong TG, Gross A, Inouye SK et al (2012) Cognitive trajectories after postoperative delirium. N Engl J Med 367:30–39
9. Pompei P, Foreman M, Rudberg MA, Inouye K, Braund V, Cassel CK (1994) Delirium in hospitalized older patients: outcomes and predictors. J Am Geriatr Soc 42:809–815
10. Mossey JM, Knott K, Craik R (1990) The effects of persistent depressive symptoms on hip fracture recovery. J Gerontol 45:M163–M168
11. Yesavage JA, Brink TL, Rose TL, Lum O, Huang V, Adey M et al (1982) Development and validation of a geriatric depression screening scale: a preliminary report. J Psychiatr Res 17:37–49
12. Alarcón T, González-Montalvo JI, Gotor P, Madero R, Otero A (2011) Activities of daily living after hip fracture: profile and rate of recovery during 2 years of followup. Osteoporos Int 22:1609–1613
13. Fredman L, Hawkes WG, Black S, Bertrand RM, Magaziner J (2006) Elderly patients with hip fracture with positive affect have better functional recovery over 2 years. J Am Geriatr Soc 54:1074–1081
14. Langer JK, Weisman JS, Rodebaugh TL, Binder EF, Lenze EJ (2015) Short term affective recovery from hip fracture prospectively predicts depression and physical functioning. Health Psychol 34:30–39
15. Visschedijk J, Achterberg W, Van Balen R, Hertogh C (2010) Fear of falling after hip fracture: a systematic review of measurement instruments, prevalence, interventions, and related factors. J Am Geriatr Soc 58:1739–1748
16. National Alliance for Caregiving (NAC) and American Association of Retired Persons (AARP) (2009) Caregiving in the U.S. Bethesda, MD: NAC, and Washington, DC: AARP
17. Neugaard B, Andresen E, McKune SL, Jamoom EW (2008) Health-related quality of life in a national sample of caregivers: findings from the behavioral risk factor surveillance system. J Happiness Stud 9:559–575
18. Svedbom A, Borgstöm F, Hernlund E, Ström O, Alekna V, Bianchi ML et al (2018) Quality of life for up to 18 months after low-energy hip, vertebral, and distal forearm fractures-results from the ICUROS. Osteoporos Int 29:557–566
19. Deimling GT, Poulshock SW (1985) The transition from family in-home care to institutional care focus on health and attitudinal issues as predisposing factors. Res Aging 7:563–576
20. Liu HY, Yang CT, Cheng HS, Wu CC, Chen CY, Shyu YI (2015) Family caregivers' mental health is associated with postoperative recovery of elderly patients with hip fracture: a sample in Taiwan. J Psychosom Res 78:452–458
21. Carretero S, Garcés J, Ródenas F, Sanjosé V (2009) The informal caregiver's burden of dependent people: theory and empirical review. Arch Gerontol Geriatr 49:74–79
22. Shyu YIL, Chen MC, Liang J, Tseng MY (2012) Trends in health outcomes for family caregivers of hip-fractured elders during the first 12 months after discharge. J Adv Nurs 68:658–666
23. Lin PC, Lu CM (2005) Hip fracture: family caregivers' burden and related factors for older people in Taiwan. J Clin Nurs 14:719–726

24. Lin PC, Lu CM (2007) Psychosocial factors affecting hip fracture elder's burden of care in Taiwan. Orthop Nurs 26:155–161
25. Falaschi P, Eleuteri S, Mitroi C, Farulla C, Martocchia A (2015) Hip fracture: relation between patient's and caregiver's psychological wellbeing. In: Abstracts of the 4th fragility fracture network congress, Rotterdam, Netherlands, pp 75–76
26. Eleuteri S, Bellanti G, Falaschi P (2016) Hip fracture: preliminary results supporting significative correlations between the psychological wellbeing of patients and their relative caregivers. J Gerontol Geriatr 64:104–111
27. Testa MA, Simonson DC (1996) Assessment of quality-of-life outcomes. N Engl J Med 334:835–840
28. World Health Organization (1984) WHO constitution. World Health Organization, Geneva
29. Roth T, Kammerlander C, Gosch M, Luger TJ, Blauth M (2010) Outcome in geriatric fracture patients and how it can be improved. Osteoporos Int 21:S615–S619
30. Randell AG, Nguyen TV, Bhalerao N, Silverman SL, Sambrook PN, Eisman JA (2000) Deterioration in quality of life following hip fracture: a prospective study. Osteoporos Int 11:460–466
31. Bertram M, Norman R, Kemp L, Vos T (2011) Review of the long-term disability associated with hip fractures. Inj Prev 17:365–370
32. Rasmussen B, Uhrenfeldt L (2014) Lived experiences of self-efficacy and wellbeing in the first year after hip fracture: a systematic review protocol of qualitative evidence. JBI Database Syst Rev Implement Rep 12:73–84
33. Garratt A, Schmidt L, Mackintosh A, Fitzpatrick R (2002) Quality of life measurement: bibliographic study of patient assessed health outcome measures. BMJ 324:1417–1421
34. Xenodemetropoulos T, Devison S, Ioannidis G, Adachi JD (2004) The impact of fragility fracture on health-related quality of life. The importance of antifracture therapy. Drugs Aging 21:711–730
35. Hutchings L, Fox R, Chesser T (2011) Proximal femoral fractures in the elderly: how are we measuring outcome? Injury 42:1205–1213
36. Liem IS, Kammerlander C, Suhmb N, Blauth M, Roth T, Gosch M et al (2013) Identifying a standard set of outcome parameters for the evaluation of orthogeriatric co-management for hip fractures. Int J Care Injured 44:1403–1412
37. Bandura A (2010) Self-efficacy. In: Weiner EB, Craighead EW (eds) The Corsini encyclopedia of psychology, 4th edn. John Wiley & Sons, Inc., Hoboken
38. Jellesmark A, Herling SF, Egerod I, Beyer N (2012) Fear of falling and changed functional ability following hip fracture among community-dwelling elderly people: an explanatory sequential mixed method study. Disabil Rehabil 34:2124–2131
39. McMillan L, Booth J, Currie K, Howe T (2013) 'Balancing risk' after fall-induced hip fracture: the older person's need for information. Int J Older People Nursing 9:249–257
40. Pesonen A, Kauppila T, Tarkkila P, Sutela A, Niinisto L, Rosenberg PH (2009) Evaluation of easily applicable pain measurement tools for the assessment of pain in demented patients. Acta Anaesthesiol Scand 53:657–664
41. Katz S, Ford AB, Moskowitz RW, Jackson BA, Jaffe MW (1963) Studies of illness in the aged. The index of ADL: a standardized measure of biological and psychosocial function. JAMA 185:914–919
42. Siddiqi N, Stockdale R, Britton AM, Holmes J (2007) Interventions for preventing delirium in hospitalized patients. Cochrane Database Syst Rev 2:CD005563
43. de Castro SMM, Ünlü Ç, Tuynman JB, Honig A, van Wagensveld BA, Steller EP et al (2014) Incidence and risk factors of delirium in the elderly general surgical patient. Am J Surg 208:26–32
44. Murray AM, Levkoff SE, Wetle TT, Beckett L, Cleary PD, Lipsitz LA et al (1993) Acute delirium and functional decline in the hospitalised elderly patient. J Gerontol Med Sci 48:M181–M186

45. Ely EW, Margolin R, Francis J, May L, Truman B, Dittus R et al (2001) Evaluation of delirium in critically ill patients: validation of the confusion assessment method for the intensive care unit (CAM-ICU). Crit Care Med 29:1370–1379
46. Nightingale S, Holmes J, Mason J, House A (2001) Psychiatric illness and mortality after hip fracture. Lancet 357:1264–1265
47. Bostrom G, Condradsson M, Rosendahl E, Nordstrom P, Gustafson Y, Littbrand H (2014) Functional capacity and dependency in transfer and dressing are associated with depressive symptoms in older people. Clin Interv Aging 9:249–257
48. Djernes JK (2006) Prevalence and predictors of depression in populations of elderly: a review. Acta Psychiatr Scand 113:372–387
49. Atay İM, Aslan A, Burç H, Demirci D, Atay T (2016) Is depression associated with functional recovery after hip fracture in the elderly? J Orthop 13:115–118
50. Folstein MF, Folstein SE, McHugh PR (1975) "Mini-mental state". A practical method for grading the cognitive state of patients for the clinician. J Psychiatr Res 12(3):189–198
51. Kelly RR, McDonald LT, Jensen NR, Sidles SJ, LaRue AC (2019) Impacts of psychological stress on osteoporosis: clinical implications and treatment interactions. Front Psych 10:200
52. Cohen S, Kamarck T, Mermelstein R (1994) A global measure of perceived stress. J Health Soc Behav 24:385–396
53. Sinoff G, Ore L, Zlotogorsky D, Tamir A (1999) Short anxiety screening test—a brief instrument for detecting anxiety in the elderly. Int J Geriatr Psychiatry 14:1062–1071
54. Fianco A, Sartori RD, Negri L, Lorini S, Valle G, Delle Fave A (2015) The relationship between burden and well-being among caregivers of Italian people diagnosed with severe neuromotor and cognitive disorders. Res Dev Disabil 39:43–54
55. Keyes CLM (2002) The mental health continuum: from languishing to flourishing in life. J Health Soc Behav 43:207–222
56. Dupuy HJ (1994) The psychological general well-being (PGWB) index. In: Wenger N (ed) Assessment of quality of life in clinical trials of cardiovascular therapies. Le Jacq, New York
57. Novak M, Guest C (1989) Application of a multidimensional caregiver burden inventory. Gerontologist 29:798–803
58. Pearlin LI, Mullan JT, Semple SJ, Skaff MM (1990) Caregiving and the stress process: an overview of concepts and their measures. Gerontologist 30:583–594
59. McCullagh E, Brigstocke G, Donaldson N, Kalra L (2005) Determinants of caregiving burden and quality of life in caregivers of stroke patients. Stroke 36:2181–2186
60. Kashner TM, Magaziner J, Pruitt S (1990) Family size and caregiving of aged patients with hip fractures. In: Biegel DE, Bulm A (eds) Aging and caregiving: theory, research and policy. Sage, Beverly Hills
61. Gambatesa M, D'Ambrosio A, D'Antini D, Mirabella L, De Capraris A, Iuso S et al (2013) Counseling, quality of life, and acute postoperative pain in elderly patients with hip fracture. J Multidiscip Healthc 6:335–346
62. Marks NF, Lambert JD, Choi H (2002) Transitions to caregiving, gender, and psychological well-being: a prospective U.S. national study. J Marriage Fam 64:657–667
63. Adams B, Aranda MP, Kemp B, Takagi K (2002) Ethnic and gender differences in distress among Anglo-American, African-American, Japanese-American, and Mexican-American spousal caregivers of persons with dementia. J Clin Geropsychol 8:279–301
64. Wallsten SS (2000) Effects of caregiving, gender, and race on the health, mutuality, and social supports of older couples. J Aging Health 12:90–111
65. Walker AJ (2000) Conceptual perspectives on gender and caregiving. In: Dwyer JW, Coward RT (eds) Gender, families and elder care. Sage, Newbury Park
66. Martin CD (2000) More than the work: race and gender differences in caregiving burden. J Fam Issues 21:986–1005
67. Lin IF, Fee HR, Wu HS (2012) Negative and positive caregiving experiences: a closer look at the intersection of gender and relationships. Fam Relat 61(2):343–358
68. Sassen S (2006) Global cities and survival circuits. In: Zimmerman MK, Litt JS, Bose CE (eds) Global dimensions of gender and carework. Stanford University Press, Stanford

69. Campbell P, Wright J, Oyebode J, Job D, Crome P, Bentham P, Jones L, Lendon C (2008) Determinants of burden in those who care for someone with dementia. Int J Geriatr Psychiatry 23:1078–1085
70. Almada AZ (2001) Gender and caregiving: a study among Hispanic and non-Hispanic white frail elders. Master's thesis, Virginia Polytechnic Institute and State University. https://vtech-works.lib.vt.edu/bitstream/handle/10919/33603/thesisjunio18.pdf. Accessed 31 Oct 2019
71. Yeates N (2012) Global care chains: a state-of-the-art review and future directions in care transnationalization research. Glob Netw 12:135–154
72. Brijnath B (2009) Familial bonds and boarding passes: understanding caregiving in a transnational context. Identities 16:83–101
73. De Regt M (2011) Intimate labors: cultures, technologies, and the politics of care. Int Rev Soc Hist 56(3):539–542
74. Mazuz K (2013) The familial dyad between aged patients and Filipina caregivers in Israel: eldercare and bodily-based practices in the Jewish home. Anthropol Aging Q 34:126–134

Part IV

Pillar III: Secondary Prevention

Fracture Risk Assessment and How to Implement a Fracture Liaison Service

14

Nicholas R. Fuggle, M. Kassim Javaid, Masaki Fujita, Philippe Halbout, Bess Dawson-Hughes, Rene Rizzoli, Jean-Yves Reginster, John A. Kanis, Cyrus Cooper, and on behalf of the IOF Capture the Fracture Steering Committee

This chapter is a component of Part 4: Pillar III.
For an explanation of the grouping of chapters in this book, please see Chapter 1: 'The multidisciplinary approach to fragility fractures around the world—an overview'.

on behalf of the IOF Capture the Fracture Steering Committee

N. R. Fuggle · C. Cooper (✉)
MRC Lifecourse Epidemiology Unit, University of Southampton, Southampton, UK
e-mail: nrf@mrc.soton.ac.uk; cc@mrc.soton.ac.uk

M. Kassim Javaid
Nuffield Department of Orthopaedics, Rheumatology and Musculoskeletal Sciences, University of Oxford, Oxford, UK
e-mail: kassim.javaid@ndorms.ox.ac.uk

M. Fujita · P. Halbout
International Osteoporosis Foundation, Geneva, Switzerland
e-mail: mfujita@iofbonehealth.org; phalbout@iofbonehealth.org

B. Dawson-Hughes
Bone Metabolism Laboratory, Jean Mayer USDA Human Nutrition Research Center on Aging at Tufts University, Boston, MA, USA
e-mail: bess.dawson-hughes@tufts.edu

R. Rizzoli
Division of Bone Diseases, Geneva University Hospitals and Faculty of Medicine, Geneva, Switzerland
e-mail: Rene.Rizzoli@unige.ch

J.-Y. Reginster
Department of Public Health, Epidemiology, and Health Economics, University of Liège, Liège, Belgium
e-mail: jyreginster@ulg.ac.be

J. A. Kanis
Centre for Metabolic Bone Diseases, University of Sheffield Medical School, Sheffield, UK
e-mail: w.j.pontefract@shef.ac.uk

© The Author(s) 2021
P. Falaschi, D. Marsh (eds.), *Orthogeriatrics*, Practical Issues in Geriatrics,
https://doi.org/10.1007/978-3-030-48126-1_14

14.1   Introduction

The fragility fracture epidemic is considerable, affecting one in three women and one in five men over the age of 50 years in the Western world [1–3]. This has significant cost to the individual (in terms of morbidity and mortality) but also accrues significant financial costs to the global health economy. Indeed, the annual cost of fragility fractures exceeded €37 billion in Europe (in 2010) [4] and $20 billion in the United States (in 1992) [5]. With the substantial burden of osteoporosis set to rise, the magnitude of this problem can only get larger.

In order to countermand the incidence of fragility fractures two main approaches are required. The first is to ensure that those with osteoporosis are adequately treated, but the second, on which we focus in this chapter, is the timely and effective identification of those at risk of fragility fractures [6].

The index fragility fracture is a vital signal to indicate the need to assess and treat osteoporosis the commencement, or at least consideration, of treatment. Despite this a large proportion of patients presenting to healthcare professionals remain needlessly at risk and untreated [4, 7] in a so-called 'Treatment Gap' [8], with estimates suggesting that a mere 20% of fractured patients are assessed and treated appropriately (though this figure varies according to country and fracture site [9]). As a result, national and international clinical guidelines [10–12] and systematic reviews from the academic community [13, 14] recommend the use of a Fracture Liaison Service (FLS) in order to effectively close this treatment gap. It is also vital to establish an individual's risk of fracture and use this parameter to determine a suitable management plan.

14.2   Fracture Risk Prediction

In 1994, the World Health Organization produced an operational definition of osteoporosis as a bone mineral density (BMD) T-score of −2.5 or lower [15] and this has subsequently become the diagnostic criterion. Indeed, there is a 1.5–2.5 fold increase in fracture risk with each standard deviation decrease in BMD [16], however, the sensitivity of BMD alone to identify those at risk of fracture is less than 50% [17, 18] and many patients sustain fractures with a T score higher than −2.5. For this reason, fracture prediction tools have been developed to aid in the identification of 'at risk' individuals.

The Fracture Risk Assessment Tool (FRAX) was developed via systematic meta-analysis of primary data from 9 geographically spread cohort studies and validated in a further 11 cohorts and was published in 2008 [19]. Key principles were used to identify variables to be included in the FRAX algorithm including:

- The variable should be intuitively linked to fracture.
- The variable should be readily clinically available.

- The variable should be (at least partly) independent of BMD.
- The variable should be associated with a risk which might be reversed by pharmacological therapy.

The clinical parameters chosen were age, sex, weight, height, previous fracture, parental hip fracture, current smoking, glucocorticoid usage, rheumatoid arthritis, secondary causes of osteoporosis, alcohol consumption and BMD (though this can be excluded in resource settings which preclude the measurement of BMD). The output is a 10-year probability of a major osteoporotic fracture (clinical spine, proximal humerus, distal forearm or hip fracture) and the 10-year probability of hip fracture. Fracture incidence varies geographically across the globe [20] and FRAX is calibrated to provide country-specific models [21].

These percentage risks can be used to inform therapeutic intervention thresholds. FRAX has been incorporated in more than 80 guidelines worldwide [21]. Examples include the guidance published by the National Osteoporosis Guidelines Group in the United Kingdom [22, 23], the National Osteoporosis Foundation (NOF) guidelines in the United States [24], The American College of Rheumatology (ACR) [25] and Scottish Intercollegiate Guidelines Network (SIGN) [26].

The Screening of Older women for the Prevention of fracture (SCOOP) trial aimed to establish the efficacy and cost-effectiveness of a community-based screening programme in primary care. A total of 12,483 women aged 70–85 years were recruited from general practice surgeries across the United Kingdom and randomised to either fracture screening using FRAX with dual X-ray absorptiometry as required or 'standard care' (as a control). The primary outcome was the proportion of individuals sustaining fragility fractures in each group and secondary outcomes included; the proportions of all fractures, the hip fracture rate, cost-effectiveness, mortality and EQ-5D in each group and the qualitative evaluation of acceptability for the participants.

The findings of the study were published in 2018. Although there was no significant difference in the primary outcome of all osteoporosis-related fractures between the two groups ($p = 0.178$, HR 0.94 (0.85–1.03) or the rate of all clinical fractures ($p = 0.83$, HR 0.94 (0.86–1.03)), the rate of hip fracture was significantly lower in the screening arm ($p = 0.002$, HR 0.72 (0.59–0.89)) [27]. As shown in Fig. 14.1, the reduction in hip fracture risk was greater than 50% for those at highest risk of fracture [28]. Later health economic analyses demonstrated that screening in this way is cost-saving [29]. In conclusion the SCOOP study suggests that adopting this screening strategy in this population had the potential to cost-effectively prevent 8000 hip fractures per year.

The use of fracture prediction tools, together with BMD measures (if available) and a population screening strategy can all assist in identifying patients at risk of primary and secondary fracture. Of course, a further method to identify and treat 'at risk' individuals is via a Fracture Liaison Service (FLS).

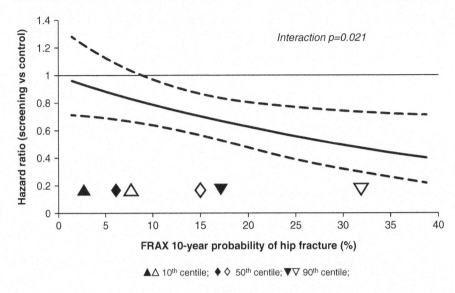

Fig. 14.1 Impact of the SCOOP screening strategy on hip fracture compared with usual care (control arm). The result is depicted as a hazard ratio, across range of FRAX 10-year hip fracture probabilities at baseline (calculated without BMD). There was an interaction of efficacy with baseline probability ($p = 0.021$). The symbols indicate the range of baseline probabilities in the whole study population (black symbols) and in the high-risk group identified by screening (white symbols) [28]

14.3   Fracture Liaison Service

14.3.1 The FLS Model

The FLS model is a coordinator-based, secondary fracture prevention service which is implemented by a healthcare system in order to ensure that those patients presenting with a fragility fracture are identified as osteoporotic and at risk of falls, and thus managed as such [11, 30, 31] (Fig. 14.2). They serve two main purposes; one, to address the aforementioned problem of 'The Treatment Gap' and two, to improve communication between healthcare providers by providing a clearly defined pathway for patients with fragility fractures. It is composed of a team of healthcare professionals including an FLS champion (usually from internal medicine or orthopaedics) and a team of junior clinicians, nurses, allied health professionals and administrators.

Through the work of a dedicated 'case-finder' (usually a clinical nurse specialist) the service will aim to identify and assess fracture patients according to predetermined protocols in the geographic locality of the FLS and can be based in either primary or secondary care.

The model used in the United Kingdom is depicted in Fig. 14.3.

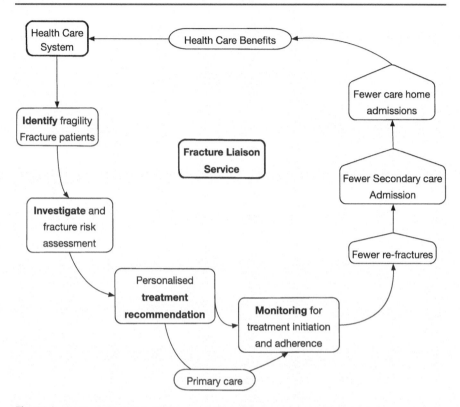

Fig. 14.2 Conceptual model of a Fracture Liaison Service

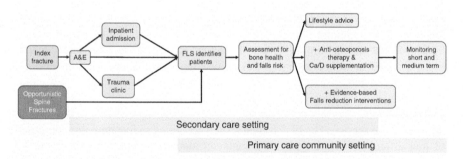

Fig. 14.3 An example of a Fracture Liaison Service model in the United Kingdom

14.3.2 Evidence for Effectiveness of FLS

In 2013, there were 57 FLS worldwide registered with the IOF Capture the Fracture® programme. In the same year, FLS coverage was assessed in 19 of 27 European countries. It was estimated that there was an FLS in less than 10% of their health-care institutions [9]. The story was even more concerning in the Asia-Pacific region with 9 out of 16 countries reporting that none of their hospitals had an FLS [32] and

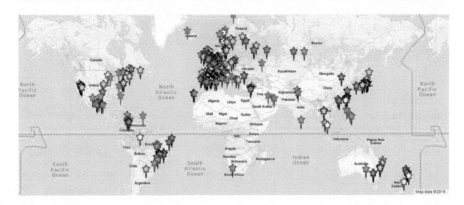

Fig. 14.4 The map of best practice recognises 327 FLS that identify over 345,000 patients every year in 41 countries

only Singapore reported an established FLS in over half their hospitals [33]. The International Osteoporosis Foundation (IOF) Capture the Fracture® (CTF) initiative has also allowed effective mapping of FLS across the globe (Fig. 14.4) and thus demonstrates an increase in uptake since the 2013 census. Indeed, in 2018 the total number of FLS had risen to 327 (identifying over 345,000 fracture patients/year) with 80 new FLS in that year alone, and three new countries registering their first FLS; The Philippines, Sri Lanka and Saudi Arabia.

Beyond coverage, it was previously considered difficult to compare 'inter-service' efficacy and performance due to the wide range of service models in use [14], however, the CTF programme (launched in 2012) has drawn up standards against which services can be assessed. This 'Best Practice Framework' is an immense aid in comparing approaches and assessing the potential patient benefit. It identifies 13 criteria and standards including patient identification, patient evaluation, post-assessment timing, vertebral fracture identification, assessment guidelines, assessment of secondary causes of osteoporosis, falls prevention services, multifaceted nature of assessment, medication initiation, medication review, communication strategy, long-term management and database curation. Each of these standards is graded as bronze, silver or gold depending on the quality of the particular facet of the service. The FLS is then scored according to five domains composed of four different fracture types (hip, inpatient, outpatient and vertebral fractures) and an organisational domain (including falls assessment and database curation).

To engage the global medical community, CTF offers the Best Practice Recognition programme where FLS can submit their service to IOF for evaluation against the BPF standards in order to receive a gold, silver or bronze star. The FLS is showcased and plotted on the CTF Map of Best Practice that displays participating FLS in the programme and their respective achievement level (Fig. 14.4). To influence change, the map can be used as a visual representation of services which are available worldwide, their achievements, as well as the areas for improvement in secondary fracture prevention [34]. The map also serves as a policy advocacy tool that can be leveraged by healthcare professionals and clinics to reach out to policy makers in order to influence changes at national levels.

Beyond the work by CTF, further analyses of the clinical and cost-effectiveness of FLS have been performed in recent years, including modelling within hypothetical cohorts.

Indeed McLellan and colleagues used a cost-effectiveness and budget-impact model (developed using 8 years of FLS data in a UK population) to show that, by implementing an FLS, 18 fractures could be prevented per year (for a hypothetical cohort of 1000 fragility fracture patients) providing an overall saving of £21,000 [35]. A similar study of a hypothetical cohort of 1000 patients in a Swedish population used a Markov micro simulation model to demonstrate that FLS implementation prevented 22 fractures with an incremental cost per QALY for FLS versus usual care of €14,029 [36].

In 2016, Hawley and colleagues examined the impact of FLS introduction or expansion on hip fracture outcomes in the United Kingdom using the Hospital Episode Statistics database. Their natural experiment included patients across 11 acute hospital trusts in England who had sustained a hip fracture between 2003 and 2013 and were aged more than 60. Using time-series analyses, 30-day and 1-year mortality and second hip fracture were examined before and after the change in fracture prevention services. Of the 33,152 primary hip fractures included in the study, 1288 (4.2%) went on to sustain a second hip fracture within 2 years, 3033 (9.5%) patients died within 30 days of their primary hip fracture and 9662 (29.8%) died within 1 year [37]. The introduction or expansion of a nurse-led fracture liaison service was protective for 30 day mortality (Hazard Ratio (HR) 0.80, 95% CI 0.71–0.91) and 1 year mortality (HR 0.84, 95% CI 0.77–0.93) (Fig. 14.5) [37]. However, there was no effect on the occurrence of second hip fracture and no account of whether patients were actually seen by the FLS. A parallel qualitative study was undertaken for the sites and identified ensuring good adherence as key for service effectiveness [38]. The findings of this study provide substantial evidence that delegating monitoring and adherence to existing primary care services blunts the effectiveness of FLSs and supports the need to include monitoring, at least in the short to medium term, within the FLS specification.

The cost-effectiveness of FLS as an intervention for hip fracture was addressed in 2017 by Leal and colleagues who used Markov models to estimate the lifetime impact of an orthogeriatrician-led FLS, nurse-led FLS and usual care. They estimated that, for a female aged 83 years, an orthogeriatrician-led service was effective at £22,709 per QALY for all costs and £12,860 per QALY for healthcare costs. For males the cost-effectiveness of healthcare costs was £14,525 per QALY. These findings demonstrate that there is a significant economic rationale for the introduction of FLS. A more recent systematic review that included any study of FLSs irrespective of study design has also demonstrated the potential benefits from introduction of an FLS [39, 40].

The workforce impact and issues surrounding the running of an FLS were assessed in a qualitative analysis of interviews with 43 health professionals in the United Kingdom, all of whom had been involved in FLS [41]. Significant themes included communication, resourcing and adherence. It was felt that fracture prevention coordinators improved communication within the multi-disciplinary team, however, communication between secondary and primary care was sometimes a challenge. It was noted that the writing of a business case (a fundamental step en route to establishing an FLS in a hospital trust in the United Kingdom) was challenging and that there was under-resourcing of FLS in some sectors. Patient

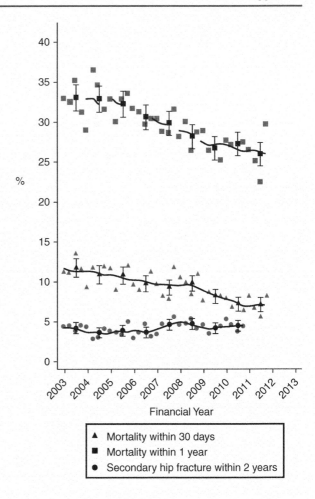

Fig. 14.5 Depicts the annual and quarterly regional mortality trends (for 30 days and 1 year) and second hip fracture (within 2 years) following initial hip fracture [37]

adherence to treatment was observed to be a weakness of the current FLS model and led to calls to improved medication monitoring.

In conclusion, an increasingly substantial body of research data supports the use of FLS by demonstrating a 50% reduction in hip fracture mortality, a 20% reduction in secondary fracture and reduced drug therapy and cost in regions served by an FLS.

14.4   How to Implement an FLS (a Step-by-Step Guide)

The key stages in the development of an FLS are developing national prioritisation, the business case, implementation and sustainability. The first step is prioritisation for FLS at the policy level nationally or regionally. This involves a national coalition of professional societies, patient groups, existing FLS champions and relevant policy makers at the regional and national level. Central to the process of prioritisation is the data pack that links current and projected burden of fragility fracture with the patient, family, health care and societal benefits and includes a formal health economic evaluation.

A FLS business case is then developed that reflects the local benefits of FLS implementation as well as the local FLS costs and inter-dependencies. This may need to be informed by pilot studies to ascertain the optimal minimally disruptive pathway for patients through the different stages of identification, investigation, treatment recommendation and monitoring [42]. Effective patient engagement is key to ensure the pathway is patient centred.

Effective staged implementation of the FLS and scaling to become sustainable requires embedding quality improvement cycles into service provision. The improvement cycles should be supported by local, regional and national and peer-peer and peer-expert forums for discussion and sharing learning. Tools to deliver these programmes of work are being developed by the Capture the Fracture working group and include national prioritisation advocacy, FLS budget impact calculators and different methods for mentoring FLSs through implementation and sustainability of their services.

A coherent multi-disciplinary team should be identified and recruited, including a lead champion for osteoporosis, orthopaedic surgeon, physicians (likely to come from specialties including geriatrics, rheumatology or endocrinology), DXA-specialist radiologists, specialist nurses, physiotherapists and an FLS coordinator. The project team should also include representation from relevant stakeholders including pharmacy, primary care physicians, health system administration, patient champions, charity sector and the health system management funders. This team will provide a holistic overview and ensure that the FLS is structured to perform the functions required by all stakeholders. An initial audit should be performed in order to provide a 'pre-FLS' baseline for future analyses of quality improvement. The data collected should include the number of individuals aged ≥50 years who attend with a hip fragility fracture, with a previous fragility fracture in the last 2 years, already receiving anti-osteoporosis medications and discharged on anti-osteoporosis medication. Additional information on length of stay, discharge destination, healthcare costs and extension to other fracture types will depend on the availability of contemporary national data.

14.4.1 Benchmarking Your Service

The processes of quality improvement described through 'Plan-Do-Study-Act' above only allow assessment of the service against itself; however, it has previously been identified that it would be helpful to compare the service to other FLS both nationally and internationally. The IOF has devised a Best Practice Framework for this purpose and FLS can register on the CTF website to be mapped and benchmarked. The 13 benchmarking criteria are graded as Level 1, 2 or 3 (3 being the best example of practice), as seen in Table 14.1 and include the following:

1. Patient identification—patients with fragility fractures may be identified (level 1), tracked through the health system and may be independently reviewed by the FLS (level 2 and 3).

Table 14.1 The Capture the Fracture® Best Practice Framework for the international benchmarking of fracture liaison services

BPF STANDARD	LEVEL 1	LEVEL 2	LEVEL 3
1. Patient Identification	Patients ID'd, **not** tracked	Patients ID'd, **are** tracked	Patients ID'd, tracked & **Independent review**
2. Patient Evaluation	**50%** assessed	**70%** assessed	**90%** assessed
3. Post Fracture Assessment Timing	Within **13-16 weeks**	Within **9-12 weeks**	Within **8 weeks**
4. Vertebral Fracture (VF) ID	Known VF assessed	Routinely assesses for VF	Radiologists identify VF
5. Assessment Guidelines	Local	Regional	National
6. Secondary Causes of Osteoporosis	**50%** of patients screened	**70%** of patients screened	**90%** of patients screened
7. Falls Prevention Services	**50%** of patients evaluated	**70%** of patients evaluated	**90%** of patients evaluated
8. Multifaceted Assessment	**50%** of patients screened	**70%** of patients screened	**90%** of patients screened
9. Medication Initiation	**50%** of patients initiated	**70%** of patients initiated	**90%** of patients initiated
10. Medication Review	**50%** assessed	**70%** assessed	**90%** assessed
11. Communication Strategy	Communicates to doctor	Communicates to doctor w/ **%50** criteria	Communicates to doctor w/ **%90** criteria*
12. Long-term Management	**1 year** follow-up		**6 month** follow-up & **1 year** follow-up
13. Database	Local	Regional	National

*Criteria: FRAX, DXA, Vertebral DXA/x-ray, primary risk factors, secondary risk factors, falls risk, current medications, medication compliance, follow-up plan, lifestyle risk-factors, time since last fracture.

2. Patient evaluation—assesses the percentage of patients with a fragilty fracture who have been evaluated for the risk of future fracture via a clinical prediction tool (FRAX®) or assessment of bone mineral density.
3. Post-fracture assessment timing—assesses how quickly patients with fragility fractures are assessed with a formal fracture risk assessment by the FLS in weeks since the fracture.
4. Vertebral fracture identification—despite being the most common fragility fracture many vertebral fractures are identified by chance (e.g. as incidental findings in radiological investigations) due to variation in clinical presentation. To achieve the highest level of practice in this criterion it is necessary to liaise with radiology to ensure that they identify and report vertebral fractures and provide a coherent pathway for these patients to access the FLS.
5. Assessment guidelines—evaluates whether the practice of the FLS is aligned to local, national or international guidance for the assessment of fragility fractures.
6. Secondary causes of osteoporosis—assesses the percentage of patients with fragility fractures who are screened for secondary causes of osteoporosis.
7. Falls prevention services—concerns the percentage of patients evaluated for referral to a falls service.
8. Multifaceted assessment—addresses the assessment (and management) of lifestyle factors which may underlie the fracture.
9. Medication initiation—includes the percentage of patients who were eligible for treatment receiving anti-osteoporosis medication.

10. Medication review—includes the percentage of patients who are on anti-osteoporosis medication who have their compliance assessed and in whom alternative medications are considered.
11. Communication strategy—assesses the quality of communication between the FLS and doctors in primary and secondary care including whether the following items are communicated; FRAX® scores, DXA outcomes, vertebral imaging, primary and secondary risk factors for fracture, falls risk, current medication and compliance, follow-up plan, lifestyle risk-factors and time since last fracture.
12. Long-term management—assesses whether medication compliance and tolerance are assessed at 6 months and 1 year after commencement.
13. Database—refers to whether the FLS contributes to a database for fragility fractures at a local, regional or national level.

It should be noted that these criteria are similar to the data collected as part of national registries, including the Australian and New Zealand Hip Fracture Registry [43].

14.4.2 Potential Barriers and How to Overcome them

In some cases, the instigation of an FLS is hampered by barriers, both perceived and real, which can potentially be overcome.

Inadequate financial resources to afford an FLS nurse specialist is one such example with a potential solution being the employment (or re-deployment) of a member of secretarial staff to take on the administrative duties which form part of the FLS nurse specialist role. Language is a potential barrier to engaging with global resources (such as those available through CTF), however, the Best Practice Framework (BPF) document is currently available in 12 major languages: English, French, Spanish, German, Portuguese, Polish, Italian, Hebrew, Russian, Slovak, Chinese (both traditional and simplified forms) and Japanese. The BPF questionnaire (which is completed by all FLS joining the Capture the Fracture program) is now available in eight languages: English, Polish, Spanish, Portuguese, Japanese, Russian, German and Slovak. A Thai version is being developed in collaboration with local FLS experts and medical association in 2019.

Lack of prior experience in running an FLS can lead to a lack of confidence and halting of an FLS initiative. This can be addressed via educational tools and direct mentorship from experienced FLS providers.

As part of the CTF Educational Programme, webinars have been organised since 2015 with the aim to engage with the FLS community of CTF and provide relevant knowledge on FLS and secondary fracture prevention. The ongoing series of webinars provide an opportunity to learn from FLS experts who have established leading FLS across the globe and contributed to development of guidelines and policy on secondary fracture prevention. To this date, 27 webinars have been organised on topics ranging from how to get mapped on CTF; global success stories of FLS

14. Sale JE, Beaton D, Posen J, Elliot-Gibson V, Bogoch E (2011) Systematic review on interventions to improve osteoporosis investigation and treatment in fragility fracture patients. Osteoporos Int 22(7):2067–2082. https://doi.org/10.1007/s00198-011-1544-y
15. Assessment of fracture risk and its application to screening for postmenopausal osteoporosis. Report of a WHO Study Group (1994). World Health Organ Tech Rep Ser 843:1–129
16. Roux C, Reginster JY, Fechtenbaum J, Kolta S, Sawicki A, Tulassay Z, Luisetto G, Padrino JM, Doyle D, Prince R, Fardellone P, Sorensen OH, Meunier PJ (2006) Vertebral fracture risk reduction with strontium ranelate in women with postmenopausal osteoporosis is independent of baseline risk factors. J Bone Miner Res 21(4):536–542. https://doi.org/10.1359/jbmr.060101
17. Schuit SC, van der Klift M, Weel AE, de Laet CE, Burger H, Seeman E, Hofman A, Uitterlinden AG, van Leeuwen JP, Pols HA (2004) Fracture incidence and association with bone mineral density in elderly men and women: the Rotterdam Study. Bone 34(1):195–202
18. Wainwright SA, Marshall LM, Ensrud KE, Cauley JA, Black DM, Hillier TA, Hochberg MC, Vogt MT, Orwoll ES (2005) Hip fracture in women without osteoporosis. J Clin Endocrinol Metab 90(5):2787–2793. https://doi.org/10.1210/jc.2004-1568
19. Kanis JA, McCloskey EV, Johansson H, Strom O, Borgstrom F, Oden A (2008) Case finding for the management of osteoporosis with FRAX—assessment and intervention thresholds for the UK. Osteoporos Int 19(10):1395–1408. https://doi.org/10.1007/s00198-008-0712-1
20. Kanis JA, Oden A, McCloskey EV, Johansson H, Wahl DA, Cooper C (2012) A systematic review of hip fracture incidence and probability of fracture worldwide. Osteoporos Int 23(9):2239–2256. https://doi.org/10.1007/s00198-012-1964-3
21. Kanis JA, Harvey NC, Cooper C, Johansson H, Oden A, McCloskey EV (2016) A systematic review of intervention thresholds based on FRAX : a report prepared for the National Osteoporosis Guideline Group and the International Osteoporosis Foundation. Arch Osteoporos 11(1):25. https://doi.org/10.1007/s11657-016-0278-z
22. Compston J, Cooper A, Cooper C, Gittoes N, Gregson C, Harvey N, Hope S, Kanis JA, McCloskey EV, Poole KES, Reid DM, Selby P, Thompson F, Thurston A, Vine N (2017) UK clinical guideline for the prevention and treatment of osteoporosis. Arch Osteoporos 12(1):43. https://doi.org/10.1007/s11657-017-0324-5
23. McCloskey EV, Johansson H, Harvey NC, Compston J, Kanis JA (2017) Access to fracture risk assessment by FRAX and linked National Osteoporosis Guideline Group (NOGG) guidance in the UK-an analysis of anonymous website activity. Osteoporos Int 28(1):71–76. https://doi.org/10.1007/s00198-016-3696-2
24. Cosman F, de Beur SJ, LeBoff MS, Lewiecki EM, Tanner B, Randall S, Lindsay R (2014) Clinician's guide to prevention and treatment of osteoporosis. Osteoporos Int 25(10):2359–2381. https://doi.org/10.1007/s00198-014-2794-2
25. Grossman JM, Gordon R, Ranganath VK, Deal C, Caplan L, Chen W, Curtis JR, Furst DE, McMahon M, Patkar NM, Volkmann E, Saag KG (2010) American College of Rheumatology 2010 recommendations for the prevention and treatment of glucocorticoid-induced osteoporosis. Arthritis Care Res (Hoboken) 62(11):1515–1526. https://doi.org/10.1002/acr.20295
26. Kanis JA, Compston J, Cooper C, Harvey NC, Johansson H, Oden A, McCloskey EV (2016) SIGN guidelines for Scotland: BMD versus FRAX versus QFracture. Calcif Tissue Int 98(5):417–425. https://doi.org/10.1007/s00223-015-0092-4
27. Shepstone L, Lenaghan E, Cooper C, Clarke S, Fong-Soe-Khioe R, Fordham R, Gittoes N, Harvey I, Harvey N, Heawood A, Holland R, Howe A, Kanis J, Marshall T, O'Neill T, Peters T, Redmond N, Torgerson D, Turner D, McCloskey E (2018) Screening in the community to reduce fractures in older women (SCOOP): a randomised controlled trial. Lancet 391(10122):741–747. https://doi.org/10.1016/s0140-6736(17)32640-5
28. McCloskey E, Johansson H, Harvey NC, Shepstone L, Lenaghan E, Fordham R, Harvey I, Howe A, Cooper C, Clarke S, Gittoes N, Heawood A, Holland R, Marshall T, O'Neill TW, Peters TJ, Redmond N, Torgerson D, Kanis JA (2018) Management of patients with high baseline hip fracture risk by FRAX reduces hip fractures-a post hoc analysis of the SCOOP study. J Bone Miner Res 33(6):1020–1026. https://doi.org/10.1002/jbmr.3411

29. Söreskog EBF, Shepstone L, Clarke S, Cooper C, Harvey I, Harvey NC, Heawood A, Howe A, Johansson H, Marshall T, O'Neill TW, Peters T, Redmond N, Torgerson D, Turner D, McCloskey E, Kanis JA, the SCOOP study (2020) Long-term cost-effectiveness of screening for fracture risk in a UK primary care setting. Osteoporos Int. https://doi.org/10.1007/s00198-020-05372-6

30. Akesson K, Marsh D, Mitchell PJ, McLellan AR, Stenmark J, Pierroz DD, Kyer C, Cooper C (2013) Capture the fracture: a best practice framework and global campaign to break the fragility fracture cycle. Osteoporos Int 24(8):2135–2152. https://doi.org/10.1007/s00198-013-2348-z

31. Mitchell PJ, Cooper C, Fujita M, Halbout P, Akesson K, Costa M, Dreinhofer KE, Marsh DR, Lee JK, Chan DD, Javaid MK (2019) Quality improvement initiatives in fragility fracture care and prevention. Curr Osteoporos Rep. https://doi.org/10.1007/s11914-019-00544-8

32. Mithal A, Bansal B, Kyer CS, Ebeling P (2014) The Asia-Pacific regional audit-epidemiology, costs, and burden of osteoporosis in India 2013: a report of international osteoporosis foundation. Indian J Endocrinol Metab 18(4):449–454. https://doi.org/10.4103/2230-8210.137485

33. Chandran M, Tan MZ, Cheen M, Tan SB, Leong M, Lau TC (2013) Secondary prevention of osteoporotic fractures--an "OPTIMAL" model of care from Singapore. Osteoporos Int 24(11):2809–2817. https://doi.org/10.1007/s00198-013-2368-8

34. Mitchell P, Åkesson K, Chandran M, Cooper C, Ganda K, Schneider M (2016) Implementation of models of care for secondary osteoporotic fracture prevention and orthogeriatric models of care for osteoporotic hip fracture. Best Pract Res Clin Rheumatol 30(3):536–558

35. McLellan AR, Wolowacz SE, Zimovetz EA, Beard SM, Lock S, McCrink L, Adekunle F, Roberts D (2011) Fracture liaison services for the evaluation and management of patients with osteoporotic fracture: a cost-effectiveness evaluation based on data collected over 8 years of service provision. Osteoporos Int 22(7):2083–2098. https://doi.org/10.1007/s00198-011-1534-0

36. Jonsson E, Borgström F, Ström C (2016) Cost effectiveness evaluation of fracture liaison services for the management of osteoporosis in Sweden. Value Health 19:A347–A766

37. Hawley S, Javaid MK, Prieto-Alhambra D, Lippett J, Sheard S, Arden NK, Cooper C, Judge A (2016) Clinical effectiveness of orthogeriatric and fracture liaison service models of care for hip fracture patients: population-based longitudinal study. Age Ageing 45(2):236–242. https://doi.org/10.1093/ageing/afv204

38. Drew S, Judge A, Cooper C, Javaid MK, Farmer A, Gooberman-Hill R (2016) Secondary prevention of fractures after hip fracture: a qualitative study of effective service delivery. Osteoporos Int 27(5):1719–1727. https://doi.org/10.1007/s00198-015-3452-z

39. Wu CH, Kao IJ, Hung WC, Lin SC, Liu HC, Hsieh MH, Bagga S, Achra M, Cheng TT, Yang RS (2018) Economic impact and cost-effectiveness of fracture liaison services: a systematic review of the literature. Osteoporos Int 29(6):1227–1242. https://doi.org/10.1007/s00198-018-4411-2

40. Wu CH, Tu ST, Chang YF, Chan DC, Chien JT, Lin CH, Singh S, Dasari M, Chen JF, Tsai KS (2018) Fracture liaison services improve outcomes of patients with osteoporosis-related fractures: a systematic literature review and meta-analysis. Bone 111:92–100. https://doi.org/10.1016/j.bone.2018.03.018

41. Judge A, Javaid MK, Leal J, Hawley S, Drew S, Sheard S, Prieto-Alhambra D, Gooberman-Hill R, Lippett J, Farmer A, Arden N, Gray A, Goldacre M, Delmestri A, Cooper C (2016) Health services and delivery research. In: Models of care for the delivery of secondary fracture prevention after hip fracture: a health service cost, clinical outcomes and cost-effectiveness study within a region of England. NIHR Journals Library. Copyright (c) Queen's Printer and Controller of HMSO 2016. This work was produced by Judge et al. under the terms of a commissioning contract issued by the Secretary of State for Health. This issue may be freely reproduced for the purposes of private research and study and extracts (or indeed, the full report) may be included in professional journals provided that suitable acknowledgement is made and the reproduction is not associated with any form of advertising. Applications for commercial reproduction should be addressed to: NIHR Journals Library, National Institute for Health Research, Evaluation, Trials and Studies Coordinating Centre, Alpha House, University of Southampton Science Park, Southampton SO16 7NS, UK, Southampton (UK). https://doi.org/10.3310/hsdr04280

42. May C, Montori VM, Mair FS (2009) We need minimally disruptive medicine. BMJ 339:b2803. https://doi.org/10.1136/bmj.b2803
43. Australian and New Zealand Hip Fracture Registry, annual report (2019)
44. Tsabasvi M, Davey S, Temu R (2017) Hip fracture pattern at a major Tanzanian referral hospital: focus on fragility hip fractures. Arch Osteoporos 12(1):47. https://doi.org/10.1007/s11657-017-0338-z
45. Senay A, Delisle J, Giroux M, Laflamme GY, Leduc S, Malo M, Nguyen H, Ranger P, Fernandes JC (2016) The impact of a standardized order set for the management of non-hip fragility fractures in a Fracture Liaison Service. Osteoporos Int 27(12):3439–3447. https://doi.org/10.1007/s00198-016-3669-5

Current and Emerging Treatment of Osteoporosis

15

Laura Tafaro and Nicola Napoli

15.1 Introduction

A fracture is a dramatic event for every patient because of pain, immobility and therefore the overall deterioration of their quality of life. Unfortunately, epidemiological data tell us that those who have suffered a fragility fracture are more at risk of suffering another in the same or other sites within a short time [1]. The goal of those treating a patient with recent fragility fracture should therefore not only be to treat the patient in the acute phase but also to prevent further fractures [2].

Interventions to increase bone mass to preventing further fragility fractures can be classified as pharmacological and non-pharmacological.

15.2 Pharmacological Treatment for All Patients with Fragility Fractures

Who are the patients that need pharmacological treatment? All European and international guidelines [3–5] do not base the need for treatment on the diagnosis of osteoporosis (based on the T-score) but on the risk of fracture, which is strongly influenced by the presence of a fragility fracture, especially vertebral or femoral fractures. A fragility fracture occurs spontaneously or following low-energy trauma in individuals with a low bone mineral density (BMD) [6].

This chapter is a component of Part 4: Pillar III.
For an explanation of the grouping of chapters in this book, please see Chapter: "The multidisciplinary approach to fragility fractures around the world—an overview".

L. Tafaro (✉)
Sant'Andrea Hospital, Sapienza University of Rome, Rome, Italy
e-mail: laura.tafaro@uniroma1.it

N. Napoli
Unit of Endocrinology and Diabetes, Campus Biomedico University of Rome, Rome, Italy

© The Author(s) 2021
P. Falaschi, D. Marsh (eds.), *Orthogeriatrics*, Practical Issues in Geriatrics,
https://doi.org/10.1007/978-3-030-48126-1_15

We do not need to apply an algorithm to decide who to treat because if our patient is a postmenopausal woman has had a fragility fracture, automatically we should consider her at high risk of further fractures. In the same way, an elderly patient with a hip fragility fracture should automatically be classified as having severe osteoporosis independently of other risk factors.

15.2.1 Bedridden Fractured Patients

Immobilisation itself causes osteopenia, indeed bedridden patients can suffer painful spontaneous fractures [7]. Secondary prevention trials usually do not include bedridden fractured patients, possibly because most common oral osteoporosis treatments are associated with esophagitis as a side effect and may increase the risk of reflux esophagitis for these patients [8]. However, a few studies on non-oral administration have shown good efficacy in patients with severe motor and intellectual disabilities [9]. Although further studies are needed, it seems to be important to treat this category of patients as well.

In conclusion, all orthogeriatric patients should start pharmacological treatment to strengthen their bone to prevent further fractures.

15.2.2 Make a Diagnosis Before Treatment

Before treatment it is important to make a differential diagnosis between primary and secondary osteoporosis because the anti-osteoporotic drug treatment would be useless if the main illness causing osteoporosis is not treated too.

In hospital, during the acute phase, it is important to investigate the osteoporosis to exclude secondary forms, by means of simple first-level blood tests (erythrocyte sedimentation rate, blood count, serum levels of protein, calcium, phosphorus, alkaline phosphatase and creatinine, 24 h urinary calcium) and some second level tests (TSH, Parathormone, 25-OH-vitamin D, serum protein electrophoresis). These tests are sufficient to exclude 90% of the secondary causes of osteoporosis. Only the evaluation of these parameters will guarantee that we are giving to the patient appropriate treatment [10].

It is important to make at any age a diagnosis of secondary causes of osteoporosis, such as hyperthyroidism and hyperparathyroidism, because these can now be treated with drugs and not only by surgery [11, 12].

15.2.3 Set Up an Appropriate and Personalised Treatment

Some studies show that anti-osteoporotic drugs are frequently interrupted within 1 month of their prescription; this happens not so much due to the occurrence of adverse events but mostly because patients have not been sufficiently informed about the importance of taking the drug and because they not receive personalised treatment [13].

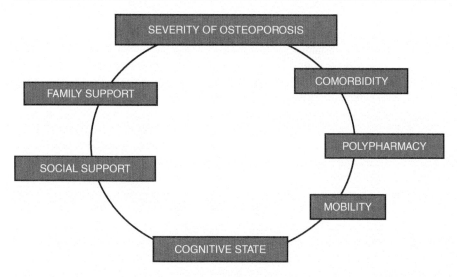

Fig. 15.1 Tailored treatment of osteoporosis in elderly people

The orthogeriatric patient with non-vertebral fracture has specific characteristics: they are normally very old (over 75 years) and present all the characteristics of frailty (reduced mobility, malnutrition, comorbidity, cognitive impairment, polypharmacy, neurosensory deficits). To improve adherence, in addition to osteoporosis severity, the degree of frailty and social family support should be considered in the choice of treatment. Osteoporosis treatment presents many choices [14], both in the route of administration and dosage frequency, so it is possible to define, together with the caregivers, a tailored treatment (Fig. 15.1). For example, subcutaneous or intramuscular administration may be easier or more complicated than oral intake depending on the patient's overall clinical and social conditions.

Sometimes, a drug recommended on the basis of severity of osteoporosis is not the most suitable for the patient. The need to renew the treatment plan every year, for an institutionalised elderly patient with a low family support, can be problematic. Depending on the complexity of the patient, a specialist management of osteoporosis therapy by a bone specialist may be necessary.

Another important point to improve adherence is that, on discharge from the orthopaedic department, the patient should be referred to a Fracture Liaison service that can also follow up the patient and change the medication in the light of the occurrence of new fractures under treatment, BMD measurement, change in clinical or social conditions and so on [15].

15.3   Non-pharmacological Treatment

15.3.1   Lifestyle and Exercise

Excessive use or abuse of alcohol should be avoided for a number of health-related risks, including bone loss. Moderate drinking during a meal (one glass of wine or beer), or only in social occasions, is harmless. Likewise, caffeine intake is harmful only when excessive amounts are ingested, although its calciuric effect should be compensated by increasing calcium intake. On the other hand, any form of nicotine use should be discouraged, although substantial negative effects of cigarette smoking on bone health are seen only in individuals with smoking histories of 30 pack-years or above.

By and large, the most important lifestyle factor to be included in managing patients with osteoporosis is physical activity. The amount and intensity of weight-bearing physical activity in young healthy individuals is a determinant of peak bone mass. Likewise, a sedentary lifestyle and prolonged bed rest lead to increased bone loss in the involutional period. Therefore, attempts should be made to encourage physical activity and implement a moderate exercise programme to minimise bone loss in elderly people.

For the older individual with vertebral fractures and severe loss of bone mass, walking may be the only feasible exercise. Swimming, which is an excellent exercise for older individuals to condition muscle tone and strength, does not appear to alter bone loss patterns appreciably because it is not a weight-bearing exercise. Bone mineral content in the spine may be increased somewhat by more vigorous programmes, individualised for target heart-rate ranges, which depend on age and the maximum predicted pulse.

Cessation of exercise results in a gradual but progressive loss of bone. When recommending exercise regimens for elderly women of unknown cardiovascular fitness with established vertebral osteoporosis, patients should be advised about the adverse effects of strenuous exercise. Extension or isometric exercises are more appropriate for these individuals because vertebral compression fractures are more apt to occur during flexion exercise. These aerobic conditioning exercise programmes should be implemented with physician advice and should also include warm-up and cool-down intervals.

15.4 Pharmacological Interventions

A wide variety of drugs have been proposed for either preventing bone loss in high-risk populations or preventing fracture and further bone loss in individuals with a previous fracture.

15.4.1 Ca and Vitamin D to All Patients in Association with Anti-osteoporotic Therapy

There have been controversies in the literature on the efficacy of calcium and vitamin D for the prevention of osteoporosis and fractures without other drugs. However, in the oldest patients, including orthogeriatric patients, all data confirm that vitamin D deficiency is very common and calcium intake is often not adequate.

So, osteoporosis guidelines recommend:

- Older people should routinely receive vitamin D supplements [16].
- In postmenopausal women with low BMD and at high risk of fractures, calcium and vitamin D should be used as an adjunct to osteoporosis therapies, otherwise the latter will be ineffective [3].

There is broad consensus that vitamin D levels should be maintained above 20 ng/mL; this would already be a good result for orthogeriatric patients, who generally have values lower than 8 ng/mL [17]. Regarding the recommended dose of vitamin D, local guidelines should be followed; the most widespread programme for the correction of vitamin D deficiency (<10 ng/mL) consists of cholecalciferol in quite high doses of 50,000 IU per week for 1 or 2 months; then continued daily, weekly or monthly doses that guarantee 1200 IU daily. The most appropriate form of vitamin D to use (cholecalciferol, calcifediol, alfacalcidol, calcitriol) depends on the patient's condition and compliance. However, hydroxylated vitamin D metabolites increase the risk of hypercalcaemia and hypercalciuria; they may therefore need to be ruled out or monitored with serial serum and urinary calcium measurement [18].

It is difficult for older patients to have an adequate calcium intake by diet alone, but it is better to improve the dietary intake before giving a calcium supplementation. Many calcium formulations are available and the most suitable one should be recommended for each patient; for example, calcium carbonate should not be prescribed for patients with dyspepsia or who use protonic pump inhibitors (PPI)—for these patients, formulations of calcium citrate are more suitable [19].

15.4.2 Choose the Safe and Effective Drug for the Orthogeriatric Patient

We have many drugs for the treatment of patients at high risk of fracture (see Table 15.1) [14], but we should choose drugs based on efficacy and safety evidence provided by targeted studies or extrapolated data in old age subgroups.

For example, the use of oestrogen, tibolone and selective oestrogen receptor modulators (SERMs) is not recommended in orthogeriatric patients because they do not fit the patient characteristics appropriate for these drugs according to the latest guidelines. Specifically, they are not usually under 60 years of age or <10 years past menopause, with low risk of deep vein thrombosis and low cardiovascular risk. Moreover, in most countries these drugs are approved for the prevention but not the treatment of osteoporosis, nor for secondary prevention of fracture [3, 14].

We can divide osteoporosis therapies into two groups: antiresorptive and anabolic.

Table 15.1 Fracture risk reduction and route of administration of antiresorptive drugs

Antiresorptive drugs	Route of administration	Fracture risk reduction			
		Vertebral	Hip	Non-vertebral	Elderly
Alendronate	Oral once daily or weekly	Yes	Yes	Yes	Yes
Risedronate	Oral once daily, weekly, or monthly	Yes	Yes	Yes	Yes
Ibandronate	Oral once monthly or intravenous every 3 months	Yes	ND[a]	ND[a]	Yes
Zoledronic acid	Intravenous once yearly	Yes	Yes	Yes	Yes
Denosumab	Subcutaneous injection every 6 months	Yes	Yes	Yes	Yes

[a]Studies not powered to observe effect on hip or non-vertebral fracture risk

15.5 Antiresorptive Therapies

The fracture risk reduction and route of administration of antiresorptive drugs are shown in Table 15.1.

15.5.1 Bisphosphonates

Bisphosphonates are chemically related to inorganic pyrophosphate, which is a potent inhibitor of calcium phosphate crystallisation and dissolution. These compounds act primarily by inhibiting osteoclast-mediated bone resorption via a variety of mechanisms. Small changes in the basic structure of the bisphosphonate can result in extensive alterations in its biological, toxicological and physiochemical characteristics in addition to its therapeutic potential for the treatment of osteoporosis. Of the bisphosphonates that have been synthesised, etidronate, clodronate, ibandronate, zoledronate, alendronate and risedronate have been available commercially for varying periods of time for the treatment osteoporosis. Others, such as neridronate, are currently being tested for use in osteoporosis.

The bisphosphonates are not all the same; their effectiveness, long-term action and safety depend on the strength of their bond with hydroxyapatite (Fig. 15.2); because of this link they have different dosages and ways of administration so it is possible to choose a personalised treatment based on the needs of the patient [20]. Another advantage is the low cost of oral therapy which makes it accessible even to patients with low economic resources.

Clodronate is currently commercially available in a variety of international locations. Clodronate does not inhibit bone mineralisation in doses recommended for osteoporosis therapy.

Fig. 15.2 Kinetic binding affinity of bisphosphonates

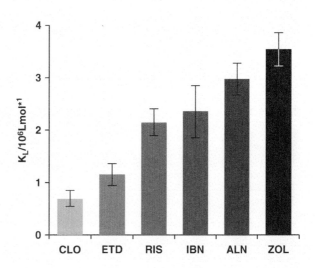

Alendronate was the first bisphosphonate to be approved by the U.S. Food and Drug Administration for the prevention and treatment of postmenopausal and glucocorticoid-induced osteoporosis and osteoporosis in men. Alendronate, an aminobisphosphonate with approximately 700 times more potency than etidronate in inhibiting bone resorption, has been shown in several controlled trials to increase bone density and reduce vertebral and hip fractures among postmenopausal women with low bone density. It also increases bone density in men and women taking glucocorticoids and in men with idiopathic osteoporosis. Data on the effectiveness of alendronate are the largest currently available for any drugs used in osteoporosis treatment.

The Fracture Intervention Trial (FIT) was the first randomised, controlled trial designed with fracture reduction as the primary outcome. In the vertebral fracture arm of FIT, 2027 women with low bone mass and at least one pre-existing vertebral fracture were randomly assigned to receive a placebo or alendronate 5 mg (raised to 10 mg at month 24) daily for 3 years [21]. They were also given 500 mg of calcium and 250 IU of vitamin D. The proportion of women with new morphometrically (radiologically) defined vertebral fracture(s) was 55% lower in those taking alendronate (8%) relative to those taking placebo (15%). Likewise, the proportion of women with clinically evident (reported during the study as adverse events) new vertebral fractures was 47% lower in the alendronate (2.3%) relative to the placebo group (5.0%). The relative risk for two or more morphometric vertebral fractures was reduced by ~90% by alendronate treatment, demonstrating that the best results are obtained in subjects at the highest risk. Importantly, the incidence of hip fractures was also reduced to 51% in women taking alendronate, an extraordinary finding considering the size of the study that was not designed to detect effects on hip fracture, a much less frequent event relative to vertebral fractures [21]. These results remain a milestone observation that has revolutionised the approach to treating osteoporosis and demonstrate the efficacy of this bisphosphonate for fracture prevention.

In the non-vertebral fracture arm of the FIT trial, 4432 postmenopausal women with femoral neck T score <-1.6, but without vertebral fractures at baseline were studied in the same fashion as for the vertebral fracture arm. At the end of the study, there was an overall statistically significant 44% reduction in new morphometrically defined vertebral fractures in the alendronate group. Although clinical vertebral fractures or hip fractures were not statistically decreased in this study population, in the subgroup of women with femoral neck T-score <-2.5 there was indeed a reduction in both clinical vertebral fractures (36%) and hip fractures (56%) in the alendronate group. This result underscores the concept that, in primary prevention, therapeutic interventions are only effective in subjects at risk. When the risk is low or absent, expecting an effect may be unreasonable. Hence, a diagnosis of osteoporosis or a full estimation of fracture risk should always be made before committing a patient to long-term therapies with a bone active drug.

Risedronate. In early postmenopausal women, 5 mg daily of risedronate for 2 years produced 5.7% and 5.4% increments of vertebral and trochanter bone density, respectively. Efficacy on vertebral fracture prevention was demonstrated in the VERT (Vertebral Efficacy with Risedronate Therapy) trial, which was conducted on 2458 postmenopausal osteoporotic (femoral neck T-score <−2.5) women with at least 1 vertebral fracture at baseline, as two separate trials in North America and in the rest of the world [22]. Relative to women receiving only vitamin D (500 IU) and calcium (1000 mg), 5 mg of risedronate daily resulted in significant increases in bone density at the lumbar spine and proximal femur, and reduced the incidence of new vertebral fractures by as much as 65% within the first year of the study and by 41% at 3 years [22]. As a secondary outcome, a significant 39% reduction in non-vertebral fractures among treated women was detected, but no significant reduction in hip fractures was noted. While the VERT trial was not powered to detect such an effect, the HIP (Hip Intervention Program) found a 30% reduction in new hip fracture in women taking risedronate (pooled data from 2.5 and 5 mg daily) [23]. In addition to the indication for prevention and therapy of postmenopausal osteoporosis, risedronate is also approved for the treatment of steroid-induced osteoporosis.

Ibandronate is a third generation, potent bisphosphonate currently available at 150 mg once a month. Bone markers of turnover were also suppressed, although with a fluctuating pattern.

Zoledronate is the most potent bisphosphonate among the ones currently available in clinical medicine. With intravenous administration, zoledronate at a yearly dose of 5 mg is currently approved for the treatment of osteoporosis, hypercalcemia of malignancy and bone metastases. The Horizon trial [24] demonstrated a 40% reduction in zoledronate-treated patients versus placebo for hip fractures, rising to more than 50% for vertebral fractures. Zoledronate treatment is also associated with 30% reduction in mortality. Recent data [25] have shown also a strong efficacy of zoledronate used every 18 months for 5 years in osteopenic post-menopausal women. Importantly, secondary analysis also proved efficacy for reducing the risk of cardiovascular diseases and mortality.

Use of zoledronate is limited by hospital setting and acute reaction symptoms.

15.5.1.1   Adverse Events

The common ones are upper gastrointestinal adverse reactions with oral dosing, acute phase reaction with intravenous dosing. The uncommon are bone, joint and muscle pain.

The rare ones are eye inflammation, femoral shaft or subtrochanteric fractures with atypical radiographic features, osteonecrosis of the jaw.

In recent years, the fear of rare side effects of bisphosphonates has increased, in particular, osteonecrosis of the jaw, an opportunistic infection with actinomyces caused by the inhibition of osteoclast activity that mostly happens after dental surgery. It is appropriate to recall the Joint Position of ASBMR which reiterates that the incidence of this event is only 1:100,000 in patients who are treated with bisphosphonates for osteoporosis while it is much higher in patients treated for bone metastases or immunosuppressed. It is however recommended to perform a dental check before starting therapy and always maintaining good oral hygiene.

Contraindications for all these drugs are hypersensitivity and hypocalcaemia. For oral drugs: oesophageal abnormalities that delay emptying, inability to remain upright; zoledronic acid should not be used in impaired renal function (creatinine clearance less than 35 mL/min).

There is a warning about the use of bisphosphonates in patients with severe renal impairment.

15.5.1.2   Technical Remark

Since their chemical structure is acidic, bisphosphonates are irritant for the oesophageal mucosa if contact is prolonged. This problem can be overcome by taking the drug with 100–200 mL of water while standing upright for 30–40 min.

An important technical remark about in patients who are taking bisphosphonates is that fracture risk be reassessed after 3–5 years:

– If the risk is still high: the patient should continue therapy.
– If the risk has become low-moderate: the patient should be considered for a temporary discontinuation of bisphosphonates (bisphosphonate holiday).

A bisphosphonate holiday should involve a reassessment of fracture risk at 2–4 year intervals and consideration of reinitiating osteoporosis therapy earlier than 5 years if there is a significant decline in BMD, a new fracture or certain other factors [3].

15.5.2   Rank Ligand Inhibitor

Denosumab is a human monoclonal antibody that specifically targets RANK Ligand, an essential mediator of osteoclast formation, function and survival. The binding of this drug to RANK ligand prevents the activation of RANK on the surface of osteoclasts and their precursors. Prevention of the RANKL/RANK interaction inhibits osteoclast formation, function and survival, thereby decreasing bone resorption and increasing bone mass and strength in both cortical and trabecular bone [26]. This drug therefore has a completely different mechanism of action from that of bisphosphonates and does not bind to bone, which is why it was more effective than bisphosphonates in the prevention of non-vertebral fractures. The effects of Denosumab on bone remodelling, reflected in bone turnover markers, reverse after 6 months [27] so it can administered only twice per year (see Table 15.2).

The positive effects of Denosumab treatment on BMD persist for 10 years (Freedom) and there is no increase in adverse effects [28]. Denosumab advantages for hip fracture patients are that it can be administered during hospitalisation in bedridden patients and doesn't have a toxicity risk in patients affected by hepatic or renal chronic failure (even with dialysis) [29]. In countries where its prescription needs a bone specialist management, family or social support is necessary.

Table 15.2 Fracture risk and route of administration of anabolic drugs

Anabolic drugs	Route of administration	Fracture risk reduction			
		Vertebral	Hip	Non-vertebral	Elderly
Teriparatide	Subcutaneous injection daily for 2 years	Yes	ND[a]	Yes	Yes
Abaloparatide (not available in Europe)	Subcutaneous injection daily for 2 years	Yes	ND[a]	Yes	Yes
Romosozumab	Subcutaneous injection monthly for 1 years	Yes	Yes[b]	Yes	Yes

[a]Studies not powered to observe effect on hip or non-vertebral fracture risk
[b]Data available only in sequential therapy with alendronate

15.5.2.1 Adverse Events

Uncommon: skin rash; rare: cellulitis, femoral shaft or subtrochanteric fractures with atypical radiographic features, osteonecrosis of the jaw.

Contraindications for Denosumab use are hypocalcaemia, pregnancy, hypersensitivity;

Warning: multiple vertebral fractures have occurred when Denosumab has been discontinued.

15.5.2.2 Technical Remark

A drug holiday is not recommended with Denosumab, administration should be not delay or stopped without subsequent antiresorptive therapy to prevent a rebound in bone turnover [30].

15.6 Anabolic Drugs

Anabolic drugs are recommended in postmenopausal women at very high risk of fracture, such as those with severe or multiple fractures. Osteoanabolic therapy has the potential to restore skeletal microstructure and uniquely transform osteoporotic bone towards normal [31]. We have two class of anabolic drugs: parathyroid hormone receptor agonist and sclerostin antibody (see Table 15.3). Teriparatide is a current therapy, whereas abaloparatide and romosozumab should be considered emerging therapies.

The fracture risk reduction and the route of administration of anabolic drugs are shown in Table 15.2.

15.6.1 Parathyroid Hormone Receptor (PTHr) Agonists: Teriparatide and Abaloparatide

The safety and efficacy of PTHr agonists have not been established beyond 2 years of treatment so the maximum duration of therapy over a patient's lifetime is 24 months.

Table 15.3 Fundamental recommendation in secondary prevention in the elderly (modified by the American Society of Bone and Mineral Research Secondary prevention Guidelines 2019)

• Offer pharmacologic therapy for osteoporosis to people aged 65 years or older with a hip or vertebral fracture, to reduce their risk of additional fractures
– Do not delay initiation of therapy for bone mineral density (BMD) testing
– Consider patients' oral health before starting therapy with bisphosphonates or denosumab
– For patients who have had repair of a hip fracture or are hospitalized for a vertebral fracture:
Oral pharmacologic therapy can begin in the hospital and be included in discharge orders
Intravenous and subcutaneous pharmacologic agents may be therapeutic options after the first 2 weeks of the postoperative period. Concerns during this early recovery period include:
Hypocalcemia because of factors including vitamin D deficiency or perioperative overhydration
Acute phase reaction of flu-like symptoms following zoledronic acid infusion, particularly in patients who have not previously taken zoledronic acid or other bisphosphonates
If pharmacologic therapy is not provided during hospitalization, then mechanisms should be in place to ensure timely follow-up.
• Initiate a daily supplement of at least 800 IU vitamin D per day for people aged 65 years or older with a hip or vertebral fracture.
• Initiate a daily calcium supplement for people aged 65 years or older with a hip or vertebral fracture who are unable to achieve an intake of 1200 mg/day of calcium from food sources.
• Because osteoporosis is a life-long chronic condition, routinely follow and re-evaluate people aged 65 years or older with a hip or vertebral fracture who are being treated for osteoporosis. Purposes include:
– Reinforcing key messages about osteoporosis and associated fractures
– Identifying any barriers to treatment plan adherence that arise
– Assessing the risk of falling
– Monitoring for adverse treatment effects
– Evaluating the effectiveness of the treatment plan; and
– Determining whether any changes in treatment should be made, including whether any antiosteoporosis pharmacotherapy should be changed or discontinued

In the registration study the hip fracture reduction for both agents was not statistically significant, probably because the numbers of hip fracture were small and the studies were inadequately powered for this endpoint; however, increased bone strength in the hip has been reported with longer term treatment [32].

These agents are much more expensive than other antiosteoporotic drugs, for this reason, they are used only in secondary treatment.

Teriparatide is a fragment of full-length PTH, it is recommended for postmenopausal women with osteoporosis at very high risk of fracture (severe or multiple fractures) [33].

In comparator studies, teriparatide was significantly more effective in:

– Protecting postmenopausal women with osteoporosis from vertebral fracture than was risedronate [34].
– Preventing new vertebral fractures in glucocorticoid-induced osteoporosis than was alendronate [35].

Its use is limited to 24 months due to a significant increase in osteosarcoma in rats given the drug for longer than this period but, since the introduction of teriparatide in 2002, in more than 1 million patients the rate of osteosarcoma has not been greater than expected [36].

Abaloparatide is a PTH-related protein analogue (PTHrP). It has a mechanism of action similar to teriparatide, but it showed a little more efficacy in preventing vertebral fractures compared with placebo, and milder adverse events than teriparatide [37].

Abaloparatide is not available in Europe because EMA refused its commercialisation on grounds of doubts about its effectiveness in reducing non-vertebral fractures and a tendency to tachycardia and palpitations.

15.6.1.1   Adverse Events

Common: nausea, dizziness, muscle cramps, increased serum or urine calcium or serum uric acid; uncommon: orthostatic hypotension. Abaloparatide causes less hypercalcemia but causes palpitations [38].

Contraindications: Hypercalcemia, hypersensitivity, nephrolithiasis.

Warnings: should not be used in children or adolescents with open epiphyses, or patients with Paget's disease of bone, previous external beam or implant radiation involving the skeleton, bone metastases, history of skeletal malignancies, other metabolic bone diseases or hypercalcaemic disorders.

15.6.2   Anti-Sclerostin Antibody: Romosozumab

Romosozumab is a monoclonal antibody that binds and inhibits sclerostin. It exerts a dual effect on bone: increased bone formation and decreased bone resorption [39]. During 2019 it was approved by FDA and EMA and in Japan for the treatment of osteoporosis in postmenopausal women at high risk of fracture.

The sequence of Romosozumab followed by an antiresorptive therapy may provide significant benefits for the treatment of osteoporosis in women at high risk for fracture [40].

Another study demonstrated that 1 year of Romosozumab followed by 1 year of Denosumab treatment in the FRAME trial led to BMD changes similar to 7 years of Denosumab treatment [41]. An increased risk of cardiovascular events was observed compared with alendronate but not compared with placebo.

15.6.2.1   Adverse Events

Common: Injection-site reaction (pain (1.6% of patients), erythema (1.3%), pruritus (0.8%), haemorrhage (0.5%), rash (0.4%) and swelling (0.3%).

Contraindications: hypersensitivity.

15.6.2.2   Technical Remark for Anabolic Agents

In patients who have completed a course of anabolic agents, it is recommended to switch to treatment with antiresorptive therapies, to maintain bone density gains [3].

15.7   Influence of Osteoporosis Medication on Fracture Healing

Pharmacologic agents that influence bone remodelling are an essential component of osteoporosis management. Because many patients are first diagnosed with osteoporosis when presenting with a fragility fracture, it is critical to understand how osteoporotic medications influence fracture healing. Vitamin D and its analogues are essential for the mineralisation of the callus and may also play a role in callus formation and remodelling that enhances biomechanical strength. In animal models, antiresorptive medications, including bisphosphonates, denosumab, calcitonin, oestrogen and raloxifene, do not impede endochondral fracture healing but may delay remodelling. Although bisphosphonates and denosumab delay callus remodelling, they increase callus volume and result in unaltered biomechanical properties. Parathyroid hormone, an anabolic agent, has demonstrated promise in animal models, resulting in accelerated healing with increased callus volume and density, more rapid remodelling to mature bone and improved biomechanical properties. Clinical data with parathyroid hormone have demonstrated enhanced healing in distal radius and pelvic fractures as well as postoperatively following spine surgery [42].

There is currently no evidence that osteoporosis treatments are detrimental for bone repair and some promising experimental evidence for positive effects on healing, notably for agents with a bone-forming mode of action, which may translate into therapeutic applications [43].

15.8   Conclusion

There is a range of good pharmacological options and indications for sequential therapy to reduce the risk of further fracture in orthogeriatric patients; despite this they are frequently undertreated. The literature shows that treatment can be started even in very old patients at high risk of fracture and may be continued for as long as the developing evidence shows efficacy and safety.

Undertreatment of patients following hip fracture is an important age-related health disparity that must be addressed by both health systems and individual clinicians. The challenge for the multidisciplinary approach to fracture patients is to abolish undertreatment, thereby enabling a real improvement of quality of life for our patients.

New guidelines on secondary fracture prevention have been recently released by an international coalition led by the American Society of Bone and Mineral Research and should be followed by treating physicians and health care providers [44] (see Table 15.3).

References

1. Lonnroos E, Kautiainen H, Karppi P, Hartikainen S, Kiviranta I, Sulkava R (2007) Incidence of second hip fractures. A population-based study. Osteoporos Int 18(9):1279–1285
2. Pioli G, Barone A, Mussi C, Tafaro L, Bellelli G, Falaschi P, Trabucchi M, Paolisso G (2014) GIOG: The management of hip fracture in the older population. Joint position statement by Gruppo Italiano Ortogeriatria (GIOG). Aging Clin Exp Res 26(5):547–553

3. Eastell R, Rosen CJ, Black DM, Cheung AM, Murad MH, Shoback D (2019) Pharmacological management of osteoporosis in postmenopausal women: an endocrine Society Clinical practice guideline. J Clin Endocrinol Metab 104(5):1595–1622

4. Eisman JA, Bogoch ER, Dell R, Harrington JT, McKinney RE Jr, McLellan A, Mitchell PJ, Silverman S, Singleton R, Siris E (2012) Making the first fracture the last fracture: ASBMR task force report on secondary fracture prevention. J Bone Miner Res 27(10):2039–2046

5. Orimo H, Nakamura T, Hosoi T, Iki M, Uenishi K, Endo N, Ohta H, Shiraki M, Sugimoto T, Suzuki T, Soen S, Nishizawa Y, Hagino H, Fukunaga M, Fujiwara S (2012) Japanese 2011 guidelines for prevention and treatment of osteoporosis--executive summary. Arch Osteoporos 7:3–20

6. Schuit SC, van der Klift M, Weel AE et al (2004) Fracture incidence and association with bone mineral density in elderly men and women: the Rotterdam Study. Bone 34:195–202

7. Wong TC, Wu WC, Cheng HS, Cheng YC, Yam SK (2007) Spontaneous fractures in nursing home residents. Hong Kong Med J 13(6):427–429

8. Crilly RG, Hillier LM, Mason M, Gutmanis I, Cox L (2010) Prevention of hip fractures in long-term care: relevance of community-derived data. J Am Geriatr Soc 58(4):738–745

9. Kaga Y, Ishii S, Kuroda I, Kamiya Y, Nakamura K, Kanemura H, Sugita K, Aihara M (2017) The efficacy of intravenous alendronate for osteoporosis in patients with severe motor intellectual disabilities. No To Hattatsu 49(2):113–119

10. Kanis JA, Burlet N, Cooper C, Delmas PD, Reginster JY, Borgstrom F et al (2008) European guidance for the diagnosis and management of osteoporosis in postmenopausal women. Osteoporos Int 19(4):399–428

11. Khan AA et al (2017) Primary hyperparathyroidism: review and recommendations on evaluation, diagnosis, and management. A Canadian and international consensus. Osteoporos Int 28(1):1–19

12. Compston JE, McClung MR, Laslie WD (2019) Osteoporosis. Lancet 393:364–376

13. Tafaro L, Nati G, Leoni E, Baldini R, Cattaruzza MS, Mei M, Falaschi P (2013) Adherence to anti-osteoporotic therapies: role and determinants of "spot therapy". Osteoporos Int 24(8):2319–2323

14. Compston JE, McClung MR, Leslie WD (2019) Osteoporosis. Lancet 393(10169):364–376

15. Walters S, Khan T, Ong T, Sahota O (2017) Fracture liaison services: improving outcomes for patients with osteoporosis. Clin Interv Aging 12:117–127

16. Lips P, Cashman K, Lamberg-Allardt C, Bischoff-Ferrari H, Obermayer-Pietsch B, Bianchi M, Stepan J, El-Hajj Fuleihan G, Bouillon R (2019) Current vitamin D status in European and Middle East countries and strategies to prevent vitamin D deficiency: a position statement of the European Calcified Tissue Society. Eur J Endocrinol 180:23–54

17. Giordano S, Proietti A, Bisaccia T, Caso P, Martocchia A, Falaschi P, Tafaro L (2018) Hypovitaminosis D: comparison between patients with hip fracture and patients with vertebral fractures. Osteoporos Int 29(9):2087–2091

18. Nuti R, Brandi ML, Checchia G, Di Munno O, Dominguez L, Falaschi P, Fiore CE, Iolascon G, Maggi S, Michieli R, Migliaccio S, Minisola S, Rossini M, Sessa G, Tarantino U, Toselli A, Isaia GC (2019) Guidelines for the management of osteoporosis and fragility fractures. Intern Emerg Med 14(1):85–102

19. Bauer DC (2014) Calcium supplements and fracture prevention. N Engl J Med 370(4):387–388

20. Russell RG, Xia Z, Dunford JE, Oppermann U, Kwaasi A, Hulley PA, Kavanagh KL, Triffitt JT, Lundy MW, Phipps RJ, Barnett BL, Coxon FP, Rogers MJ, Watts NB, Ebetino FH (2007) Bisphosphonates: an update on mechanisms of action and how these relate to clinical efficacy. Ann N Y Acad Sci 1117:209–257

21. Black DM, Cummings SR, Karpf DB, Cauley JA, Thompson DE, Nevitt MC, Bauer DC, Genant HK, Haskell WL, Marcus R, Ott SM, Torner JC, Quandt SA, Reiss TF, Ensrud KE (1996) Randomised trial of effect of alendronate on risk of fracture in women with existing vertebral fractures. Fracture Intervention Trial Research Group. Lancet 348(9041):1535–1541

22. Harris ST, Watts NB, Genant HK, CD MK, Hangartner T, Keller M, Chesnut CH 3rd, Brown J, Eriksen EF, Hoseyni MS, Axelrod DW, Miller PD (1999) Effects of risedronate treatment on vertebral and nonvertebral fractures in women with postmenopausal osteoporosis: a randomized controlled trial. Vertebral Efficacy With Risedronate Therapy (VERT) Study Group. JAMA 282(14):1344–1352

23. MR MC, Geusens P, Miller PD, Zippel H, Bensen WG, Roux C, Adami S, Fogelman I, Diamond T, Eastell R, Meunier PJ, Reginster JY, Hip Intervention Program Study Group (2001) Effect of risedronate on the risk of hip fracture in elderly women. Hip Intervention Program Study Group. N Engl J Med 344(5):333–340

24. Black DM, Delmas PD, Eastell R, Reid IR, Boonen S, Cauley JA, Cosman F, Lakatos P, Leung PC, Man Z, Mautalen C, Mesenbrink P, Hu H, Caminis J, Tong K, Rosario-Jansen T, Krasnow J, Hue TF, Sellmeyer D, Eriksen EF, Cummings SR, HORIZON Pivotal Fracture Trial (2007) Once-yearly zoledronic acid for treatment of postmenopausal osteoporosis. N Engl J Med 356(18):1809–1822

25. Reid IR, Horne AM, Mihov B, Stewart A, Garratt E, Wong S, Wiessing KR, Bolland MJ, Bastin S, Gamble GD (2018) Fracture prevention with zoledronate in older women with osteopenia. N Engl J Med 379(25):2407–2416

26. Cummings SR, San Martin J, McClung MR et al (2009) Denosumab for prevention of fractures in postmenopausal women with osteoporosis. N Engl J Med 361:756–765

27. McClung MR, Boonen S, Törring O, Roux C, Rizzoli R, Bone HG, Benhamou CL, Lems WF, Minisola S, Halse J, Hoeck HC, Eastell R, Wang A, Siddhanti S, Cummings SR (2012) Effect of denosumab treatment on the risk of fractures in subgroups of women with postmenopausal osteoporosis. J Bone Miner Res 27(1):211–218

28. Bone HG, Wagman RB, Brandi ML et al (2017) 10 years of denosumab treatment in postmenopausal women with osteoporosis: results from the phase 3 randomised FREEDOM trial and open-label extension. Lancet Diabetes Endocrinol 5:513–523

29. Chen CL, Chen NC, Liang HL, Hsu CY, Chou KJ, Fang HC, Lee PT (2015) Effects of denosumab and calcitriol on severe secondary hyperparathyroidism in dialysis patients with low bone mass. J Clin Endocrinol Metab 100(7):2784–2792

30. Cummings SR, Ferrari S, Eastell R et al (2018) Vertebral fractures after discontinuation of denosumab: a post hoc analysis of the randomized placebo-controlled FREEDOM trial and its extension. J Bone Miner Res 33:190–198

31. Dempster DW, Zhou H, Ruff VA, Melby TE, Alam J, Taylor KA (2018) Longitudinal effects of teriparatide or zoledronic acid on bone modeling- and remodeling-based formation in the SHOTZ Study. J Bone Miner Res 33:627–633

32. Black DM, Greenspan SL, Ensrud KE et al (2003) The effects of parathyroid hormone and alendronate alone or in combination in postmenopausal osteoporosis. N Engl J Med 349:1207–1215

33. Macdonald HM, Nishiyama KK, Hanley DA, Boyd SK (2011) Changes in trabecular and cortical bone microarchitecture at peripheral sites associated with 18 months of teriparatide therapy in postmenopausal women with osteoporosis. Osteoporos Int 22:357–362

34. Kendler DL, Marin F, Zerbini CAF, Russo LA, Greenspan SL, Zikan V, Bagur A, Malouf-Sierra J, Lakatos P, Fahrleitner-Pammer A, Lespessailles E, Minisola S, Body JJ, Geusens P, Moricke R, Lopez-Romero P (2018) Effects of teriparatide and risedronate on new fractures in post-menopausal women with severe osteoporosis (VERO): a multicentre, double-blind, doubledummy, randomised controlled trial. Lancet 391(10117):230–240

35. Saag KG, Zanchetta JR, Devogelaer JP et al (2009) Effects of teriparatide versus alendronate for treating glucocorticoid-induced osteoporosis: thirty six month results of a randomized, double-blind, controlled trial. Arthritis Rheum 60:3346–3355

36. Black DM, Rosen CJ (2016) Postmenopausal osteoporosis. N Engl J Med 374(3):254–262

37. Miller PD, Hattersley G, Riis BJ et al (2016) Effect of abaloparatide vs placebo on new vertebral fractures in postmenopausal women with osteoporosis: a randomized clinical trial. JAMA 316:722–733

38. Barrionuevo P, Kapoor E, Asi N, Alahdab F, Mohammed K, Benkhadra K, Almasri J, Farah W, Sarigianni M, Muthusamy K, Al Nofal A, Haydour Q, Wang Z, Murad MH (2019) Efficacy of pharmacological therapies for the prevention of fractures in postmenopausal women: a network meta-analysis. J Clin Endocrinol Metab 104(5):1623–1630

39. Cosman F, Crittenden DB, Adachi JD et al (2016) Romosozumab treatment in postmenopausal women with osteoporosis. N Engl J Med 375:1532–1543

40. Saag K, Petersen J, Brandi M, Karaplis A, Lorentzon M, Thomas T, Maddox J, Fan M, Meisner P, Grauer A (2017) Romosozumab or alendronate for fracture prevention inwomen with osteoporosis. N Engl J Med 377:1417–1427

41. Cosman F, Crittenden DB, Ferrari S, Khan A, Lane NE, Lippuner K, Matsumoto T, Milmont CE, Libanati C, Grauer A (2018) FRAME study: the foundation effect of building bone with 1 year of romosozumab leads to continued lower fracture risk after transition to denosumab. J Bone Miner Res 33(7):1219–1226

42. Hegde V, Jo JE, Andreopoulou P, Lane JM (2016) Effect of osteoporosis medications on fracture healing. Osteoporos Int 27(3):861–871

43. Goldhahn J, Féron JM, Kanis J, Papapoulos S, Reginster JY, Rizzoli R, Dere W, Mitlak B, Tsouderos Y, Boonen S (2012) Implications for fracture healing of current and new osteoporosis treatments: an ESCEO consensus paper. Calcif Tissue Int 90(5):343–353. https://doi.org/10.1007/s00223-012-9587-4

44. Conley RB, Adib G, Adler RA, Åkesson KE, Alexander IM, Amenta KC, Blank RD, Brox WT, Carmody EE, Chapman-Novakofski K, Clarke BL, Cody KM, Cooper C, Crandall CJ, Dirschl DR, Eagen TJ, Elderkin AL, Fujita M, Greenspan SL, Halbout P, Hochberg MC, Javaid M, Jeray KJ, Kearns AE, King T, Koinis TF, Koontz JS, Kužma M, Lindsey C, Lorentzon M, Lyritis GP, Michaud LB, Miciano A, Morin SN, Mujahid N, Napoli N, Olenginski TP, Puzas JE, Rizou S, Rosen CJ, Saag K, Thompson E, Tosi LL, Tracer H, Khosla S, Kiel DP (2019) Secondary fracture prevention: consensus clinical recommendations from a multistakeholder coalition. J Bone Miner Res. https://doi.org/10.1002/jbmr.3877

How Can We Prevent Falls?

16

Hubert Blain, Stéphanie Miot, and Pierre Louis Bernard

16.1 Epidemiology of Falls

Falls represent a major health problem in subjects aged 65 or older because of their high prevalence and the severity of their physical, functional, psychological and financial consequences. Indeed, approximately 30% of people living in the community aged over 65 years and 50% of those older than 80 experience at least one fall every year and one-third of fallers are repeated fallers. Falls result in injuries that require medical attention in 30%, fractures in 5%, a hip fracture (HF) in 1% or another major injury in 5–6%. Every year, around 50 million falls occur in Europe amongst community-dwelling older people, 2.3 million persons aged 65 years or older attend emergency departments for a fall-related injury, 1.4 million are admitted to hospital and 36,000 die from falls. Falls induce psychological consequences in patients, including fear of falling and loss of confidence that can result in self-restricted activity levels, reduction in physical function and social interactions, and put a major strain on the family. With the ageing of the population, fall has become the third leading cause of years living with disability in older subjects and one of the main causes of admission to a nursing home [1].

This chapter is a component of Part 4: Pillar III.
For an explanation of the grouping of chapters in this book, please see Chapter 1: "The multidisciplinary approach to fragility fractures around the world—an overview".

H. Blain (✉) · S. Miot
Department of Internal Medicine and Geriatrics, University Hospital of Montpellier,
Montpellier University, Centre Antonin Balmes, Montpellier Cedex 5, France
e-mail: h-blain@chu-montpellier.fr; s-miot@chu-montpellier.fr

P. L. Bernard
Euromov, University of Montpellier, Montpellier, France
e-mail: pierre-louis.bernard@umontpellier.fr

© The Author(s) 2021
P. Falaschi, D. Marsh (eds.), *Orthogeriatrics*, Practical Issues in Geriatrics,
https://doi.org/10.1007/978-3-030-48126-1_16

Falls represent also a major health problem in nursing homes, half of residents experiencing at least one fall every year. Fallers are most often women and repeated fallers in nursing homes. Indeed, falls prevalence is about 2 and 1.5 falls per person-year in institutionalised men and women, respectively [2, 3]. Falls are a major cause of hospital admission in nursing homes patients, 7.5–15% of residents being admitted to hospital every year after a fall and hip fractures accounting for 10% of overall admissions [3]. Falls also account for up to 70% of accidents in hospitalised patients; approximately 30% of falls occurring in inpatients result in physical injury, with 4–6% resulting in serious injury [4].

The health care expenditure for treating fall-related injuries in the European Union is estimated to be €25 billion each year, fractures accounting for about 1–1.5% of health care expenditure. The ageing of the population could result in annual fall-related expenditures exceeding €45 billion by the year 2050 [1]. Persons aged 80 years or older account for almost 50% of all fall-related emergency department visits and 66% of total costs [5]. The costs of long-term care at home and in nursing homes show the largest age-related increases and account together for 54% of the fall-related costs in older people [6]. Fractures, especially HF, that are most often caused by a fall from a standing position, account for up to 80% of the fall-related healthcare costs [1]. About 10% of patients are hospitalised for a second injury in the year after the HF [7], and the major concerns of people after a hip fracture are the fear of falling and of re-fracturing [8].

For all the above reasons, falls prevention is now widely recognised as one of the main priorities to promote active and healthy ageing in older subjects (http://profound.eu.com/wp-content/uploads/2016/12/Silver-Paper-Executive-Summary-Final.pdf).

Most guidelines for the prevention of falls in older people [AGS/BGS Clinical Practice Guideline Prevention of Falls in Older Person-2010 (https://sbgg.org.br/wp-content/uploads/2014/10/2010-AGSBGS-Clinical.pdf); Stopping Elderly Accidents, Death, and Injury (STEADI) initiative, Center for Disease Control and Prevention (https://www.cdc.gov/steadi/index.html); [9] recommend to assess regularly the older patients' risk for a fall and to propose interventions adapted to the risk of falling, considering that patients with repeated or injurious falls, especially those who have experienced a hip fracture, are at the highest risk of new incident falls and fractures.

16.2   How to Assess Older Patients' Risk of Falling

Subjects aged 65 or older at increased risk of falling can be screened:

– *By themselves or their caregivers using simple questions*
    For the experts of the STEADI programme, subjects with a history of fall in the previous year, who feel unsteady when standing or walking, or subjects who scored 4/12 points or more on the stay independent brochure (https://www.cdc.gov/steadi/pdf/STEADI-Brochure-StayIndependent-508.pdf) should be considered at increased risk of falling and should require further assessment provided by a general practitioner [10, 11].

– *By healthcare providers using simple questions and tests*

Three simple questions:

The STEADI initiative recommends healthcare providers to include in the routine examination of patients 70 and older three questions: Have you fallen in the past year? Do you feel unsteady when standing or walking? Do you worry about falling? If the patient answers no to all these key screening questions, he/she can be considered at low risk of falling. If the patient answers "yes" to any of these key screening questions, further assessment is needed to distinguish subjects at moderate or high risk of falling. The AGS/BGS 2010 and the 2013 NICE guidelines (https://www.nice.org.uk/guidance/cg161) recommend accordingly that all older persons who are under the care of a health professional (or their caregivers) should be asked at least once a year about falls, frequency of falling and difficulties in gait, balance and muscle strength. This routine assessment is especially important in patients with multimorbidities that may induce falls, such as Parkinson's disease, kidney, vision and cognitive impairment, incontinence, depression or with polypharmacy [12–14] and in patients admitted to the emergency room or hospitalised. Indeed, nearly half of hip fracture patients have visited the emergency room (ER) or have been admitted to hospital in the year prior to fracture, a quarter of them for a previous fall [15]. Unfortunately, very few of the patients visiting the ER or hospital receive falls counselling [15], which is a major missed opportunity since patient-centred interventions can reduce incident falls and fracture in older people presenting to the ED after a fall [16] or a fracture [17].

– *Simple physical tests*:

AGS/BGS-2010 and 2013 NICE guidelines recommend to assess balance and gait using simple tests such as the timed up and go test (TUG) and the 'turn 180°' test (TT). These tests are indeed easy to perform in any setting and their administration requires no special equipment. Cut-off values for abnormal results remain however discussed (the risk of falling is increased when the TUG is >15 s (threshold for sarcopenia) [18] and a TUG >20 s indicates a significant gait disorder). The one-leg stand test can also easily been used, with the same limits (the risk of falling is low when >10 s and high when <5 s) (https://www.nice.org.uk/guidance/cg161; [19]). Other tests such as the Berg balance test, the Tinetti scale, the functional reach and the dynamic gait test need equipment or clinical expertise. Dual-task testing can also be used since patients who reduce their walking speed when performing a second task are more prone to falls. People with a difference of 4.5 s or more between the TUG test (simple task) and the dual manual task TUG test (TUG test while carrying a glass of water in one hand) or who need 14.7 s or over to perform the cognitive TUG (TUG test while counting backward in threes from a random start point) are at risk of falling, especially in case of Parkinson's disease [20].

A low muscle strength is a significant but less consistent risk of falls or injurious falls than gait and balance impairments. Muscle strength can be assessed using grip strength, which requires specific equipment [19] or more easily by measuring the chair rising performance [21]. Time to perform five chair-rising stands can be considered as normal when <12 s and may be a sign of sarcopenia when >15 s [18].

The STEADI algorithm recommends to use the TUG, the 30-s chair stand and the four-stage balance test to identify people with gait/strength/balance disturbances, although cut-off values are not indicated (https://www.cdc.gov/steadi/index.html).

The Short Physical Performance Battery (SPPB), which includes sit-to-stand performance, walking speed and balance performance, can also be used since it demonstrates a significant association with fall history [21]. The Physiological Profile Assessment (PPA), which involves a series of simple tests of vision, peripheral sensation, muscle force, reaction time, postural sway and the Timed Up and Go test can also identify people at risk for falls [22].

The Downton Fall Risk Index (DFRI) that is a composite index of five groups of fall risk factors including previous falls, medications (tranquilisers, sedatives, diuretics, antihypertensives, antiparkinsonian drugs, antidepressants), sensory disability (visual or hearing impairment, impaired motor skills (reduced muscle strength or loss of function in a limb), cognitive disability (orientation to time, place, and person) and walking ability (unsafe gait) has been shown to predict hip fracture [23].

16.2.1 Definition of Older People at Low, Moderate or High Risk of Falling

In order to be pragmatic and based on the three above questions (history of falls and injurious falls, fear of falling or feeling of unsteadiness) and the three simples tests (TUG, one-leg stand and five chair-rising) that take less than 5 min to be asked and performed, it can be proposed that:

- People at low risk of falling are those without any history of fall in the 12 last months, fear of falling or feeling of unsteadiness and without balance (e.g. one-leg stand test >10 s), gait (e.g. timed up and go test <12 s) and muscle strength (e.g. five sit-to-stand test in <12 s) problem.
- People at high risk of falling are those 1. with a history of repeated or injurious falls in the six previous months or 2. with a fear of falling or a feeling of unsteadiness or a history of one fall in the 12 last months associated with a significant balance (e.g. one-leg stand test <5 s)or gait (e.g. timed up and go test >20 s) or muscle strength problem (e.g. five sit-to-stand test in >15 s).
- People at moderate risk of falling are those who are nor at low or high risk of falling. There is a continuum among patients at moderate risk of falling, approaching low risk when the number of risk factors is low and high risk when the number of risk factors is high.

16.3 Fall Prevention Intervention in Patients with Low Risk of Falling

Education and exercise should be offered in older subjects at low risk of falling since people with high activity and performance are, with those with the lowest activity/worst physical performances, the subjects at the highest risk of falls [24].

Education: The STEADI initiative provides educational materials and brochures for family caregivers (https://www.cdc.gov/steadi/pdf/steadi-CaregiverBrochure.pdf) including the following educational messages: (1) A healthcare provider should be told right away in case of fall, unsteadiness or fear of falling; (2) medications, including over-the-counter medications and supplements, should be regularly reviewed by a healthcare provider or a pharmacist, especially in case of dizziness or sleepiness; (3) the interest of taking vitamin D supplements to improve bone, muscle and nerve health should be regularly discussed with an healthcare provider; (4) physical activities that improve balance and lower limbs muscle strength (like Tai Chi) should be regularly performed to prevent falls and also to improve well-being and confidence; (5) eyes should be checked by a health provider at least once a year to optimise vision (e.g. to update eyeglasses, if needed, and to optimise the treatment of condition like glaucoma or cataracts); (6) feet should be checked by a health provider at least once a year to a allow a safe and comfortable walking (to provide well-fitting shoes discuss with good support inside and outside, and ask whether seeing a foot specialist is advised). Counselling is also (7) home safety should be optimised by keeping floors clutter-free, removing small throw rugs or using double-sided tape to keep the rugs from slipping, by adding grab bars in the bathroom next to and inside the tub, and next to the toilet, and having handrails and lights installed on all staircases. A checklist is also available to find and fix hazards at home on the STEADI site (https://www.cdc.gov/steadi/pdf/steadi-Brochure-CheckForSafety-508.pdf).

Community exercise programmes to maintain or improve balance and strength: The programmes with the best evidence are the Otago Exercise Programme (OEP), Tai Chi, the Falls Management Exercise programme (FaME -sometimes called PSI), Lifestyle-integrated Functional Exercise (LiFE) and the Ossebo programme [25]. On the whole, physical activity in older people may reduce the risk of fall-related injuries by 32–40%, including severe falls requiring medical care or hospitalisation, and improves physical function in older people without or with frailty or Parkinson's disease (http://bachlab.pitt.edu/sites/default/files/DiPietro2019.pdf). The effect on the rate of falls of resistance exercise (without balance and functional exercises), dance or walking is uncertain [26]. The NICE guidelines recommend to promote the participation of older people at low risk of falls in exercise programmes, considering also the psychological and social values of such exercise programmes in addition to their physical benefits (https://www.nice.org.uk/guidance/cg161).

Systematic vitamin D ± calcium supplements should not be recommended in subjects with low or moderate risk of falling since their effectiveness to prevent fractures or falls is not demonstrated [27, 28]. High-dose vitamin D may even have adverse effects on fall risk [29].

16.4   Multifactorial Interventions in Patients with Moderate Risk of Falling

A targeted intervention programme should be offered in patients at moderate risk of falling including.

Education: Interventions that aim to increase knowledge/education about fall prevention alone seem not be able to reduce significantly the rate of falls. The NICE guidelines recommend however to implement measures to enhance "fall awareness" in older people at moderate or high risk of falling and healthcare professionals (https://www.nice.org.uk/guidance/cg161). The education material provided by the STEADI initiative described previously for people at low or moderate risk of falling can be used by patients at high risk of falling and their caregivers (https://www.cdc.gov/steadi/materials.html). The Prevention of Falls Network for Dissemination (ProFouND) that is an European Commission funded initiative dedicated to the dissemination and implementation of best practice in falls prevention across Europe has also produced documents to influence policy and increase awareness of falls for health and social care authorities, the commercial sector, NGOs and the general public (http://profound.eu.com/).

Exercises supervised by a physiotherapist or in a community fall prevention programme: Exercise when challenging, progressive, regular and conducted in the long term is indeed effective to prevent falls and falls requiring medical attention and fractures (no proof for HF specifically) in older persons living in the community (http://profound.eu.com/wp-content/uploads/2016/12/Falls-Intervention-Factsheets-FinalV2.pdf; [26, 30]).

Exercises that allow to develop and mobilise sufficient attention resources to recover a stable posture following an external perturbation such as dual-task training, and exercises to improve floor-rise ability, should be included in clinical practice [31]. Tai Chi is effective to reduce falls in people at low or moderate risk of falling and there is no evidence that walking or brisk walking reduces the risk of falling [32].

Whole body vibration, through its ability of enhancing balance, improving leg and plantar flexor muscle strength, and reducing fall rate may also help reduce the risk of fracture [33, 34].

On the whole, dedicated falls prevention programmes conducted in people living in the community at low to moderate risk of falling decrease falls and fall-related injury rates by 20–40% and are cost-effective [32, 35, 36].

Modification/progressive withdrawal of fall risk-increasing drugs (FRIDs): Polypharmacy is a risk factor of falling. The most common FRIDs are—psychotropic drugs, such as sedatives, hypnotics, antidepressants, antipsychotic medications, antiepileptics, opioids and other drugs which can cause sedation, delirium or impaired balance and coordination (including those that induce hyponatremia)—cardiovascular drugs and other drugs which can cause or worsen orthostatic hypotension (such as anticholinergic drugs) and induce cardiac arrhythmias (such as drugs at risk of GT prolongation) [37–39].

A meta-analysis of randomised-controlled interventions aiming to prevent falls in the elderly living in the community showed that slow withdrawal of psychotropics and prescribing modification programmes for primary care physicians significantly reduce the risk of falling [32, 40].

Vision optimisation: Visual control plays a role in the assessment of the risks in the environment and in the effectiveness of protective responses to avoid a fall explaining why poor vision is associated with a risk of fall-related injuries including HF [41, 42]. Cataract surgery on the first affected eye and replacement of multifocal glasses by single lens glasses are effective in reducing the falling rate in older people living in the community [32].

Treatment of foot problems: Physical examination should include feet and footwear check and foot problems should be addressed. Indeed, one trial conducted in 305 participants has shown that multifaceted podiatry, and foot and ankle exercises reduce significantly the rate of falls in people with disabling foot pains [32].

Vitamin D supplementation at patients at risk of vitamin D deficit: The STEADI guidelines recommend vitamin D and calcium supplementation in all patients, whatever their risk of falling. Taking vitamin D supplements, however, does not appear to reduce falls in most community-dwelling older people, but may do so in those who have low vitamin D blood levels [32, 43]. Vitamin D deficiency indeed, especially when sufficiently deep to induce elevated PTH, predisposes both to falls and HF [44]. Thus, people at moderate risk of falling who are at risk of vitamin D deficits (low outdoor activity, high fat mass) should be offered vitamin D supplements without any vitamin D serum measurement during the winter season (https://www.has-sante.fr/jcms/c_1525705/fr/avis-de-la-has-concernant-l-evaluation-du-risque-de-chutes-chez-le-sujet-age-autonome-et-sa-prevention). Calcium supplementation is not recommended in patients at moderate risk of falls [45].

16.5 Multifactorial Falls Risk Assessment and Interventions in Patients with High Risk of Falling

The AGS/BGS 2010/ [46] and STEADI initiative recommend to offer a multifactorial fall prevention programme in complex patients with an history of recurrent or injurious falls or with a fall with significant balance, gait, or muscle strength disorders (https://www.nice.org.uk/guidance/cg161; https://www.cdc.gov/steadi/pdf/steadi-Algorithm-508.pdf). Indeed, this kind of programme that identifies modifiable risk factors and propose a personalised fall prevention programme reduces the number of falls in randomised controlled trials (RCTs) (https://www.cochranelibrary.com/cdsr/doi/10.1002/14651858.CD012221.pub2/full) and in pre-post-intervention studies [47]. The NICE recommends that individualised multifactorial assessment and intervention should be performed by healthcare professionals with appropriate skills and experience, normally in the setting of a specialist falls service (most often called falls clinics) with clinic-level quality improvement strategies (eg, case management), multifactorial assessment and treatment (e.g. comprehensive geriatric assessment) (https://www.nice.org.uk/guidance/cg161).

According to the STEADI initiative and the NICE guidelines, the management of patients at risk of falling starts with the management of conditions that alter gait, balance and mobility such as postural dizziness and postural hypotension, cognitive impairment, metabolic abnormalities such as hypoglycaemia [48] or hyponatraemia [49], sleep disturbances [50], muscle weakness and urinary incontinence [47] and conditions that induce fainting. Insertion of a pacemaker should be considered for older people with frequent falls associated with cardioinhibitory carotid sinus hypersensitivity, or sinus node dysfunction, conditions which cause sudden changes in heart rate and blood pressure [32, 51]. Multifaceted podiatry and foot and ankle exercises reduce significantly the rate of falls in people with disabling foot pains [32]. A falls and fracture successful multifactorial intervention programmes in older people at high risk of falling should also comprise, besides education (see above):

Modification/progressive withdrawal of fall risk-increasing drugs (FRIDs): As indicated previously, progressive withdrawal of fall risk-increasing drugs reduces the risk of falling [32, 40]. Polypharmacy and fall-risk increasing drugs remain however prevalent in patients discharged from orthogeriatric care after surgery for a hip fracture [52, 53]. FRIDs are present in two-thirds of patients visiting fracture liaison services [54], benzodiazepines and opioids being more specific risk factors of HF [55]. This suggests the interest to conduct interventions on drug use at discharge of patients admitted to hospital for a falls-related injury [52, 53].

Vision optimisation: Any history of cataracts, macular degeneration, glaucoma or visual loss should be identified in people at high risk of falling and those people should be referred to an eye doctor when no eye examination has occurred during the past year. Vision assessment and referral are therefore a component of successful multifactorial falls prevention programmes, especially when associated with home hazard intervention [32, 56].

Exercises: As indicated previously, programmes that combine balance and moderate intensity strength training either alone or with other interventions, especially vision assessment and treatment and environmental assessment and modification, are effective to prevent falls, fall-related fractures and other types of injurious falls https://www.nice.org.uk/guidance/cg161; [26, 32, 36, 57–60]). Tai Chi is not recommended in patients at high risk of falling [32].

Exercises improving medial-lateral stability are especially recommended in patients at high risk of falling and fracture since sideways falls are associated with a sixfold increased risk for hip fracture [61, 62]. Exercises enhancing anterior–posterior postural control are also warranted, given that forward falls can also result in hip impact [63]. Exercises to help reduce the hip impact during the descent stage of falling and therefore make landing safer may include exercises of forward or backward axial rotation of the torso and pelvis during descent [64] and exercises to strengthen upper extremity muscles to make protective responses during falls more effective [65, 66].

The NICE and ProFouND initiative recommend that the exercise programme in patients at high risk of falling should be individually prescribed and monitored by professionals, such as physiotherapists, sport scientists and specialist exercise instructors, who are appropriately trained in delivering falls prevention exercise programmes (http://profound.eu.com/wp-content/uploads/2016/12/Falls-Intervention-Factsheets-FinalV2.pdf; https://www.nice.org.uk/guidance/cg161).

Evidence from the 2018 PAGAC Scientific Report indicates that older people who have sustained hip fracture should benefit from weight-bearing, multicomponent activity [67]. The meta-analysis of RCT by Lee et al. reported that progressive resistance exercise significantly improved overall physical function (mobility, balance, lower limb strength or power and performance tasks) after hip fracture surgery [68].

When associated with orthogeriatric co-management and physician consultations, group exercise and vibration-therapy over a 18-month period can reduce the re-fracture rate, improve balance and mobility and reduce costs in fragility hip fracture patients [69].

Home hazard intervention: The majority of fall-related injuries occur while older people move around home. Interventions to improve home safety, such as night-lights or bathroom grab bars, appear to be effective to reduce falls, especially in people who fall at home or have received treatment in hospital following a fall (https://www.nice.org.uk/guidance/cg161), and especially when carried out by suitably trained healthcare professionals, such as occupational therapists [32]. Indeed, home assessment visits by occupational therapists prior to hospital discharge for patients recovering from hip fracture can reduce the number of readmissions to hospital, increase functional independence at 6 months and may reduce the risk of falls in the first 30 days after discharge [70].

Assuming that home safety measures reduce fall-related hip fractures in accordance with the reduction of the rate of falls, a home safety intervention to prevent falls could be cost-effective in impaired elderly people living in the community [71].

NICE and ProFouND guidelines recommend to seeking opportunities from the Information and Communication Technologies (ICT) sector to provide solutions for fall-detection and prevention (http://profound.eu.com/wp-content/uploads/2016/12/Falls-Intervention-Factsheets-FinalV2.pdf; https://www.nice.org.uk/guidance/cg161).

Vitamin D and calcium: Screening of vitamin D deficiency by measuring serum total 25(OH)D is recommended in individuals with a history of falls or nontraumatic fracture and in patients at risk of vitamin D deficiency, such as patients with diseases affecting vitamin D metabolism and absorption, and osteoporosis [72]. Measuring blood 25OHVitamin D in recurrent fallers or after a fall-related fracture helps to guide the vitamin D deficits correction. Vitamin D and calcium supplementation may reduce falls in patients with increased risk for falls and a vitamin D deficiency [32, 43, 45].

Osteoporosis screening and treatment if needed: Bone health should be assessed in patients at high risk of falls, and especially in those with sarcopenia or with an history of fracture [73]. A low bone mineral density, a poor physical function and falls are indeed the strongest independent risk factors for a subsequent nonvertebral fracture [74].

The NICE and more recently the European guidelines recommend to perform a BMD and calculate the FRAX risk (calculation without BMD if DXA is not possible) in patients at high risk of falling in order to determine if an osteoporosis treatment is required (https://www.nice.org.uk/guidance/cg161; [75]). Nevertheless, life expectancy should be taken into account when assessing the appropriateness of DXA in fallers, as osteoporosis treatments require at least 12 months to decrease the fracture risk [75].

16.6   Fall Assessment and Prevention in Care Settings

The 2016 NICE guidelines do not recommend to use fall risk prediction tools to assess the risk of falling in inpatients, but rather to consider that all hospitalised patients aged 65 years or older are at high risk of falling as well as patients aged 50 and older with underlying conditions (https://www.nice.org.uk/guidance/cg161;). Some tools with good sensitivity and specificity can however been used to screen patients particularly at risk of falling at hospital, including the STRATIFY tool that assesses five factors (patients who present or not to hospital with a fall or who has fallen on the ward since admission; patients agitated, visually impaired, in need of especially frequent toileting, with poor transfer and mobility, living in a nursing home or not) [76] and the Hendrich II Fall Risk Model that consists of eight variables including (confusion/disorientation/impulsivity, symptomatic depression, altered elimination, dizziness/vertigo, gender, any administered anti-epileptics, benzodiazepines and the "get up and go" test) [77].

Similarly, risk assessment tools do not add significant value to nurses' judgment for identifying individuals at high risk of falls in daily practice [78]. Indeed, most of nursing home residents are at high risk of falling since a fall history, gait and balance instability, cognitive and functional impairment, sedating and psychoactive medications and multimorbidity are significant risk factors of falling in nursing home residents [3].

If the same guidance relating to community-dwelling older adults at high risk of falling presented above applies to acute and long-term care settings (http://profound.eu.com/), the evidence for effective falls prevention interventions in acute and subacute wards and in nursing homes is more limited [3, 79, 80].

The NICE guidelines underline the fact that architects should take into account improvements to the inpatient environment to prevent falls when designing new setting for older people (https://www.nice.org.uk/guidance/cg161). The clinical effectiveness of compliant flooring at preventing serious fall-related injuries among long-term care residents remains discussed [81]. International evidence suggests that physical restraints may increase the risk of falling by limiting mobility in this group of frail elderly persons [82].

A key component for falls prevention in care settings and for physical restraint reduction in nursing homes is the implementation of a proactive organisational strategy that includes leadership, individualised patient education programmes combined with staff education and training, careful monitoring with audit, reminders and feedback to staff, provision of equipment, supportive risk management and change agent [57, 79, 83].

16.7 Fall Assessment and Prevention in Patients with Cognitive Impairments

Almost two-thirds of people with dementia living in the community fall annually, i.e. a rate that is twice that of the population without cognitive impairment [84]. Falls are a major cause of injury to cognitively impaired older people [85]. The high prevalence and morbidity of falls in dementia are in part due to the relationship between low performance in attention and executive function and gait slowing, instability and future falls [86].

This explains why some recent falls prevention programmes in cognitively impaired older people include, in addition to the above conventional measures, the prescription of walking aids and training programmes targeting identified gait abnormalities and appropriate to the individuals' cognitive capacity, non-pharmaceutical and pharmaceutical strategies to increase attention, cognitive training and behavioural change/modulation to improve planning, judgment, inhibitory control and flexibility/problem-solving skills in order to improve safely mobilisation during challenging circumstances [87]. Thus, cognitive training, dual-task training and virtual reality modalities are promising strategies to improve mobility in older adults with cognitive impairment and dementia [86]. In the advanced stage of dementia, recurrent falls can be sentinel events indicating the need for a palliative approach to care with a focus on symptom management, comfort and dignity.

16.8   Falls Clinics and Fracture Liaison Services

Falls clinics are one approach by which older people with high levels of falls risk can be managed. Falls clinics, that are however too seldom in the world, offer detailed multidisciplinary assessment and make recommendations or implement a range of targeted falls and falls injury-prevention strategies based on the assessment findings. Several pre–post clinic intervention studies and randomised controlled-studies have indicated substantial reductions in falls and related injuries (between 30 and 77%) in high falls–risk populations, and improvements in other outcomes such as balance and mobility, physical functioning, fear of falling and engagement with falls prevention interventions [47, 88, 89]. The number of patients to see in a fall clinic to prevent a fall or an injurious fall has been found to be 5 and 6, respectively [89].

As indicated previously, a fragility fracture is one of the strongest risk factor for a subsequent nonvertebral fracture [74, 90]. Fracture liaison services (FLS) working together with geriatric units specialised with falls prevention are probably the most efficient way of addressing primary and secondary prevention of fracture including the assessment of both bone health and falls risk [75, 91, 92], especially in frail older patients [93].

16.9   Conclusion

Falls are a major public health problem in the elderly population. Some simple questions related to fall and fall-related injury in the previous months, feeling of unsteadiness and fear of falling, and some simple tests that aim to assess balance/gait and muscle strength (e.g. timed up and go and sit-to-stand tests) may help distinguish people at low, moderate or high risk of falling. Balance and strength exercises and education are recommended to reduce falls in people whatever the risk of falls. A multifactorial falls and fracture risk assessment and prevention should be offered to older people at high risk of falls, i.e. those who present for medical attention because of a fall, especially after a fracture or who are recurrent fallers. This multifactorial falls risk assessment and prevention should be offered by a healthcare professional with appropriate skills and experience, normally in the setting of a falls clinic, in link with a fall liaison service in case of fall-related fracture. Individualised, targeted multifactorial interventions comprise the management of specific causes of gait/balance and muscle strength disturbances, prescription of vitamin D supplements when blood level of vitamin D is low and of BMD and FRAX risk calculation in order to determine recommendations for osteoporosis treatment, measures to improve home safety (at best delivered by an occupational therapist), a review of medications, vision optimisation, insertion of a pacemaker in case of carotid sinus hypersensitivity and multifaceted podiatry. Because falls and fracture are most often preventable, it is now crucial to overcome limited awareness and usage of solutions to prevent and monitor falls and osteoporosis and make these available (Action Group A2 of the European Innovation Partnership on Active and Healthy Ageing (EIP on AHA)) (https://ec.europa.eu/eip/ageing/actiongroup/index/a2_en).

References

1. EuroSafe, Amsterdam (2015) Falls among older adults in the EU-28: key facts from the available statistics. https://eupha.org/repository/sections/ipsp/Factsheet_falls_in_older_adults_in_EU.pdf
2. Rapp K, Becker C, Cameron ID, König HH, Büchele G (2012) Epidemiology of falls in residential aged care: analysis of more than 70,000 falls from residents of bavarian nursing homes. J Am Med Dir Assoc 13(2):187.e1–187.e6
3. Vlaeyen E, Coussement J, Leysens G, Van der Elst E, Delbaere K, Cambier D, Denhaerynck K, Goemaere S, Wertelaers A, Dobbels F, Dejaeger E, Milisen K, Center of Expertise for Fall and Fracture Prevention Flanders (2015) Characteristics and effectiveness of fall prevention programs in nursing homes: a systematic review and meta-analysis of randomized controlled trials. J Am Geriatr Soc 63(2):211–221
4. Krauss MJ, Evanoff B, Hitcho E et al (2005) A case–control study of patient, medication, and care-related risk factors for inpatient falls. J Int Gen Med 20:116–122
5. Hanley A, Silke C, Murphy J (2011) Community-based health efforts for the prevention of falls in the elderly. Clin Interv Aging 6:19–25
6. Hartholt KA, Polinder S, Van der Cammen TJ, Panneman MJ, Van der Velde N, Van Lieshout EM, Patka P, Van Beeck EF (2012) Costs of falls in an ageing population: a nationwide study from the Netherlands (2007–2009). Injury 43(7):1199–1203
7. Cabalatungan S, Divaris N, McCormack JE, Huang EC, Kamadoli R, Abdullah R, Vosswinkel JA, Jawa RS (2018) Incidence, outcomes, and recidivism of elderly patients admitted for isolated hip fracture. J Surg Res 232:257–265. https://doi.org/10.1016/j.jss.2018.06.054
8. Yoo JI, Lee YK, Koo KH, Park YJ, Ha YC (2018) Concerns for older adult patients with acute hip fracture. Yonsei Med J 59(10):1240–1244. https://doi.org/10.3349/ymj.2018.59.10.1240
9. Falls and fracture prevention strategy in Scotland 2019–2024. https://www.gov.scot/publications/national-falls-fracture-prevention-strategy-scotland-2019-2024/pages/6/
10. Nithman RW, Vincenzo JL (2019) How steady is the STEADI? Inferential analysis of the CDC fall risk toolkit. Arch Gerontol Geriatr 83:185–194. https://doi.org/10.1016/j.archger.2019.02.018

11. Phelan EA, Mahoney JE, Voit JC, Stevens JA (2015) Assessment and management of fall risk in primary care settings. Med Clin North Am 99(2):281–293
12. Bowling CB, Bromfield SG, Colantonio LD, Gutiérrez OM, Shimbo D, Reynolds K, Wright NC, Curtis JR, Judd SE, Franch H, Warnock DG, McClellan W, Muntner P (2016) Association of reduced eGFR and albuminuria with serious fall injuries among older adults. Clin J Am Soc Nephrol 11(7):1236–1243. https://doi.org/10.2215/CJN.11111015
13. Paul SS, Harvey L, Canning CG, Boufous S, Lord SR, Close JC, Sherrington C (2017 Mar) Fall-related hospitalization in people with Parkinson's disease. Eur J Neurol 24(3):523–529. https://doi.org/10.1111/ene.13238
14. Stevens JA (2013) The STEADI Tool Kit: a fall prevention resource for Health Care Providers. IHS Prim Care Provid 39(9):162–166
15. Pierrie SN, Wally MK, Churchill C, Patt JC, Seymour RB, Karunakar MA (2019) Pre-hip fracture falls: a missed opportunity for intervention. Geriatr Orthop Surg Rehabil 10:2151459319856230. https://doi.org/10.1177/2151459319856230. eCollection 2019
16. Barker A, Cameron P, Flicker L, Arendts G, Brand C, Etherton-Beer C, Forbes A, Haines T, Hill AM, Hunter P, Lowthian J, Nyman SR, Redfern J, Smit V, Waldron N, Boyle E, MacDonald E, Ayton D, Morello R, Hill K (2019) Evaluation of RESPOND, a patient-centred programme to prevent falls in older people presenting to the emergency department with a fall: a randomised controlled trial. PLoS Med 16(5):e1002807. https://doi.org/10.1371/journal.pmed.1002807
17. Inderjeeth CA, Raymond WD, Briggs AM, Geelhoed E, Oldham D, Mountain D (2018) Implementation of the Western Australian Osteoporosis Model of Care: a fracture liaison service utilising emergency department information systems to identify patients with fragility fracture to improve current practice and reduce re-fracture rates: a 12-month analysis. Osteoporos Int 29(8):1759–1770. https://doi.org/10.1007/s00198-018-4526-5
18. Cruz-Jentoft AJ, Sayer AA (2019) Sarcopenia. Lancet 393(10191):2636–2646. https://doi.org/10.1016/S0140-6736(19)31138-9
19. Cöster ME, Karlsson M, Ohlsson C, Mellström D, Lorentzon M, Ribom E, Rosengren B (2018) Physical function tests predict incident falls: a prospective study of 2969 men in the Swedish osteoporotic fractures in men study. Scand J Public Health 29:1403494818801628. https://doi.org/10.1177/1403494818801628
20. Vance RC, Healy DG, Galvin R, French HP (2015) Dual tasking with the timed "up & go" test improves detection of risk of falls in people with Parkinson disease. Phys Ther 95(1):95–102
21. Kim JC, Chon J, Kim HS, Lee JH, Yoo SD, Kim DH, Lee SA, Han YJ, Lee HS, Lee BY, Soh YS, Won CW (2017) The association between fall history and physical performance tests in the community-dwelling elderly: a cross-sectional analysis. Ann Rehabil Med 41:239–247
22. Lord SR, Menz BH, Tiedemann A (2003) A physiological profile approach to falls risk assessment and prevention. Phys Ther 83:237–252
23. Nilsson M, Eriksson J, Larsson B, Odén A, Johansson H, Lorentzon M (2016) Fall risk assessment predicts fall-related injury, hip fracture, and head injury in older adults. J Am Geriatr Soc 64(11):2242–2250. https://doi.org/10.1111/jgs.14439
24. Orwoll ES, Fino NF, Gill TM, Cauley JA, Strotmeyer ES, Ensrud KE, Kado DM, Barrett-Connor E, Bauer DC, Cawthon PM, Lapidus J, Osteoporotic Fractures in Men (MrOS) Study Research Group (2018) The relationships between physical performance, activity levels and falls in older men. J Gerontol A Biol Sci Med Sci. https://doi.org/10.1093/gerona/gly248
25. El-Khoury F, Cassou B, Latouche A, Aegerter P, Charles MA, Dargent-Molina P (2015) Effectiveness of two year balance training programme on prevention of fall induced injuries in at risk women aged 75–85 living in community: Ossébo randomised controlled trial. BMJ 351:h3830. https://doi.org/10.1136/bmj.h3830
26. Sherrington C, Fairhall NJ, Wallbank GK, Tiedemann A, Michaleff ZA, Howard K, Clemson L, Hopewell S, Lamb SE (2019) Exercise for preventing falls in older people living in the community. Cochrane Database Syst Rev 1:CD012424. https://doi.org/10.1002/14651858. CD012424.pub2

27. Bolland MJ, Grey A, Avenell A (2018) Effects of vitamin D supplementation on musculoskeletal health: a systematic review, meta-analysis, and trial sequential analysis. Lancet Diabetes Endocrinol 6(11):847–858. https://doi.org/10.1016/S2213-8587(18)30265-1

28. Khaw KT, Stewart AW, Waayer D, Lawes CMM, Toop L, Camargo CA Jr, Scragg R (2017) Effect of monthly high-dose vitamin D supplementation on falls and non-vertebral fractures: secondary and post-hoc outcomes from the randomised, double-blind, placebo-controlled ViDA trial. Lancet Diabetes Endocrinol 5(6):438–447. https://doi.org/10.1016/S2213-8587(17)30103-1

29. Lewis JR, Sim M, Daly RM (2019) The vitamin D and calcium controversy: an update. Curr Opin Rheumatol 31(2):91–97. https://doi.org/10.1097/BOR.0000000000000584

30. Zhao R, Feng F, Wang X (2017) Exercise interventions and prevention of fall-related fractures in older people: a meta-analysis of randomized controlled trials. Int J Epidemiol 46(1):149–161. https://doi.org/10.1093/ije/dyw142

31. Brown LA, Shumway-Cook A, Woollacott MH (1999) Attentional demands and postural recovery: the effects of aging. J Gerontol A Biol Sci Med Sci 54(4):M165–M171

32. Gillespie LD, Robertson MC, Gillespie WJ, Sherrington C, Gates S, Clemson LM, Lamb SE (2012) Interventions for preventing falls in older people living in the community. Cochrane Database Syst Rev 9:CD007146

33. Bemben D, Stark C, Taiar R, Bernardo-Filho M (2018) Relevance of whole-body vibration exercises on muscle strength/power and bone of elderly individuals. Dose Response 16(4):1559325818813066. https://doi.org/10.1177/1559325818813066

34. Jepsen DB, Thomsen K, Hansen S, Jørgensen NR, Masud T, Ryg J (2017) Effect of whole-body vibration exercise in preventing falls and fractures: a systematic review and meta-analysis. BMJ Open 7(12):e018342. https://doi.org/10.1136/bmjopen-2017-018342

35. Davis JC, Robertson MC, Ashe MC, Liu-Ambrose T, Khan KM, Marra CA (2010) International comparison of cost of falls in older adults living in the community: a systematic review. Osteoporos Int 21(8):1295–1306

36. Tricco AC, Thomas SM, Veroniki AA, Hamid JS, Cogo E, Strifler L, Khan PA, Robson R, Sibley KM, MacDonald H, Riva JJ, Thavorn K, Wilson C, Holroyd-Leduc J, Kerr GD, Feldman F, Majumdar SR, Jaglal SB, Hui W, Straus SE (2017) Comparisons of interventions for preventing falls in older adults: a systematic review and meta-analysis. JAMA 318(17):1687–1699

37. de Vries M, Seppala LJ, Daams JG, van de Glind EMM, Masud T, van der Velde N, EUGMS Task and Finish Group on Fall-Risk-Increasing Drugs (2018) Fall-risk-increasing drugs: a systematic review and meta-analysis: I. Cardiovascular drugs. J Am Med Dir Assoc 19(4):371.e1–371.e9. https://doi.org/10.1016/j.jamda.2017.12.013. Epub 2018 Feb 12

38. Seppala LJ, Wermelink AMAT, de Vries M, Ploegmakers KJ, van de Glind EMM, Daams JG, van der Velde N, EUGMS Task and Finish Group on Fall-Risk-Increasing Drugs (2018a) Fall-risk-increasing drugs: a systematic review and meta-analysis: II. Psychotropics. J Am Med Dir Assoc 19(4):371.e11–371.e17. https://doi.org/10.1016/j.jamda.2017.12.098

39. Seppala LJ, van de Glind EMM, Daams JG, Ploegmakers KJ, de Vries M, Wermelink AMAT, van der Velde N, EUGMS Task and Finish Group on Fall-Risk-Increasing Drugs (2018b) Fall-risk-increasing drugs: a systematic review and meta-analysis: III. Others. J Am Med Dir Assoc 19(4):372.e1–372.e8. https://doi.org/10.1016/j.jamda.2017.12.099. Epub 2018 Mar 2

40. Musich S, Wang SS, Ruiz J, Hawkins K, Wicker E (2017) Falls-related drug use and risk of falls among older adults: a study in a US Medicare population. Drugs Aging 34(7):555–565. https://doi.org/10.1007/s40266-017-0470-x

41. Dargent-Molina P, Favier F, Grandjean H, Baudoin C, Schott AM, Hausherr E, Meunier PJ, Bréart G (1996) Fall-related factors and risk of hip fracture: the EPIDOS prospective study. Lancet 348(9021):145–149

42. Zettel JL, McIlroy WE, Maki BE (2008) Gaze behavior of older adults during rapid balance-recovery reactions. J Gerontol A Biol Sci Med Sci 63(8):885–891

43. Dhaliwal R, Aloia JF (2017) Effect of vitamin D on falls and physical performance. Endocrinol Metab Clin N Am 46(4):919–933

44. Dretakis K, Igoumenou VG (2019) The role of parathyroid hormone (PTH) and vitamin D in falls and hip fracture type. Aging Clin Exp Res 31:1501. https://doi.org/10.1007/s40520-019-01132-7

45. Grossman DC, Curry SJ, Owens DK, Barry MJ, Caughey AB, Davidson KW, Doubeni CA, Epling JW Jr, Kemper AR, Krist AH, Kubik M, Landefeld S, Mangione CM, Silverstein M, Simon MA, Tseng CW, US Preventive Services Task Force (2018) Vitamin D, calcium, or combined supplementation for the primary prevention of fractures in community-dwelling adults: US Preventive Services Task Force Recommendation Statement. JAMA 319(15):1592–1599. https://doi.org/10.1001/jama.2018.3185

46. NICE (National Institute for Health and Care Excellence) (2013) Falls in older people: assessing risk and prevention. https://www.nice.org.uk/guidance/cg161

47. Blain H, Dabas F, Mekhinini S, Picot MC, Miot S, Bousquet J, Boubakri C, Jaussent A, Bernard PL (2019) Effectiveness of a programme delivered in a falls clinic in preventing serious injuries in high-risk older adults: a pre- and post-intervention study. Maturitas 122:80–86. https://doi.org/10.1016/j.maturitas.2019.01.012

48. Shah VN, Wu M, Foster N, Dhaliwal R, Al Mukaddam M (2018) Severe hypoglycemia is associated with high risk for falls in adults with type 1 diabetes. Arch Osteoporos 13(1):66. https://doi.org/10.1007/s11657-018-0475-z

49. Corona G, Norello D, Parenti G, Sforza A, Maggi M, Peri A (2018) Hyponatremia, falls and bone fractures: a systematic review and meta-analysis. Clin Endocrinol 89(4):505–513. https://doi.org/10.1111/cen.13790. Epub 2018 July 12

50. Cauley JA, Hovey KM, Stone KL, Andrews CA, Barbour KE, Hale L, Jackson RD, Johnson KC, LeBlanc ES, Li W, Zaslavsky O, Ochs-Balcom H, Wactawski-Wende J, Crandall CJ (2019) Characteristics of self-reported sleep and the risk of falls and fractures: the Women's Health Initiative (WHI). J Bone Miner Res 34(3):464–474. https://doi.org/10.1002/jbmr.3619

51. Brenner R, Ammann P, Yoon SI, Christen S, Hellermann J, Girod G, Knaus U, Duru F, Krasniqi N, Ramsay D, Sticherling C, Lippuner K, Kühne M (2017) Reduction of falls and fractures after permanent pacemaker implantation in elderly patients with sinus node dysfunction. Europace 19(7):1220–1226. https://doi.org/10.1093/europace/euw156

52. Correa-Pérez A, Delgado-Silveira E, Martín-Aragón S, Rojo-Sanchís AM, Cruz-Jentoft AJ (2019) Fall-risk increasing drugs and prevalence of polypharmacy in older patients discharged from an orthogeriatric unit after a hip fracture. Aging Clin Exp Res 31(7):969–975. https://doi.org/10.1007/s40520-018-1046-2

53. Munson JC, Bynum JP, Bell JE, Cantu R, McDonough C, Wang Q, Tosteson TD, Tosteson AN (2016) Patterns of prescription drug use before and after fragility fracture. JAMA Intern Med 176(10):1531–1538. https://doi.org/10.1001/jamainternmed.2016.4814

54. Vranken L, Wyers CE, Van der Velde RY, Janzing HM, Kaarsemaker S, Geusens PP, Van den Bergh JP (2018) Comorbidities and medication use in patients with a recent clinical fracture at the Fracture Liaison Service. Osteoporos Int 29(2):397–407. https://doi.org/10.1007/s00198-017-4290-y

55. Machado-Duque ME, Castaño-Montoya JP, Medina-Morales DA, Castro-Rodríguez A, González-Montoya A, Machado-Alba JE (2018) Association between the use of benzodiazepines and opioids with the risk of falls and hip fractures in older adults. Int Psychogeriatr 30(7):941–946. https://doi.org/10.1017/S1041610217002745

56. Sotimehin AE, Yonge AV, Mihailovic A, West SK, Friedman DS, Gitlin LN, Ramulu PY (2018) Locations, circumstances, and outcomes of falls in patients with Glaucoma. Am J Ophthalmol 192:131–141. https://doi.org/10.1016/j.ajo.2018.04.024

57. Hofmeyer MR, Alexander NB, Nyquist LV, Medell JL, Koreishi A (2002) Floor-rise strategy training in older adults. J Am Geriatr Soc 50(10):1702–1706

58. Huang ZG, Feng YH, Li YH, Lv CS (2017) Systematic review and meta-analysis: Tai Chi for preventing falls in older adults. BMJ Open 7(2):e013661

59. Rimland JM, Abraha I, Dell'Aquila G, Cruz-Jentoft A, Soiza R, Gudmusson A, Petrovic M, O'Mahony D, Todd C, Cherubini A (2016) Effectiveness of non-pharmacological interventions

to prevent falls in older people: a systematic overview. The SENATOR Project ONTOP Series. PLoS One 11(8):e0161579

60. Strouwen C, Molenaar EALM, Münks L, Keus SHJ, Zijlmans JCM, Vandenberghe W, Bloem BR, Nieuwboer A (2017) Training dual tasks together or apart in Parkinson's disease: results from the DUALITY trial. Mov Disord 32(8):1201–1210

61. Greenspan SL, Myers ER, Maitland LA, Resnick NM, Hayes WC (1994) Fall severity and bone mineral density as risk factors for hip fracture in ambulatory elderly. JAMA 271:128–133

62. Rogers MW, Mille ML (2003) Lateral stability and falls in older people. Exerc Sport Sci Rev 31(4):182–187

63. Yang Y, Mackey DC, Liu-Ambrose T, Feldman F, Robinovitch SN (2016) Risk factors for hip impact during real-life falls captured on video in long-term care. Osteoporos Int 27(2):537–547. https://doi.org/10.1007/s00198-015-3268-x

64. Robinovitch SN, Inkster L, Maurer J, Warnick B (2003) Strategies for avoiding hip impact during sideways falls. J Bone Miner Res 18(7):1267–1273

65. De Goede KM, Ashton-Miller JA (2003) Biomechanical simulations of forward fall arrests: effects of upper extremity arrest strategy, gender and aging-related declines in muscle strength. J Biomech 36(3):413–420

66. Sran MM, Stotz PJ, Normandin SC, Robinovitch SN (2010) Age differences in energy absorption in the upper extremity during a descent movement: implications for arresting a fall. J Gerontol A Biol Sci Med Sci 65(3):312–317. https://doi.org/10.1093/gerona/glp153

67. King AC, Whitt-Glover MC, Marquez DX, Buman MP, Napolitano MA, Jakicic J, Fulton JE, Tennant BL, 2018 Physical Activity Guidelines Advisory Committee* (2019) Physical activity promotion: highlights from the 2018 Physical Activity Guidelines Advisory Committee systematic review. Med Sci Sports Exerc 51(6):1340–1353. https://doi.org/10.1249/MSS.0000000000001945

68. Lee SY, Yoon BH, Beom J, Ha YC, Lim JY (2017) Effect of lower-limb progressive resistance exercise after hip fracture surgery: a systematic review and meta-analysis of randomized controlled studies. J Am Med Dir Assoc 18(12):1096.e19–1096.e26. https://doi.org/10.1016/j.jamda.2017.08.021

69. Cheung WH, Shen WY, Dai DL, Lee KB, Zhu TY, Wong RM, Leung KS (2018) Evaluation of a multidisciplinary rehabilitation programme for elderly patients with hip fracture: a prospective cohort study. J Rehabil Med 50(3):285–291. https://doi.org/10.2340/16501977-2310

70. Lockwood KJ, Harding KE, Boyd JN, Taylor NF (2019) Predischarge home visits after hip fracture: a randomized controlled trial. Clin Rehabil 33(4):681–692. https://doi.org/10.1177/0269215518823256

71. Kunigkeit C, Stock S, Müller D (2018 Nov 9) Cost-effectiveness of a home safety intervention to prevent falls in impaired elderly people living in the community. Arch Osteoporos 13(1):122. https://doi.org/10.1007/s11657-018-0535-4

72. Charoenngam N, Shirvani A, Holick MF (2019) Vitamin D for skeletal and non-skeletal health: what we should know. J Clin Orthop Trauma 10(6):1082–1093. https://doi.org/10.1016/j.jcot.2019.07.004. Epub 2019 Jul 13. Review

73. Blain H, Rolland Y, Beauchet O, Annweiler C, Benhamou CL, Benetos A, Berrut G, Audran M, Bendavid S, Bousson V, Briot K, Brazier M, Breuil V, Chapuis L, Chapurlat R, Cohen-Solal M, Cortet B, Dargent P, Fardellone P, Feron JM, Gauvain JB, Guggenbuhl P, Hanon O, Laroche M, Kolta S, Lespessailles E, Letombe B, Mallet E, Marcelli C, Orcel P, Puisieux F, Seret P, Souberbielle JC, Sutter B, Trémollières F, Weryha G, Roux C, Thomas T, Groupe de recherche et d'information sur les ostéoporoses et la Société française de gérontologie et gériatrie (2014) Usefulness of bone density measurement in fallers. Joint Bone Spine 81:403–408

74. Adachi JD, Berger C, Barron R, Weycker D, Anastassiades TP, Davison KS, Hanley DA, Ioannidis G, Jackson SA, Josse RG, Kaiser SM, Kovacs CS, Leslie WD, Morin SN, Papaioannou A, Prior JC, Shyta E, Silvia A, Towheed T, Goltzman D (2019) Predictors of imminent non-vertebral fracture in elderly women with osteoporosis, low bone mass, or a history of fracture, based on data from the population-based Canadian Multicentre Osteoporosis Study (CaMos). Arch Osteoporos 14(1):53. https://doi.org/10.1007/s11657-019-0598-x

75. Blain H, Masud T, Dargent-Molina P, Martin FC, Rosendahl E et al (2016) A comprehensive fracture prevention strategy in older adults: the European Union Geriatric Medicine Society (EUGMS) statement. Eur Geriatr Med 7:519–525

76. Aranda-Gallardo M, Morales-Asencio JM, Canca-Sanchez JC, Barrero-Sojo S, Perez-Jimenez C, Morales-Fernandez A, de Luna-Rodriguez ME, Moya-Suarez AB, Mora-Banderas AM (2013) Instruments for assessing the risk of falls in acute hospitalized patients: a systematic review and meta-analysis. BMC Health Serv Res 13:122

77. Zhang C, Wu X, Lin S, Jia Z, Cao J (2015) Evaluation of reliability and validity of the Hendrich II fall risk model in a Chinese hospital population. PLoS One 10(11):e0142395. https://doi.org/10.1371/journal.pone.0142395. eCollection 2015

78. Holte HH, Underland V, Hafstad E (2015) Review of systematic reviews on prevention of falls in institutions. NIPH systematic reviews: executive summaries. Report from Norwegian Knowledge Centre for the Health Services (NOKC) 2015; No. 13

79. Hill AM, McPhail SM, Waldron N, Etherton-Beer C, Ingram K, Flicker L, Bulsara M, Haines TP (2015) Fall rates in hospital rehabilitation units after individualised patient and staff education programmes: a pragmatic, stepped-wedge, cluster-randomised controlled trial. Lancet 385(9987):2592–2599

80. Roigk P, Becker C, Schulz C, König HH, Rapp K (2018) Long-term evaluation of the implementation of a large fall and fracture prevention program in long-term care facilities. BMC Geriatr 18(1):233. https://doi.org/10.1186/s12877-018-0924-y

81. Mackey DC, Lachance CC, Wang PT, Feldman F, Laing AC, Leung PM, Hu XJ, Robinovitch SN (2019) The Flooring for Injury Prevention (FLIP) Study of compliant flooring for the prevention of fall-related injuries in long-term care: a randomized trial. PLoS Med 16(6):e1002843. https://doi.org/10.1371/journal.pmed.1002843

82. Morley JE (2010) Clinical practice in nursing homes as a key for progress. J Nutr Health Aging 14:586–593

83. Köpke S, Mühlhauser I, Gerlach A, Haut A, Haastert B, Möhler R, Meyer G (2012) Effect of a guideline-based multicomponent intervention on use of physical restraints in nursing homes: a randomized controlled trial. JAMA 307(20):2177–2184

84. Close JC, Wesson J, Sherrington C, Hill KD, Kurrle S, Lord SR, Brodaty H, Howard K, Gitlin LN, O'Rourke SD, Clemson L (2014) Can a tailored exercise and home hazard reduction programme reduce the rate of falls in community dwelling older people with cognitive impairment: protocol paper for the i-FOCIS randomised controlled trial. BMC Geriatr 14:89. https://doi.org/10.1186/1471-2318-14-89

85. Taylor ME, Delbaere K, Lord SR, Mikolaizak AS, Brodaty H, Close JC (2014) Neuropsychological, physical, and functional mobility measures associated with falls in cognitively impaired older adults. J Gerontol A Biol Sci Med Sci 69(8):987–995. https://doi.org/10.1093/gerona/glt166

86. Montero-Odasso M, Speechley M (2018) Falls in cognitively impaired older adults: implications for risk assessment and prevention. J Am Geriatr Soc 66(2):367–375. https://doi.org/10.1111/jgs.15219

87. Zhang W, Low LF, Schwenk M, Mills N, Gwynn JD, Clemson L (2019) Review of gait, cognition, and fall risks with implications for fall prevention in older adults with dementia. Dement Geriatr Cogn Disord 48(1–2):17–29. https://doi.org/10.1159/000504340

88. Gomez F, Curcio CL, Brennan-Olsen SL, Boersma D, Phu S, Vogrin S, Suriyaarachchi P, Duque G (2019 Jul 29) Effects of the falls and fractures clinic as an integrated multidisciplinary model of care in Australia: a pre-post study. BMJ Open 9(7):e027013. https://doi.org/10.1136/bmjopen-2018-027013

89. Palvanen M, Kannus P, Piirtola M, Niemi S, Parkkari J, Järvinen M (2014) Effectiveness of the Chaos Falls Clinic in preventing falls and injuries of home-dwelling older adults: a randomised controlled trial. Injury 45(1):265–271

90. Roux C, Briot K (2017) Imminent fracture risk. Osteoporos Int 28(6):1765–1769. https://doi.org/10.1007/s00198-017-3976-5

91. Pflimlin A, Gournay A, Delabrière I, Chantelot C, Puisieux F, Cortet B, Paccou J (2019) Secondary prevention of osteoporotic fractures: evaluation of the Lille University Hospital's Fracture Liaison Service between January 2016 and January 2018. Osteoporos Int 30:1779. https://doi.org/10.1007/s00198-019-05036-0

92. Pioli G, Bendini C, Pignedoli P, Giusti A, Marsh D (2018) Orthogeriatric co-management—managing frailty as well as fragility. Injury 49(8):1398–1402. https://doi.org/10.1016/j.injury.2018.04.014. Epub 2018 Apr 20

93. Liu LK, Lee WJ, Chen LY, Hwang AC, Lin MH, Peng LN, Chen LK (2015) Association between frailty, osteoporosis, falls and hip fractures among community-dwelling people aged 50 years and older in Taiwan: results from I-Lan Longitudinal Aging Study. PLoS One 10(9):e0136968. https://doi.org/10.1371/journal.pone.0136968. eCollection 2015

Part V
Cross-Cutting Issues

Nursing in the Orthogeriatric Setting

17

Julie Santy-Tomlinson, Karen Hertz,
Charlotte Myhre-Jensen, and Louise Brent

17.1   Introduction

The aims of this chapter are to provide an overview of the role of nurses in the multidisciplinary orthogeriatric team and help medical, surgical practitioners and therapists to understand the potential of the nursing team to foster collaboration in achieving best outcomes for patients. The call to action issued by the Fragility Fracture Network [1] describes four pillars of fragility fracture care, all of which involve expert nursing: (1) multidisciplinary co-management in the acute fracture episode; (2) post-acute rehabilitation; (3) secondary prevention after every fragility fracture and (4) the formation of multidisciplinary national alliances. These pillars support the need for nursing education, collaboration between nurses and their supporting local, national and global associations and the development of education,

This chapter is a component of Part 5: Cross-cutting issues.
For an explanation of the grouping of chapters in this book, please see Chapter 1: "The multidisciplinary approach to fragility fractures around the world—an overview".

J. Santy-Tomlinson (✉)
Orthopaedic Nursing, Odense University Hospitals and University of Southern Denmark,
Odense, Denmark
e-mail: juliesanty@tomlinson15.karoo.co.uk

K. Hertz
University Hospitals of North Midlands, Stoke-on-Trent, UK
e-mail: Karen.Hertz@uhnm.nhs.uk

C. Myhre-Jensen
Department of Orthopaedic Surgery and Traumatology, Odense University Hospital,
Odense, Denmark
e-mail: Charlotte.Myhre.Jensen@rsyd.dk

L. Brent
National Office of Clinical Audit, Dublin, Ireland
e-mail: louisebrent@noca.ie

clinical guidance and resources that can be adapted and adopted in any part of the world so that best practice nursing care can be achieved. In some countries, regions and/or localities, the concept of orthogeriatric nursing has yet to be fully recognised. Even so, the principles of orthogeriatric care and management can be applied in any setting with consideration of the context of local practice, culture and resources.

17.2 Nursing Care Quality

Orthogeriatric patients have complex health care needs, many of which can be met by skilled, compassionate nursing. Nursing involves autonomous and collaborative care that includes the promotion of health as well as prevention of illness and supporting recovery during ill health and following injury and surgery. Nursing also embodies advocacy, promotion of safety, leadership and participation in shaping health policy [2]. Nurses make a unique contribution to orthogeriatric care because they spend the most time with patients and develop a therapeutic relationship with individuals and their families while acting as coordinators of care. They understand the patient experience of the fracture and its care through qualitative exploration of experiences. These experiences are often described as difficult and painful, leading to significant decrease in quality of life, and are fraught with restrictions and insecurity [3, 4], although patient experiences in resource-poor countries have yet to be studied or documented.

Hip fracture audit, where it takes place, has had a significant impact on the quality of medical and surgical care, but with a limited focus on nursing. It is essential that indicators of the value of nursing care are developed and measured [5]. The overall contribution of health care delivery is often measured in terms of health status, outcomes, readmissions rates, length of stay, complication rates and mortality [6], but these do not always help to capture the specific contribution of nursing care.

Nurse-sensitive quality indicators include patient comfort and quality of life, complication rates, safety, empowerment and satisfaction. More specific clinical indicators can include healthcare-associated infection, pressure ulcers, falls and drug administration errors [7]. Pain management, delirium, pressure ulcers, hydration and nutrition, constipation, prevention of secondary infections and venous thromboembolism (VTE), rehabilitation and remobilisation are all nursing care priorities [5] but evidence-based nurse management strategies need to co-exist with medical and therapist models of care. This includes reducing the risk of complications and mortality, improving recovery, maintaining function and improving patient experiences. Preventing harm and patient safety, focused on avoiding adverse events, are multidisciplinary concerns that vary depending on the country and its resources. Nurses, through their extended contact with patients, remain central to recognising risk and alerting other team members. Nursing quality indicators should also take into consideration the local context and available resources.

17.3 Acute Care

The high prevalence, complexity of needs, length of stay and cost, often make hip fracture care the focus of practice development. The skills and knowledge needed to look after patients with hip fractures, however, also apply to the management of all older people with fractures and include fundamental aspects of nursing care for the adult as well as specialised interventions for older people [8, 9]. A hip fracture is a sudden traumatic event, threatening many aspects of patients' lives and a forceful reminder of their mortality [10]. Care is dominated by restoring function, so physical care attracts the most attention and the primary goal of nursing is to maximise mobility and preserve optimal function whilst also prioritising psychosocial factors so that patients can participate in their rehabilitation [11].

Emergency care following hip fracture usually takes place in Emergency Departments that are noisy, busy and overstimulating, making them inappropriate care environments for vulnerable older people in a state of personal and physical crisis. Avoiding the impact of this situation requires consideration of three principles [12]:

- Timeliness—avoiding unnecessary and unwanted delay.
- Effectiveness—aiming for optimal outcomes using the best available evidence.
- Patient-centeredness—care that is respectful of and responsive to individual needs.

This is equally true of the hospital ward and perioperative environment which are rarely designed to meet the needs of frail older people.

17.3.1 Complexity and Frailty

Trauma care for older people must follow the same principles as for all age groups but the normal and abnormal changes of ageing, compounded by active comorbidities, mean that morbidity and mortality are increased concerns [13].

Trauma/orthopaedic services evolved to treat all adult patients, irrespective of age, following all types of musculoskeletal injury. However, there has been less focus on the complex needs of those who are older and frail but have also sustained a fracture. Highly skilled nursing is needed that is tailored to the needs of the older person. This must encompass expert care of both the older person and the individual with a musculoskeletal condition/injury.

These "complex patients" present with multiple problems including; comorbidity, multimorbidity, poly-pathology, dual diagnosis and multiple chronic conditions [14] with multiple interlocking problems related to both breadth (range) and depth (severity) [15]. In the orthogeriatric patient there are three main facets of complexity; the person, the fracture and the care environment—all of which have a significant impact on patient care outcomes and are influenced by nursing care (see Fig. 17.1).

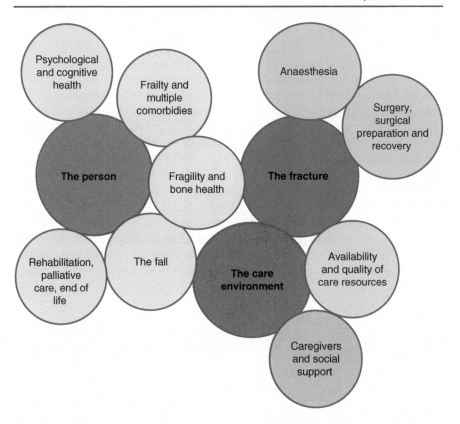

Fig. 17.1 The complexity of nursing care needs for hospitalised patients with hip fracture (adapted from Hertz & Santy-Tomlinson 2017 [16])

Complexity and frailty are linked. As described in Chap. 4, frailty is a distinctive health state in which multiple body systems gradually lose their in-built reserves; incidence increases with age and is associated with negative outcomes such as falls, hospitalisation, poor functional outcomes and death [17]. Dramatic changes in their physical and mental well-being after any event which challenges a frail person's health, such as an injury or surgery leads to increased vulnerability and diminished resistance to stressors [18]. Frailty can be physical or psychological or a combination of the two elements when physical frailty is coupled with cognitive impairment [19]. Frailty is known to be a dynamic state, varying in severity with capacity to be made better and worse. It is not an inevitable part of ageing; but is a long-term condition that is linked with falls and fractures.

The identification of frailty is an interdisciplinary responsibility, but nurses need to recognise it in patient assessment so that care can be planned accordingly [20]. In collaboration with the orthogeriatric team, a validated assessment tool may identify frailty and its contributing factors as part of the multidisciplinary assessment process (see Chap. 4).

Sarcopenia, reduced muscle mass and strength, is an additional driver for specialised nursing care for orthogeriatric patients, increasing fracture risk as it contributes to falls and is associated with lower bone mineral density, partly due to reduced forces of muscle on bone [17]. This combination of problems affects balance, gait and overall ability to perform tasks of daily living, highlighting the link between frailty, falls and fragility. Just as osteoporosis predicts the future risk of fracture, sarcopenia is a powerful predictor of future disability and need for specialised nursing care to reverse or manage decline.

17.3.2 Nursing Assessment and Management of Pain

Frequent, accurate pain assessment is essential. Pain in older people is often underreported by patients and ignored by health care professionals. Unmanaged or undermanaged pain increases the risk of delirium, impaired mobility, chronic pain and poorer long-term function [21]. Cognitive impairment increases the risk of pain not being recognised. The individual and highly variable nature of pain and an individual's response to it make accurate assessment central to nursing care that facilitates individualised pain management and monitoring. If pain is poorly controlled, mobilisation will be delayed, increasing the risk of complications of prolonged immobility, increased dependency and delirium.

Verbal reports of pain are valid and reliable in patients with mild to moderate dementia or delirium but the assessment of pain in a patient with more severe cognitive impairment may be more difficult. It has been shown that cognitively impaired and acutely confused patients receive less analgesia than their unimpaired counterparts. Using specific assessment tools can help staff to understand the individual needs of a person with dementia and encourages families to share patient information, characteristics and behaviour that enable staff to better understand their pain experience and needs [22]. For pain assessment to be effective it must be carried out frequently and recorded accurately, just like vital signs or the administration of medication and other interventions. Pain management must provide sufficient relief to allow nursing care to be performed with least distress to the patient followed by reassessment and appropriate administration of analgesia.

As nurses become increasingly responsible for more advanced patient care interventions, non-medical prescribing will permit nurses to assess pain and to formulate a patient-centred plan for pain management. In some settings, advanced practitioners with enhanced skills can prescribe a range of medications including opioid and non-opioid analgesics to enable a faster response to patient needs. Administration pre-operatively of nerve blocks for patients with hip fracture is becoming increasingly common, minimising the need for opiates which have multiple risk factors in older and frail patients and have been shown to have a significant positive effect on the pain experience [23].

17.3.3 Nursing Assessment and Management of Delirium

Delirium is a common and serious condition in older surgical patients, with an incidence of up to 60% following hip fracture. It is identifiable by its sudden onset, fluctuating course and effect on consciousness and perception. The consequences of delirium can include [24]:

- Increased rates of complications.
- Increased length of hospital stay.
- Increased risk of dementia.
- More care and support needs following discharge.
- Increased risk of death.

Assessment of delirium has two focuses:

1. Identification of those at highest risk.
2. Identification of those developing symptoms of delirium.

Delirium is avoidable and the severity can be reduced through nursing interventions as the nursing team are most likely to recognise the signs of delirium discussed in Chap. 11. Good communication with patients, family and carers can help practitioners to recognise risk of delirium and subtle changes that suggest both delirium and its underlying causes, enabling them to co-ordinate multidisciplinary interventions.

Patients with or at risk of delirium and their carers need information about delirium and what they might experience, encouraging them to report changes and inconsistencies in behaviour as there are several nursing interventions which may prevent delirium [25] as well as contribute to effective general nursing care of all older people:

- An environment that helps to re-orientate patients; large-face clocks and calendars, well-lit areas with clear signage.
- Gentle re-orientation by introducing team members and with explanations of time and place; family/friends should be encouraged to visit and be supported in modifying their own communication.
- Dehydration, hypoxia and constipation prevention and management.
- Supported mobilisation to give more control.
- Recognition and management of infections.
- Assessment and management of pain.
- Ensure dentures are fitting correctly and encourage patients to eat.
- Resolve reversible causes of sensory impairment e.g. hearing and visual aids.
- Facilitating sleep and rest.

17.3.4 Pressure Ulcer Prevention

Pressure ulcers (PUs) are serious complications of immobility, hospitalisation and surgery which increase the need for nursing care and extend hospital stay. Patients with hip fracture are at high risk, so prevention and management are central to patient safety. PU prevention is largely a nursing responsibility, but a multidisciplinary approach is needed to manage all risk factors.

Assessment of the skin on admission should be followed by frequent reassessment. PUs can develop rapidly, so prompt and repeated assessment of risk using an appropriate and validated tool is essential in identifying the intrinsic and extrinsic factors that may lead to PUs. Identification of specific risk factors can then assist in planning and delivering appropriate interventions for prevention [26]. Examples of intrinsic and extrinsic factors are listed in Table 17.1.

Prevention strategies must be individualised to the patient's skin condition and risk factors and based on evidence-based guidelines [27]. Interventions should include:

- Head to toe skin assessment at least once during each nursing shift.
- Pressure relieving/redistributing support surfaces on beds and chairs, including in the home.
- Off-loading of bony prominences, especially the sacrum and heels.
- Frequent re-positioning based on assessment of the individual's tissue tolerance to pressure, including use of the 30-degree tilt to ensure off-loading of bony prominences.
- General skin care; careful washing and drying of the skin (especially following incontinence) and the use of emollient therapy to help promote the skin barrier function.
- Effective management of pain to promote movement and mobilisation.
- Nutrition and hydration.

Table 17.1 Common pressure ulcer risk factors for patients following hip fracture and surgery

Extrinsic
• Pressure—Bony prominences—Especially heels
• Shear
• Friction
• Skin moisture
Intrinsic
• Immobility
• Surgery
• Ageing, dry and damaged skin
• Concurrent medical conditions: e.g. diabetes, cardiovascular, respiratory, neurological
• Malnutrition
• Dehydration

- Carefully selected support surfaces on beds and chairs;
  - Foam mattresses to redistribute pressure and reduce friction in patients at medium risk of PUs.
  - For patients at high to very high risk, dynamic pressure reducing equipment such as alternating pressure mattresses for all patients until their mobility has improved enough for them to be able to change their own position.
  - Once remobilisation is in progress, these principles should also be applied to seating.

17.3.5 Nutrition, Hydration, Acute Kidney Injury and Constipation

Nutrition and hydration are fundamental to recovery and are the responsibility of the whole team, but the nursing team is central to adequate dietary and fluid intake because of their extended presence. Routine care must include assessment of nutritional status on admission, nutritional intake following admission, nurse-based strategies to improve calorific intake and, where appropriate, referral for dietetic advice (see Chap. 18). Team communication should maximise nutrition and fluid intake in close collaboration with patients/families. Minimal duration of preoperative fasting is a priority [8] so nurses need to be able to assess the likely time of commencement of surgery.

Fluid management in older people can be difficult; they may self-regulate fluid to try to control urinary incontinence/frequency and difficulties in accessing toilet facilities. Close monitoring of fluid balance is an essential aspect of nursing care to prevent or identify acute kidney injury. Patients' acceptance of drinks is often poor and nursing interventions to promote adequate fluid intake should include:

- Accurate administration of prescribed IV and parenteral fluids.
- Avoidance of long periods of fasting, including interdisciplinary commitment to ensuring the timing of older patients' surgery is managed and transparent.
- Assisting with oral fluid intake with regard for patient preferences and monitoring fluid intake/output.
- Appropriate toilet signage, regular toileting and other measures to enable patients to maintain continence.
- Close observation of vital signs and other indicators of health deterioration.

Renal function is affected by the ageing process as well as ill health. Acute kidney injury (AKI) is a significant cause of death in hospitalised older people: a sudden episode of kidney failure or damage that happens rapidly and is normally the consequence of acute illness, trauma or surgery and leads to reduced renal function [28].

Nurses can identify those at risk of AKI:

- Age 65 years or over.
- History of acute kidney injury.
- Chronic kidney disease.
- Symptoms of urological conditions.
- Chronic conditions such as heart failure, liver disease and diabetes mellitus.
- Neurological or cognitive impairment or disability (which may limit independent fluid intake).
- Sepsis.
- Hypovolaemia.
- Oliguria (urine output less than 0.5 mL/kg/h).
- Nephrotoxic drug use within the last week (especially if hypovolaemic) e.g. non-steroidal anti-inflammatory drugs (NSAIDs), angiotensin-converting enzyme (ACE) inhibitors, angiotensin II receptor antagonists (ARBs) and diuretics.
- Exposure to iodinated contrast agents within the past week.
- Cancer and cancer therapy.
- Immunocompromise (e.g. HIV infection).
- Toxins (e.g. some herbal remedies, poisonous plants and animals).

Risk should be documented and discussed within the MDT and an enhanced plan of care initiated. In at-risk patients baseline assessment of blood creatinine should be conducted with daily monitoring in the peri-operative period and continued regularly throughout admission. Medication review should be conducted pre-operatively and, in the peri-operative period, identification of nephrotoxic drugs and those that may significantly reduce BP during acute illness.

Management of AKI depends on the cause. Nursing interventions include:

1. Identifying those at risk/presenting with AKI, reporting to senior clinicians.
2. Accurate recording and documentation of fluid balance.
3. Maintaining fluid intake.
4. Acting as a conduit of information between the MDT and the patient and family. In the frailest patients, where the risk of AKI is highest, patient/carer involvement is essential in ensuring adequate fluid intake.

Constipation can be acute or chronic and is a common complication following fracture and during periods of ill health/immobility. Prevention should be considered early in the care pathway. Prevention of constipation from a nursing perspective should involve:

- Regular assessment of bowel function including frequency and consistency of defaecation.
- Providing and encouraging a palatable fibre-rich diet and prevention of dehydration.
- Careful but early use of prescribed aperients.

17.3.6 Healthcare Associated Infection

17.3.6.1 Pneumonia: Nursing Assessment, Prevention and Management

Nursing interventions to prevent pneumonia reflect general good nursing practice for the older people:

- Universal infection prevention precautions.
- Good pain relief to facilitate coughing, deep breathing and mobility.
- Early, regular mobilisation; encouraging activity out of bed.
- Prevention of aspiration risks.
- Encourage patients to sit in a chair for meals.
- Monitoring of dysphagia and swallow and cough reflexes.
- Thickener in drinks or modified diets as appropriate.
- Education of family/carers about the risk and preventive strategies in use.
- Reporting of signs and symptoms of respiratory problems to medical practitioners.

Patients with pneumonia need to be closely monitored by the nursing team for further deterioration. Adequate nutrition is central to supporting recovery and enteral feeding may be needed, although nasogastric feeding can increase the risk of aspiration. Hydration, early mobilisation, encouraging deep breathing and coughing, regular changes of position, chest physiotherapy and nebulisers to moisten secretions can also assist in recovery.

17.3.6.2 Urinary Tract Infection: Nursing Assessment, Prevention and Management

Prevention, recognition and management of urinary tract infection (UTI) are the responsibility of the whole team, but are a fundamental nursing role. Strategies for prevention, risk reduction and recognition of UTI include:

- Avoiding indwelling urinary catheters as much as possible.
- Insertion and removal of urinary catheters under aseptic conditions.
- Using a closed drainage catheter bag system.
- Compliance with infection prevention precautions when inserting, handling and removing catheters.
- Meticulous perineal hygiene.
- Removal of indwelling urinary catheters as soon as possible.
- Reducing the risk of dehydration.
- Early mobilisation to reduce urinary stasis.
- Monitoring for signs of developing infection; particularly delirium, fever and tachycardia.
- Obtain a urine sample for microbiological analysis and referral to medical staff if symptoms of urinary tract infection are present.

17.3.7 Venous Thromboembolism: Nursing Interventions for Prevention

Following hip fracture there is a high risk of venous thromboembolism (VTE). Although prevention and medical management of VTE are considered in Chap. 7, the nursing role in prevention includes assessment of risk on admission and when the patient's condition changes using a risk assessment tool. Nursing specific measures that contribute to the prevention of VTE include:

• Restoration of mobility.
• Supporting early mobilisation and leg exercises to activate the calf muscle pump.
• Maintaining adequate hydration.
• Patient and carer information about the causes, prevention and the need to comply with prophylaxis, especially on discharge/transfer.
• Observation of patients for signs and symptoms of deep vein thrombosis and pulmonary embolism.

Nursing interventions for prophylaxis focus on mechanical measures, particularly graduated compression "anti-embolic" stockings. Stockings can, however, contribute to lower limb compartment syndrome, skin ulceration and common peroneal nerve palsy and should not be used in patients with cardiac or vascular disease, fragile skin or limb shape/deformity preventing correct fit. Safe use of compression stockings includes making sure that stockings are correctly fitted, checking to make sure the fit is not affected by changes in leg shape due to oedema and ensuring stocking are removed regularly for hygiene purposes, assessment of neurovascular status of the limb and checking for skin problems [29].

17.4 Rehabilitation, Discharge and Continuing Care

Independence in physical function and quality of life drive multidisciplinary rehabilitation. Effective rehabilitation is important as it promotes independence and supports patients in reaching their potential. Rehabilitation in the hospital setting and beyond tend to be largely a nursing role, alongside therapists, because of the need to support rehabilitation as part of 24 h and extended care in a collaborative, supportive culture with patient motivation in mind. There is limited evidence, however, regarding the value of different care strategies in supporting rehabilitation and discharge and which team members can best provide such care.

Early supported multidisciplinary rehabilitation can reduce hospital stay, improve early return to function and impact positively on both readmission rates and the level of public-funded home care required [30]. Community rehabilitation schemes facilitate early discharge of less frail patients to their own home. Ongoing rehabilitation allows them to continue to improve functionally and progress towards their goals after discharge, although in many settings this is not provided.

From admission, patients should be offered a formal, acute, orthogeriatric or orthopaedic ward-based hip fracture programme that includes the following [31]:

- Comprehensive multidisciplinary geriatric/orthogeriatric assessment and continuous review.
- Rapid preoperative optimisation of fitness for surgery.
- Early identification of individual goals for rehabilitation; to recover mobility and independence and facilitate return to pre-fracture residence and long-term well-being.
- Liaison or integration with related services, particularly mental health, falls prevention, bone health, primary care and social services.
- Clinical and service governance responsibility for all stages of the pathway of care and rehabilitation, including those aspects delivered in the community.

Patients with hip fracture have a lower perception of readiness for hospital discharge than other medical–surgical groups [32]. Improvements are needed in nursing practice so that patients feel adequately prepared for discharge and achieve the best possible outcomes. Discharge planning in acute hospitals is multidisciplinary, but nurses take responsibility for much of this, particularly patient and family education, coordination and liaising with follow-on care providers.

The responsibility for care after discharge is often delegated to the patient and their family along with the general practitioner and, sometimes, community care staff. The patient and their caregivers must be able to understand the discharge instructions so that they can recall aftercare instructions and remember to follow them. Providing patients with written discharge instructions has proven to be valuable, as has the provision of information in electronic formats via a smart phone or tablet applications and other devices [33]. Supporting oral information/education with written/electronic information on discharge helps older people with perception, visual, auditory and/or cognitive problems to manage the complex multiple messages.

In an ideal world, patients should have the option to receive rehabilitative care in a specialist rehabilitation setting. This is not an option in most resource-poor settings and is rarely the case even in settings with better resources. The fundamental goal of orthogeriatric care is to discharge the patient to either independent or supported living in their own home or to alternative accommodation where post-discharge care can be provided either permanently or temporarily. Patients and families need intensive support when returning to a community setting or moving to residential care following discharge. Issues that need to be considered include the prevention of future falls, the continued management of bone fragility and secondary fracture prevention as well as the need for continued progress towards optimum achievement of rehabilitation. Post-discharge services vary significantly globally, and the availability of specialist community nursing resources is even more of a challenge than in the hospital setting.

Nurses must be aware of the possibility and effects of care giver burden especially since the majority of orthogeriatric patients require physical care after discharge. Care giver burden is defined as "the physical, emotional and financial responses of a caregiver to the changes and demands caused by providing help to another person with a physical or mental disability" [34]. Continued support of care givers should be in place following hospital discharge. Ongoing communication and contact are vital in ensuring care giver burden is minimised. The ability of informal care to meet the care needs of patients is limited, so longer term plans may need to be in place if care needs are prolonged or carers are not able to cope [35].

17.5 Palliative and End of Life Care

Hip fractures can herald decline in function and independence and may indicate the beginning of the end of life. Such decline leads to a variety of experiences and symptoms that increase patient need for carefully planned sensitive nursing care. Palliative care is defined by the World Health Organization [36] as: "an approach that improves the quality of life of patients and their families facing the problems associated with life-threatening illness, through the prevention and relief of suffering by means of early identification and impeccable assessment and treatment of pain and other problems, physical, psychosocial and spiritual". This approach should be available for people who are struggling to recover from a hip fracture whether they are likely to be at the end of their lives or require intensive support for management of symptoms and experiences when outcomes from the acute care episode are poor.

The fundamental aims of palliative care include [36]:

- Providing adequate pain relief and minimising discomfort by providing symptom relief.
- Affirming life and regarding dying as a normal process.
- Intending neither to hasten nor postpone death.
- Integrating the psychological and spiritual aspects of patient care.
- Offering a support system to help patients live as actively as possible until death.
- Offering to provide a system of support to help the family cope during the patient's illness and death and in their own bereavement.
- Working collaboratively as a team to address the needs of patients and their families, including bereavement counselling, if indicated.
- Enhancing quality of life and positively influencing the course of illness.
- Applicable early in the course of illness, in conjunction with other therapies that are intended to prolong life, such as chemotherapy or radiation therapy, and includes those investigations needed to better understand and manage distressing clinical complications.

This philosophy allows for physical, psychological, social and emotional care for patients and their families when the patient does not have the physical resilience to fully recover from/survive the trauma of the injury. Typically, palliative care is provided by an MDT who focuses on the assessment and treatment of pain and other symptoms whilst ensuring that care is enhanced by patient-centred communication and decision-making across the continuum of care settings, from hospital to home.

Identifying patients for whom a palliative care approach is most appropriate is difficult and is influenced by cultural issues. Nurses play a key role in helping the patient throughout this process. Following hip fracture, patients may have multiple co-morbidities that can additionally limit life, but most recover well from surgery and have good functional outcomes and subsequent quality of life. Appropriate models of end of life care are currently a matter of considerable discussion and debate. Palliative care has not previously been a natural consideration in orthopaedic care, so this is a matter for continuing debate and discussion rather than something that is currently integrated into practice [13].

The patient and family must be included in making decisions that ensure ongoing care and treatment is appropriate to the patient's needs. Good nursing care for those at the end of their life should include physical, emotional and psychological aspects of care along with spiritual support [37]. The process of dying creates multiple emotions and feelings for all involved: the patient, family, carers and the care providers [36]. It is the responsibility of the MDT, through good communication with patients and families, to identify those who were frail pre-fracture and for whom the fall, fracture, surgery and hospitalisation experience may lead to the "winding down" of the body at the end of life.

17.6   Secondary Prevention, Health Improvement and Health Promotion

The nursing team are in an ideal position to recognise and act on the need for bone health assessment and identification of those whose fracture requires investigation for osteoporosis (see Chap. 14) as they have the most sustained contact with patients. This, however, is not a simple process since most patients will be unaware of the influence of bone health on their current fracture. Early in the care trajectory it may be a shock to them that the cause of the fracture may be fragile bone due to osteoporosis. While there is, therefore, an opportunity for nurses in any care setting to instigate bone health assessment referral, this needs to be discussed in a sensitive manner with patients and carers. Nurses need to be able to discuss the reasons for referral for bone health assessment with patients as soon as possible after the fracture has occurred so that patients and their families can be prepared for the next steps. Conversations that introduce the topic of bone health and osteoporosis can be conducted during normal nursing care activities in a manner which enables patients to gradually acknowledge the need for them to consider their bone health. To do this, nurses working in acute settings need to have enough understanding of the processes involved in bone health assessment and the treatment of osteoporosis so that they can effectively educate and counsel patients and their families.

17.7   Nursing Resources, Education and Leadership

There is a global shortage of nurses owing to changing demographics, political ideologies and financial austerity and recruitment and retention problems. The availability of appropriately educated and skilled nurses to provide both fundamental and specialist care is a major concern. A large international study [38] demonstrated that an increase in a nurses' workload by one patient, from eight to nine patients per qualified nurse, increased the likelihood of an inpatient dying within 30 days of admission by 7%. Under-resourcing nursing teams leads to insufficient capacity for the team to undertake actions to prevent morbidity and mortality. Studies have indicated that this "missed care" is associated with one or more adverse patient outcomes including; medication errors, urinary-tract infections, falls, pressure injuries, critical incidents, quality of care and patient readmissions. The quality of studies relating to missed care is, however, weak and the link between missed care and mortality is yet to be explored in more robust research [19]. Most of the research has, however, considered high resource settings, while in lower resource settings the impact of limited resources on patients and communities has yet to be explored. In many settings the number of qualified nurses is severely limited and skills development focuses on nursing assistants and other team members.

Unless the nursing resource is protected and grows, the added nursing value needed to continue to improve outcomes and the quality of care for patients with fragility fractures globally will not happen. Sahota and Currie [39] pointed out that: "...looking after hip fracture patients well is a lot cheaper than looking after them badly", the nursing resource is significant in this, meaning that it is important for the multidisciplinary community, through organisations such as the Fragility Fracture Network (FFN), to lobby governments and health and social care providers of to ensure that nurses are able to do undertake their role effectively, aligning the profession to the fourth pillar in the FFN call to action [1].

Nurses work in a professional culture of constant skills and knowledge development through learning and reflection. Many nurses working in orthogeriatric settings, however, are more likely to have been educated solely in the care of adults with musculoskeletal problems rather than to meet the complex needs of older people. Multiple "orthogeriatric" specialist skills that combine orthopaedic care expertise with the care of older people are needed that are based on an in-depth knowledge of the theory underpinning care. Few nurses working with patients with fragility fractures have undertaken education beyond that of their initial nursing qualification and they rely on knowledge and skills developed through generic, rather than specialist, education. This education and skills gap can result in care which does not meet all needs. Specialist orthogeriatric nursing education could have a positive impact on patient outcomes [19]. Many nurses working in orthogeriatric settings are better prepared educationally for the care of adults with musculoskeletal problems than to meet the complex needs of older people. Multiple specialist "orthogeriatric" nursing skills are needed as well as fundamental adult nursing skills. Specialist nursing qualifications in orthogeriatric care do not currently exist, so nurses are obliged to be reflective self-led learners who are able to extend their own knowledge of both caring for patients following trauma and the complex care of older people together through reflection.

Multidisciplinary orthogeriatric care can be fragmented and less effective if it is not managed or coordinated effectively; nurses' 24-h presence and detailed knowledge of patient pathways make them ideal care co-ordinators. The complex nursing care requirements of orthogeriatric patients mean that they should have their care led by those who are experts in the field with an intuitive understanding of need. In some settings care and its coordination are led by a specialist nurse or coordinator such as a hip fracture nurse specialist, elderly/elder care nurse specialist, trauma nurse coordinator, nurse practitioner or advanced nurse practitioner. In some countries, multidisciplinary collaborative working has supported the development of advanced nursing roles often operationalised as clinical nurse specialists, nurse practitioners or physicians' assistants who have a variety of skills that are complementary to the MDT and enhance patient care. Care should be supervised and managed by those who have enhanced experience, skills and knowledge in working with older people following fracture so that they perceive care needs holistically and from individual perspectives.

References

1. Fragility Fracture Network (2018) Global call to action on fragility fractures. https://www. fragilityfracturenetwork.org/cta/
2. International Council of Nurses (ICN) (2010) Definition of nursing. Geneva: ICN. http://www. icn.ch/who-we-are/icn-definition-of-nursing/. Accessed 6 May 2016
3. Ziden L, Scherman H, Wenestam MH, C-G. (2010) The break remains—elderly people's experiences of a hip fracture 1 year after discharge. Disabil Rehabil 32(2):103–113
4. Kondo A, Sada K, Ito Y, Yamaguchi C et al (2014) Difficulties in life after hip fracture and expected hospital supports for patients and families. Int J OrthopTrauma Nurs 18(4):191–204
5. MacDonald V, Butler Maher A, Mainz H et al (2018) Developing and testing an international audit of quality indicators for older adults with fragility hip fracture. Orthop Nurs 37(2):115–121
6. Pitzul K, Munce S, Perrier L et al (2017) Scoping review of potential quality indicators for hip fracture patient care. BMJ Open 7:e014769. https://doi.org/10.1136/bmjopen-2016-014769
7. Heslop L, Liu S (2014) Nursing-sensitive indicators: a concept analysis. J Adv Nurs 70(11):2469–2482. http://www.ncbi.nlm.nih.gov/pmc/articles/PMC4232854/. Accessed 6 May 2016
8. Meehan AJ, Hommel A, Hertz K et al (2016) Care of the older adult with fragility hip fracture. In: Boltz M, Capezuti E, Fulmer T, Zwicker D (eds) Evidence-based geriatric nursing protocols for best practice. Springer, New York
9. Meehan A, Maher A, Brent L et al (2019) The International Collaboration of Orthopaedic Nursing (ICON): best practice nursing care standards for older adults with fragility hip fracture. Int J Orthop Trauma Nurs 32:3–26
10. Geszar B et al (2017) Hip fracture; an interruption that has consequences four months later. A qualitative study. Int J Orthop Trauma Nurs 26:43–48

11. Jensen CM, Hertz K, Mauthner O (2018) Orthogeriatric nursing in the emergency and peri-operative in-patient setting. In: Hertz K, Santy-Tomlinson J (eds) Fragility fracture nursing. Springer, Cham, pp 53–65
12. Weissenberger-Leduc M, Zmaritz M (2013) Nursing care for the elderly with hip fracture in an acute care hospital. Wien Med Wochenschr 163(19–20):468–475
13. Hertz K, Santy-Tomlinson J (2014) Fractures in the older person. In: Clarke S, Santy-Tomlinson J (eds) Orthopaedic and trauma nursing: an evidence-based approach to musculoskeletal care. Wiley Blackwell, Oxford, pp 236–250
14. Manning E, Gagnon M (2017) The complex patient: a concept definition. Nurs Health Sci 19:13–21
15. Rankin J, Regan S (2004) Complex needs: the future of social care. Institute for Public Policy Research/Turning Point, London. http://www.ippr.org/files/images/media/files/publication/2011/05/Meeting_Complex_Needs_full_1301.pdf?noredirect=1. Accessed 6 May 2016
16. Hertz K, Santy-Tomlinson J (2017) The nursing role. In: Falaschi P, Marsh D (eds) Orthogeriatrics. Springer, Cham, pp 131–144
17. Marques A, Queiros C (2018) Frailty, sarcopenia and falls. In: Hertz K, Santy-Tomlinson J (eds) Fragility fracture nursing. Springer, Cham, pp 15–26
18. Morley J, Vellas B, van Kan G, Anker S et al (2013) Frailty consensus: a call to action. J Am Med Dir Assoc 14(6):392–397
19. Brent L, Hommel A, Maher AB, Hertz K, Meehan AJ, Santy-Tomlinson J (2018) Nursing care of fragility fracture patients. Injury 49(8):1409–1412
20. Maxwell C, Wang J (2017) Understanding frailty: a nurse's guide. Nurs Clin N Am 52:349–361
21. Bjorkelund KB, Hommel A, Thorngren KG et al (2011) The influence of perioperative care and treatment on the 4-month outcome in elderly patients with hip fracture. AANA J 79(1):51–61
22. Alzheimer's Society (UK) (2010) This is me. London Alzheimer's Society/Royal College of Nursing. https://www.alzheimers.org.uk/site/scripts/download_info.php?downloadID=399. Accessed 6 May 2016
23. Obideyi A, Srikantharajah I, Grigg L, Randall A (2008) Nurse administered fascia iliaca compartment block for pre-operative pain relief in adult fractured neck of femur. Acute Pain 10(3–4):145–149
24. Cross J (2018) Nursing the patient with altered cognitive function. In: Hertz K, Santy-Tomlinson J (eds) Fragility fracture nursing. Springer, Cham, pp 109–124
25. NICE (National Institute for Health and Care Excellence) (2014) Delirium (QS63). www.nice.org.uk/guidance/qs63. Accessed 6 May 2016
26. NPIAP-EPUAP-PPPIA (National Pressure Injury Advisory Panel/European Pressure Ulcer Advisory Panel/Pan Pacific Pressure Injury Alliance) (2019) Prevention and Treatment of Pressure Ulcers/Injuries: Quick Reference Guide. 3rd Edition file:///C:/Users/tomli/Downloads/ggg-quick-reference-guide-version29dec2019-secured.pdf
27. Hommel A, Bjorkelund KB, Thorngren K-G, Ulander K (2007) A study of a pathway to reduce pressure ulcers in patients with a hip fracture. J Orthop Nurs 11(3–4):151–159
28. NICE (National Institute for Health and Care Excellence) (2014) Acute kidney injury: Quality standard www.nice.org.uk/guidance/qs76
29. Wellington B, Flynn S, Duperouzel W (2015) Anti-embolic stockings for the prevention of VTE in orthopaedic patients: a practice update. Int J Orthop Trauma Nurs 19(1):45–49
30. Dyer S et al (2017) Rehabilitation following hip fracture. In: Falaschi P, Marsh D (eds) Orthogeriatrics. Springer, Cham, pp 145–163
31. Barberi S, Mielli L (2018) Rehabilitation and discharge. In: Hertz K, Santy-Tomlinson J (eds) Fragility fracture nursing. Springer, Cham, pp 125–113
32. Brent L, Coffrey A (2013) Patient's perceptions of their readiness for discharge following hip fracture surgery. Int J Orthop Trauma Nurs 17:190–198
33. Jensen CM, Overgaard S, Wiil UK, Clemensen J (2019) Can tele-health support self-care and empowerment? A qualitative study of hip fracture patients' experiences with testing an "App". SAGE Open Nurs 5:1–11

34. Pearlin LI, Mullan JT, Semple SJ, Skaff MM (1990) Caregiving and the stress process: an overview of concepts and their measures. Gerontologist 30(5):583–594
35. Falaschi P, Eleuteri S (2017) The psychological health of patients and their caregivers. In: Falaschi P, Marsh D (eds) Orthogeriatrics. Springer, Cham, pp 201–211
36. World Health Organization (2014) Global atlas of palliative care at the end of life. www.who.int/nmh/Global_Atlas_of_Palliative_Care.pdf
37. Brent L, Santy-Tomlinson J, Hertz K (2018) Family partnerships, palliative care and end of life. In: Hertz K, Santy-Tomlinson J (eds) Fragility fracture nursing. Springer, Cham, pp 137–146
38. Aiken L, Sloane D, Bryneel L, Van den Heede K et al (2014) Nurse staffing and education and hospital mortality in nine European countries: a retrospective observational study. Lancet 383(993):1824–1830
39. Sahota O, Currie C (2008) Hip fracture care: all change. Editorial. Age Ageing 37:128–129

Nutritional Care of the Older Patient with Fragility Fracture: Opportunities for Systematised, Interdisciplinary Approaches Across Acute Care, Rehabilitation and Secondary Prevention Settings

18

Jack J. Bell, Ólöf Guðný Geirsdóttir, Karen Hertz,
Julie Santy-Tomlinson, Sigrún Sunna Skúladóttir,
Stefano Eleuteri, and Antony Johansen

This chapter is a component of Part 5: Cross-cutting Issues.
For an explanation of the grouping of chapters in this book, please see Chapter 1: 'The multidisciplinary approach to fragility fractures around the world—an overview'.

J. J. Bell (✉)
The Prince Charles Hospital and School of Human Movement and Nutrition Sciences,
University of Queensland, St Lucia, QLD, Australia
e-mail: Jack.Bell@health.qld.gov.au

Ó. G. Geirsdóttir · S. S. Skúladóttir
Faculty of Food Science and Nutrition, School of Health, University of Iceland,
Reykjavík, Iceland
e-mail: ogg@hi.is

K. Hertz
Royal Stoke University Hospital, Stoke-on-Trent, UK
e-mail: karen.hertz@uhns.nhs.uk

J. Santy-Tomlinson
Orthopaedic Nursing, Odense University Hospitals/University of Southern Denmark,
Odense, Denmark
e-mail: juliesanty@tomlinson15.karoo.co.uk

S. Eleuteri
Department of Psychology, Sapienza University of Rome A, Rome, Italy
e-mail: stefano.eleuteri@uniroma1.it

A. Johansen
Trauma Unit, University Hospital of Wales, Cardiff, UK

National Hip Fracture Database, Royal College of Physicians, London, UK
e-mail: antony.johansen@wales.nhs.uk

P. Falaschi, D. Marsh (eds.), *Orthogeriatrics*, Practical Issues in Geriatrics,
https://doi.org/10.1007/978-3-030-48126-1_18

18.1   Background

Increasing numbers of fragility fractures in ageing populations represent a substantial and significant pressure on patients, carers, healthcare systems and societies around the world [1]. Frail older people with fragility fractures require comprehensive, orthogeriatric care [2]. Co-existing chronic diseases confound acute interventions and efforts to improve recovery in rehabilitation, and have a negative impact on patient outcomes, long-term survival and quality of life.

An interdisciplinary approach to the management of the presenting fracture and pre-existing co-morbidities will improve outcomes. Preventing future fractures and additional harmful diagnoses should also be a priority for treating teams in the acute, rehabilitation and secondary prevention settings [1]. Individualised care is a core component of orthogeriatric care. However, this must be underpinned by interdisciplinary actions and systems that support timely and appropriate delivery of care.

Nutrition-related diagnoses are key predictors of initial and secondary fragility fractures and are among the most harmful co-morbidities in older orthopaedic patients across acute, rehabilitation and community settings. Nutrition interventions are core components of primary and secondary fracture prevention and have been shown to improve outcomes in the acute and rehabilitation settings.

Many models of nutrition care focus on highly individualised assessments and interventions provided by dietitians or medical nutrition specialists [3]. The high prevalence of protein–energy malnutrition and other nutrition-related diagnoses is well described across many orthogeriatric settings, and there are strong associations between nutrition-related diagnoses and patient and healthcare outcomes. Despite this, in many orthopaedic settings timely access to specialist clinical nutrition care is limited or absent [4]. Increases in diagnosis and referral rates, patient complexity, healthcare costs and service demands, combined with reduced lengths of stay and unsustainable health expenditure growth, suggest that it will not be possible to provide all patients identified at risk of a nutrition-related diagnosis with individual access to specialist nutrition services [3]. This chapter therefore presents a call to action. Systematised, interdisciplinary nutrition care actions are urgently required across the pillars of acute care, rehabilitation and secondary fracture prevention [1].

18.2   SIMPLE or Specialised Nutrition Care?

Models in which interdisciplinary healthcare workers provide early, supportive nutrition care across the three pillars may be best placed to deliver high value nutrition support. Such models include the Systematised, Interdisciplinary Malnutrition Program for impLementation and Evaluation (SIMPLE), the More-2-Eat program and a multidisciplinary, multimodal nutrition care model applied in hip fracture by Bell et al. [3, 5, 6]. These models suggest that patients are triaged into three groups: those not at risk and appropriate for standard care, those who are at risk or malnourished but do not require specialised nutrition care and those who are likely to benefit from a nutrition care specialist.

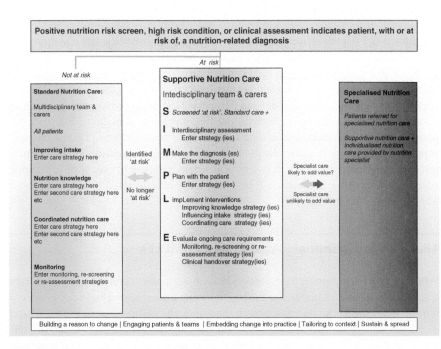

Fig. 18.1 Nutritional care of the older patient with fragility fracture

These models have focused on implementing nutrition care in the acute setting for patients with, or at risk of, protein–energy malnutrition. This has included the use of action reflection cycles to collect relevant data justifying change, then progressively developing, implementing, evaluating and iteratively improving chosen nutrition care activities [7, 8].

Figure 18.1 provides a SIMPLE illustration of how to support nutrition care of the older patient with fragility fracture. This is considerate of key nutrition care models internationally [3, 5, 9–11], and supports different members of orthogeriatric teams to contribute to systematised, interdisciplinary nutrition care for patients with, or at risk of a nutrition-related diagnosis, globally.

Specific strategies have not been identified, so that local teams can tailor the approach across a variety of nutrition-related diagnoses, frameworks and contexts. Systematised and interdisciplinary care nutrition actions are encouraged, but local processes should still inform referral for specialist nutrition advice when this is likely to add value. Conversely, if referral is unlikely to add value, for example when ongoing specialist intervention is unlikely to add benefit or improve what matters to the patient, supportive nutrition care should be the priority [12, 13].

The underlying themes along the bottom of the model highlight that successful and sustained nutrition care requires the engagement of local patients and teams using a knowledge translation approach; a 'cut and paste' approach to process changes will not yield the same outcomes [7, 11, 14].

18.3 Screening for Nutrition Risk (SIMPLE)

Nutritional risk increases substantially with age, multimorbidity and fragility fracture, and screening and/or assessment should be routine across orthopaedic settings. A two-step approach, with 'first pass' nutrition screening, followed by a detailed assessment by a qualified health professional, is often applied as an efficient approach to making a nutrition-related diagnosis [15]. In high-risk settings, such as acute hip fracture units (with a high proportion of patients at malnutrition risk), the poor sensitivity of common screening tools and the need for prompt nutrition care, support proceeding straight to detailed assessment and intervention [15]. Nutrition screening to identify patients at risk of a nutrition deficiency, excess or imbalance state should be quick and easy and designed to be administered by diverse people with limited or no training [16].

18.4 Interdisciplinary Assessment (S/MPLE)

Where patients are identified at nutrition risk, appropriately trained interdisciplinary team members should undertake further nutrition assessment. The lack of distinction between screening and assessment measures, the diversity of nutrition-related diagnoses and factors contributing to their development and the presence of confounding co-morbid conditions have resulted in the absence of any gold standards for nutrition screening or diagnosis [17–19]. Not surprisingly, a range of nutrition screening and assessment tools have been applied or recommended in orthogeriatric settings; Table 18.1 applies an ABCDEF anagram to highlight nutrition assessment measures, screening tools and malnutrition diagnostic criteria commonly reported, observed, applied or recommended for use in orthogeriatric settings [4, 10, 15–38] (Table 18.1). Local treating teams should select measures, tools and diagnostic criteria that have proven concurrent and predictive validity in the population in which they are to be applied, and that are feasible for local implementation [19, 21, 39, 40].

The ease of retrospective access and cut-off measures have led to the continued practice of using single-point nutrition outcomes measures, such as BMI or albumin, in clinical and research settings [17, 22]. Single measures may be appropriate for some specific nutrition-related diagnoses, for example some vitamin deficiency states. However, applying single measures for the definition of protein–energy malnutrition should probably be avoided. Protein–energy malnutrition has traditionally been assumed to apply to 'stick thin' patients with low BMIs. However, there is now a clear imperative to screen for malnutrition in overweight and obese as well as underweight older people [41]. Protein–energy malnutrition is evident across BMI ranges and the risks of increased morbidity and mortality associated with rapid loss of muscle mass are now becoming recognised across under-, overweight and obese BMI categories [42, 43]. Serum albumin and other markers of visceral protein status are also not reliable as a standalone malnutrition markers in acutely unwell orthogeriatric populations [18, 44]. Inflammation is today considered the major reason for

Table 18.1 Nutrition assessment measures, screening tools and malnutrition diagnostic criteria commonly applied or recommended for use in orthogeriatric settings

Nutrition assessment measures	
A: Anthropometry and body composition	*D: Dietary intake assessment*
Weight/weight changes	Food history
Height	24 h recall
BMI	Food records
Circumference measures	Diets and dietary restrictions e.g.: Special diet I Poor diet I Monotonous diet
Skinfold measures	*E: Environmental and psycho-social assessment*
Bioelectrical impedance analysis (BIA)	Social status, i.e. poverty, low education
Dual-energy X-ray absorptiometry (DXA)	Living alone
	Functional status
B: Biochemical measurement	Depression
Albumin	Declined cognitive function
Prealbumin	*F: Functional measures*
Insulin-like growth factor-1	Walking test for distance or time
Retinol binding protein	Grip strength
Transferrin	Delayed cutaneous hypersensitivity
Glucose/HBA1C	Total lymphocyte count
Liver function tests	*Other:*
Renal function tests	Sarcopaenia consensus criteria
Electrolytes	Frailty scores
C: Clinical history	
Physiological contributors to wasting	
Physiological contributors to cachexia	
e.g. COPD, heart failure, some cancers	
Screening tools for protein-energy malnutrition	
Mini Nutrition Assessment [23]	Mini Nutrition Assessment- Short Form [27]
Malnutrition screening tool [24]	Malnutrition Universal Screening Tool [10]
Nutrition Risk Screening 2002 [25]	Prognostic nutrition index [28]
Rainey-MacDonald Nutrition Index [26]	Simplified Nutrition Appetite Questionnaire [29]
Criteria for protein-energy malnutrition diagnosis	
ASPEN/Academy Criteria (2012) [30]	GLIM criteria [33]
ESPEN criteria (2015) [31]	ICD 10 criteria [34]
Mini Nutrition Assessment [23]	Mini Nutrition Assessment- Short Form [27]
Subjective Global Assessment [32]	

reduced serum levels of visceral proteins, and inflammation due to disease or ageing is well recognised as a contributor to the development of malnutrition [44]. Inflammation is also a predictor of sepsis, longer hospital stay and readmission and mortality, so it is not surprising that studies report associations between low visceral proteins and poor patient and healthcare outcomes.

Differences in study designs, populations, evidence-based outcomes, guidelines and consensus recommendations preclude making specific macro- or micronutrient recommendations. Consequently, local teams should consider latest evidence and relevant national or international recommendations for macro- and micronutrients. As a start point, ageing-related inefficiencies in absorption and utilisation suggest considering an energy intake target of 30 kcal/kg bodyweight daily in older patients, and at least 1 g/kg protein with individual adjustment for nutritional status, physical activity level, disease status and tolerance [45, 46].

Dehydration should also be closely monitored as this can be causative for fracture incidence and a substantial and significant contributor to subsequent harm [47]. Unless a clinical comorbidity requires a different approach consensus daily recommendations suggest 1.6 L for women and 2.0 L for men with normal physical activity in a moderate climate [46, 48].

In summary, in many settings, a positive nutrition risk screen simply informs a referral for a thorough assessment and diagnosis by an appropriately trained nutrition care specialist, prior to commencing nutrition care interventions. A SIMPLE alternative is recommended; orthogeriatric teams need to action opportunities for systematised nutrition care from the point of risk identification. These may consider opportunities for timely nutrition diagnoses, goal setting, interventions and evaluation processes.

18.5   Make the Diagnosis/(es) (SIMPLE)

A broad array of nutrition-related diagnoses are observed across orthogeriatric settings and can result from deficiency, excess or imbalance states that lead to adverse effects on body form, function, clinical outcomes, healthcare systems and community costs (Table 18.2) [34].

Cachexia, sarcopaenia, frailty and osteoporosis are of particular interest, given their prevalence trajectories and likely impact on outcomes globally. Concurrent diagnoses, for example of obesity and malnutrition, are also worthy of special attention. The most outstanding single diagnosis in terms of reported prevalence, incidence and harm imposed on patient and healthcare systems is protein–energy malnutrition. In many settings globally, the skeleton continues to hide in the hospital closet; undervalued, under-recognised, and consequently, undertreated [49, 50].

Protein–energy malnutrition (malnutrition) is an ICD-coded condition that can be treated using medical nutrition therapy [34]. Its prevalence varies across orthogeriatric settings, reflecting differences in screening and diagnostic tools, as well as real differences in the populations observed. Estimates suggest that less than 1 in 3 non-complex elective orthogeriatric inpatients are at risk of malnutrition, whilst up to two-thirds of hip fracture patients will have a diagnosis of protein–energy malnutrition by the time they are discharged from acute or rehabilitation care settings [36, 50]. Although differences in design and tools again make comparisons difficult, the reported prevalence appears higher in studies from low- and middle-income counties than in high-income countries [51, 52].

Table 18.2 Common nutrition-related diagnoses observed or reported within and across global orthogeriatric settings—with ICD-10 Diagnostic Code [34]

Undernutrition
- Protein–energy malnutrition—serve E43/moderate E44/unspecified E46
- Starvation related underweight—E43
- Anorexia of ageing—R63.0
- Wasting—M62.5
- Cachexia/disease-related malnutrition—R64
- Nutritional marasmus—E41
- Sarcopenia—M62.84
- Frailty—R54
- Dehydration—E86.0

Micronutrient deficiency -E56.9
- Vitamin D deficiency—E55
- Vitamin B12 deficiency—E53.8/intrinsic factor deficiency D51.0
- Iron deficiency—E61.1/anaemia D50

Overnutrition
- Overweight—E66.3
- Obesity—E66.9
- Fatty liver disease/non-alcoholic steatohepatitis—K76.0
- Excessive alcohol intake—F10.99

Nutrition imbalance states/metabolic disorders/autoimmune
- Osteopenia—M85.80
- Osteoporosis—M81.0/with fracture M80.0
- Diabetes mellitus—DM1 E10/DM2 E11
- Acute kidney injury—Unspecified N17.9
- Chronic kidney disease—Unspecified N18.9
- Irritable bowel syndrome—K58
- Refeeding syndrome—Endocrine, nutritional and metabolic disease E00-E89/disorder of electrolyte and fluid balance E87. 8

Protein–energy malnutrition is recognised as the most costly comorbidity in hip fracture, the one most likely to increase length of stay and a strong independent predictor of post discharge mortality [53, 54]. Table 18.3 highlights associations between protein–energy malnutrition and outcomes observed across orthopaedic specified studies and those including older, multimorbid populations including those with fragility fractures [18, 54–63].

Recent updates to key orthogeriatric evidence-based recommendations, guidelines and registry datasets suggest positive, albeit belated, recognition of the need for timely identification, treatment and monitoring of nutrition care across the acute, rehabilitation and secondary prevention orthogeriatric settings globally.

A thorough assessment will also identify the aetiology, or root cause, of the nutrition-related diagnosis or diagnoses being assessed [9]. A comprehensive list of all potential aetiologies observed in orthogeriatric settings is beyond the remit of this chapter, however, Table 18.4 provides some potential starting points for consideration [17, 37, 50].

Efforts to identify a primary aetiology for a nutrition-related diagnosis in older, multimorbid inpatients are difficult, and perhaps over-simplistic [64]. For example, protein–energy malnutrition may be attributable to wasting, cachexia or a combination

Table 18.3 Association between protein-energy malnutrition and outcomes in orthogeriatric settings

Affected	Outcome
Patient	Altered body composition /sarcopaenia
	Reduced mobility/frailty/falls
	Post-operative complications
	Increased infection risk
	Pressure injuries
	Wound complications
	Functional impairment/apaty
	Psychological effects/tendency to depression, anxiety, impaired social function
	Delirium
	Reduced quality of life
	Unfavourable discharge destination
	Life expectancy
Healthcare system	Increased hospital-acquired complications
	Infections/wound dehiscence
	Pressure injuries
	Harmful falls
	Delirium
	Increased length of stay
	Increased healthcare costs
	Unfavourable discharge
	Unplanned hospital readmissions
	Increased requirements for rehabilitation
	Increased requirements for long term care
Society	Increased caregiver burden
	Increased societal healthcare costs

of these [30]. This is further confounded by the complex relationships and substantial overlap in variables applied for the purposes of screening and diagnosing protein–energy malnutrition, wasting, cachexia, sarcopaenia, frailty, osteoporosis and other nutrition-related diagnoses [65]. It is therefore unsurprising that malnutrition is considered a 'wicked' problem [66, 67] (Table 18.5). A pragmatic approach would consider whether administration of nutritional intervention is likely to improve outcomes; if so then the aetiology is likely to include a nutritional component and locally tailored nutrition interventions should be provided.

Once diagnoses and aetiologies have been articulated, these should be documented in the appropriate care record. Proper documentation is critical to providing quality standard care, communication with other professions and recording diagnosis that can have effects on other medical diagnosis or treatment [68]. Documentation also supports service planning and review processes, and in many settings also influences resource allocation.

Multidisciplinary clinicians should ensure that patients are aware of positive nutrition risk screens. Open and honest discussion about consequent nutrition-related diagnoses and a shared decision-making approach to treatment (and no treatment) options should be considered within a sensitive approach that allows patients or carers to control the amount of information they receive [46, 69].

Table 18.6 (continued)

Education	• Dietary counselling • Inclusion of nutrition curriculum in interdisciplinary training and education • Informed consent discussions • Mobile Health (mHealth) applications nutrition component in ward rounds, huddles, case conferences, interdisciplinary care planning meetings	• Nutrition-related diagnosis and education provided to patients, caregivers and health professionals • Nutrition specialist representation in advocacy and governance roles • Quality improvement, research and development shared goal setting and treatment planning • Standards, policies, guidelines • Traditional and social media marketing
Psychosocial	• Group interventions • Shared mealtimes/dining rooms • Social support networks	• Wellness/lifestyle/mindfulness/cognitive behaviour therapy programs
Monitoring	• Audits (nutrition care included in orthogeriatric audits; nutrition-specific audits/sprints) Anthropometric monitoring • Biochemistry/pathology/vitamin/mineral assays • Food intake monitoring • Nutrition re-screening	• Nutrition re-assessments • Patient-reported experience and outcomes measures (PROMS/PREMS) • Physical and functional re-assessment
Clinical handover/care across the continuum	• Discharge summaries/clinical handover documents • mHealth apps • Nutrition specific fields in eHealth records and systems	• Referrals for ongoing care • Self-management processes

18.7.3 Interventions Leading to Coordinated Nutrition Care Across Disciplines and Settings

It is well recognised that dietitians, nutritionists and medical nutrition specialists are experts in nutrition care. However, in many settings, access to nutrition care experts is limited outside of acute care facilities or tertiary rehabilitation settings. In some healthcare settings, dietitians and medical nutrition specialists may be best placed to coordinate nutrition care across disciplines and settings, but this may not always be an option. Appropriately educated patients and their family, friends and social networks are also often ideally placed to provide supportive nutrition care.

Of focus though are the many interdisciplinary healthcare workers that orthogeriatric patients interface with across the three pillars of orthogeriatric care who may be able to provide supportive nutrition care processes. Where available, dietetic (or nutrition) assistants are particularly well best placed; but dietetic assistants are also not available in many settings even though they have been shown to reduce mortality in hip fracture [87].

As described in Chap. 17, the best-placed profession to oversee, lead and implement interventions to coordinate nutrition care is therefore nursing. Nurses are usually the main professional group providing care to patients and the best-placed professional group to coordinate systematised or interdisciplinary nutrition care processes where specialist care is not available or is unlikely to add benefit. Nurses also have the most significant amounts of repeat-contact with patients and carers in different settings, whether over the full 24-h period in acute and rehabilitation settings, or in other situations such as secondary prevention settings and home care.

Nurses also witness patients' eating and drinking activities, have a strong understanding of barriers and enablers to nutrition intake, and are likely to be best placed to understand where the patient 'fits' within a social–ecological setting. This makes them ideal coordinators and champions of nutritional aspects of care. Nurses are often in the best position to conduct primary nutritional screening and assessment that identifies those in need of nutritional support to be provided solely by nurses or in collaboration with other members of the orthogeriatric team, or specialist care where accessible and likely to add benefit. In settings where dietitian, nutritionist or medical nutrition specialist resources are limited, nurses can provide excellent nutritional care to most patients whilst allowing nutrition specialists to focus on the most in need of their expertise.

Most, if not all of the strategies listed in Table 18.6 are considered to sit squarely in remit of nursing-led essential care [88]. Although it is difficult to identify an evidence base for such fundamental aspects of nursing care, such nurse-led interventions are likely to have a positive impact on nutritional status [89]. These fundamental aspects of nursing care are the responsibility of the whole nursing team, but require co-ordination and leadership so that they are a priority. In many settings, nursing professionals are well placed to guide allocation of resources, alterations to institutional structures and organisational process reform.

A call to action is therefore made to global and local nursing leadership to engage patients, interdisciplinary teams and broad stakeholders to deliver high-value nutrition care across the three pillars of orthogeriatrics.

18.8 Evaluating Ongoing Care Requirements (SIMPLE)

Patients with or at risk of a nutrition-related diagnosis will routinely require nutrition monitoring or re-assessment strategies. Processes for re-screening should also be considered for those not currently at risk. What needs to be monitored, how often, and by whom will depend on many factors, perhaps most notably the nutrition diagnosis in question, and resource constraints. This makes it challenging to provide definitive recommendations for clinical handover across the care pathway.

Local treating teams need to work with patients to identify the best opportunities for ongoing nutritional monitoring and evaluation. Discussions may consider the availability of access to specialist nutrition outpatient or community services and the potential benefits, costs and opportunity costs of these. Other alternatives for consideration could include general practitioners, nurse practitioners, mHealth programs, group programs or self-monitoring.

Finally, clinical audits of care delivery positively influence patient and healthcare outcomes. Table 18.7 provides a summative recap of potential opportunities for

Table 18.7 Evaluating nutritional care of the older patient with fragility fracture

	Nutrition care opportunity	Audit opportunity
S	Screen for nutrition risk	Proportion of patients screened using a valid nutrition screening tool
I	Interdisciplinary assessment	On admission nutrition assessment completed Weight documented within 72 h of admission
M	Make diagnosis (es)	Proportion of patients with a documented nutrition diagnosis using a tool with adequate concurrent and predictive validity
P	Plan with the patient—Goal setting and informed consent	Documented or patient-reported informed consent discussion regarding diagnosis and treatment plan
L	impLement interventions using systems and teams	Documented or patient-reported provision of: Nutrition education Food intake strategy(ies) Nutrition care plan
E	Evaluate ongoing care options	Nutrition audit report

systematised, interdisciplinary nutrition care approaches across acute care, rehabilitation and secondary prevention orthogeriatric settings, and how these may be evaluated [3].

18.9 Recommended Further Reading

- Bell JJ et al (2018) Rationale and developmental methodology for the SIMPLE approach: a Systematised, Interdisciplinary Malnutrition Pathway for impLementation and Evaluation in hospitals. Nutr Diet 75(2):226–234
- King PC et al (2019) "I wouldn't ever want it": a qualitative evaluation of patient and caregiver perceptions toward enteral tube feeding in hip fracture inpatients. J Parenter Enteral Nutr 43(4):526–533
- Volkert D et al (2019) ESPEN guideline on clinical nutrition and hydration in geriatrics. Clin Nutr 38(1):10–47

References

1. Dreinhöfer KE et al (2018) A global call to action to improve the care of people with fragility fractures. Injury 49(8):1393–1397
2. Pioli G, Giusti A, Barone A (2008) Orthogeriatric care for the elderly with hip fractures: where are we? Aging-Clin Exp Res 20(2):113–122
3. Bell JJ et al (2018) Rationale and developmental methodology for the SIMPLE approach: a Systematised, Interdisciplinary Malnutrition Pathway for impLementation and Evaluation in hospitals. Nutr Diet 75(2):226–234
4. Jensen GL et al (2013) Recognizing malnutrition in adults: definitions and characteristics, screening, assessment, and team approach. J Parenter Enter Nutr 37(6):802–807
5. Keller H et al (2018) Update on the Integrated Nutrition Pathway for Acute Care (INPAC): post implementation tailoring and toolkit to support practice improvements. Nutr J 17(1):2
6. Bell JJ et al (2014) Multidisciplinary, multi-modal nutritional care in acute hip fracture inpatients—results of a pragmatic intervention. Clin Nutr 33(6):1101–1107

7. Bell JJ et al (2014) Developing and evaluating interventions that are applicable and relevant to inpatients and those who care for them; a multiphase, pragmatic action research approach. BMC Med Res Methodol 14:98
8. Graham ID et al (2006) Lost in knowledge translation: time for a map? J Contin Educ Heal Prof 26(1):13–24
9. Writing Group of the Nutrition Care Process/Standardized Language Committee (2008) Nutrition care process and model part I: the 2008 update. J Am Diet Assoc 108(7):1113–1117
10. Elia M (2003) Screening for malnutrition: a multidisciplinary responsibility. Development and Use of the Malnutrition Universal Screening Tool (MUST) for Adults, ed. B.A.f.P.a.E. Nutrition. BAPEN, Redditch
11. Laur C et al (2017) Changing nutrition care practices in hospital: a thematic analysis of hospital staff perspectives. BMC Health Serv Res 17(1):498
12. Queensland Clinical Senate (2016) Value-based healthcare—shifting from volume to value. 2016 [cited 2017 September 27]. https://www.health.qld.gov.au/__data/assets/pdf_file/0028/442693/qcs-meeting-report-201603.pdf
13. Palmer S, Raftery J (1999) Opportunity cost. BMJ 318(7197):1551
14. Laur C et al (2018) The Sustain and Spread Framework: strategies for sustaining and spreading nutrition care improvements in acute care based on thematic analysis from the More-2-Eat study (Report). BMC Health Serv Res 18(1):930
15. Bell JJ et al (2014) Quick and easy is not without cost: implications of poorly performing nutrition screening tools in hip fracture. J Am Geriatr Soc 62(2):237–243
16. Bell J et al (2014) Mobilising nutrition diagnoses beyond protein-energy malnutrition in patients with acute hip fracture. Nutr Diet 71(S1):35
17. Bell JJ (2014) Identifying and overcoming barriers to nutrition care in acute hip fracture inpatients, PhD thesis. School of Human Movement and Nutrition Sciences. The University of Queensland
18. Bell JJ et al (2014) Concurrent and predictive evaluation of malnutrition diagnostic measures in hip fracture inpatients: a diagnostic accuracy study. Eur J Clin Nutr 68(3):358–362
19. Elia M, Stratton RJ (2011) Considerations for screening tool selection and role of predictive and concurrent validity. Curr Opin Clin Nutr Metab Care 14(5):425–433
20. Bell JJ et al (2013) Quick and easy in theory but costly in practice? Implications of poorly performing nutrition screening tools in hip fracture. Clin Nutr 32(Suppl 1):s76
21. Marshall WJ (2008) Nutritional assessment: its role in the provision of nutritional support. J Clin Pathol 61(10):1083–1088
22. Bell JJ (2018) Nutrition support in orthopaedics. In: Hickson M, Smith S, editors. Advanced nutrition and dietetics in nutrition support. John Wiley and Sons, Oxford
23. Guigoz Y, Vellas B (1999) The mini nutritional assessment (MNA) for grading the nutritional state of elderly patients: presentation of the MNA, history and validation. Nestle Nutr Workshop Ser Clin Perform Programme 1:3–11; discussion 11–12
24. Ferguson M et al (1999) Development of a valid and reliable malnutrition screening tool for adult acute hospital patients. Nutrition 15(6):458–464
25. Kondrup J et al (2003) Nutritional risk screening (NRS 2002): a new method based on an analysis of controlled clinical trials. Clin Nutr 22(3):321–336
26. Rainey-Macdonald CG et al (1983) Validity of a two-variable nutritional index for use in selecting candidates for nutritional support. J Parenter Enter Nutr 7(1):15–20
27. Kaiser MJ et al (2009) Validation of the Mini Nutritional Assessment short-form (MNA-SF): a practical tool for identification of nutritional status. J Nutr Health Aging 13(9):782–788
28. Buzby GP et al (1980) Prognostic nutritional index in gastrointestinal surgery. Am J Surg 139(1):160–167
29. Kruizenga HM et al (2005) Development and validation of a hospital screening tool for malnutrition: the short nutritional assessment questionnaire (SNAQ). Clin Nutr 24(1):75–82
30. White JV et al (2012) Consensus statement: Academy of Nutrition and Dietetics and American Society for Parenteral and Enteral Nutrition: characteristics recommended for the

identification and documentation of adult malnutrition (undernutrition). J Parenter Enteral Nutr 36(3):275–283

31. Cederholm T et al (2015) Diagnostic criteria for malnutrition—an ESPEN Consensus Statement. Clin Nutr 34(3):335–340
32. Detsky AS et al (1987) What is subjective global assessment of nutritional status? J Parenter Enteral Nutr 11(1):8–13
33. Cederholm T et al (2019) GLIM criteria for the diagnosis of malnutrition - a consensus report from the global clinical nutrition community. Clin Nutr 38(1):1–9
34. World Health Organisation (2010) International Statistical Classification of Diseases and Related Health Problems 10th Revision. https://icd.who.int/browse10/2016/en
35. Stratton RJ, Green CJ, Elia M (2003) Disease-related malnutrition: an evidence-based approach to treatment. CABI Publishing, Wallingford
36. Barker LA, Gout BS, Crowe TC (2011) Hospital malnutrition: prevalence, identification and impact on patients and the healthcare system. Int J Environ Res Public Health 8(2):514–527
37. Bell J (2018) Nutrition screening and assessment in hip fracture. In: Preedy V, Patel VB, editors. Handbook of famine, starvation, and nutrient deprivation: from biology to policy. Springer International Publishing, Cham, pp 1–22
38. NICE (2012) NICE Quality Standard 24: Quality Standard for Nutrition Support in Adults. NICE: UK
39. Bowen DJ et al (2009) How we design feasibility studies. Am J Prev Med 36(5):452–457
40. Proctor E et al (2011) Outcomes for implementation research: conceptual distinctions, measurement challenges, and research agenda. Admin Pol Ment Health 38(2):65–76
41. Ng WL et al (2019) Evaluating the concurrent validity of body mass index (BMI) in the identification of malnutrition in older hospital inpatients. Clin Nutr 38(5):2417–2422
42. Ness SJ et al (2018) The pressures of obesity: the relationship between obesity, malnutrition and pressure injuries in hospital inpatients. Clin Nutr 37(5):1569–1574
43. Soeters PB, Schols AMWJ (2009) Advances in understanding and assessing malnutrition. Curr Opin Clin Nutr Metab Care 12(5):487–494
44. Soeters PB, Wolfe RR, Shenkin A (2019) Hypoalbuminemia: pathogenesis and clinical significance. JPEN J Parenter Enteral Nutr 43(2):181–193
45. Alix E et al (2007) Energy requirements in hospitalized elderly people. J Am Geriatr Soc 55(7):1085–1089
46. Volkert D et al (2019) ESPEN guideline on clinical nutrition and hydration in geriatrics. Clin Nutr 38(1):10–47
47. Renneboog B et al (2006) Mild chronic hyponatremia is associated with falls, unsteadiness, and attention deficits. Am J Med 119(1):71.e1–71.e8
48. EFSA Panel on Dietetic Products, Nutrition and Allergies (2010) Scientific opinion on dietary reference values for water. EFSA J 8(3):1459
49. Butterworth CE (1994) The skeleton in the hospital closet. Nutrition 10(5):435–441; discussion 435, 441
50. Bell JJ et al (2013) Barriers to nutritional intake in patients with acute hip fracture: time to treat malnutrition as a disease and food as a medicine? Can J Physiol Pharmacol 91(6):489–495
51. Margetts BM et al (2003) Prevalence of risk of undernutrition is associated with poor health status in older people in the UK. Eur J Clin Nutr 57(1):69–74
52. Kabir ZN et al (2006) Mini Nutritional Assessment of rural elderly people in Bangladesh: the impact of demographic, socio-economic and health factors. Public Health Nutr 9(8):968–974
53. Nikkel LE et al (2012) Impact of comorbidities on hospitalization costs following hip fracture. J Bone Joint Surg Am 94(1):9–17
54. Bell JJ et al (2016) Impact of malnutrition on 12-month mortality following acute hip fracture. ANZ J Surg 86(3):157–161
55. Diekmann R, Wojzischke J (2018) The role of nutrition in geriatric rehabilitation. Curr Opin Clin Nutr Metab Care 21(1):14–18
56. Tana C et al (2019) Impact of nutritional status on caregiver burden of elderly outpatients. A cross-sectional study. Nutrients 11(2):281

57. Goisser S et al (2015) Malnutrition according to mini nutritional assessment is associated with severe functional impairment in geriatric patients before and up to 6 months after hip fracture. J Am Med Dir Assoc 16(8):661–667

58. Malafarina V et al (2018) Nutritional status and nutritional treatment are related to outcomes and mortality in older adults with hip f555racture. Nutrients 10(5)

59. Mazzola P et al (2017) Association between preoperative malnutrition and postoperative delirium after hip fracture surgery in older adults. J Am Geriatr Soc 65(6):1222–1228

60. Freijer K et al (2013) The economic costs of disease related malnutrition. Clin Nutr 32(1):136–141

61. Curtis LJ et al (2017) Costs of hospital malnutrition. Clin Nutr 36(5):1391–1396

62. Sharma Y et al (2018) Economic evaluation of an extended nutritional intervention in older Australian hospitalized patients: a randomized controlled trial. BMC Geriatr 18(1):41–41

63. Elia M (2015) The cost of malnutrition in England and potential cost savings from nutritional interventions (short version): A report on the cost of disease-related malnutrition in England and a budget impact analysis of implementing the NICE clinical guidelines/quality standard on nutritional support in adults. NHS

64. Writing Group of the Nutrition Care Process/Standardized Language Committee (2008) Nutrition care process part II: using the International Dietetics and Nutrition Terminology to document the nutrition care process. J Am Diet Assoc 108(8):1287–1293

65. Cederholm T et al (2017) ESPEN guidelines on definitions and terminology of clinical nutrition. Clin Nutr 36(1):49–64

66. Rittel HWJ, Webber MM (1973) Dilemmas in a general theory of planning. Policy Sci 4(2):155–169

67. Young AM (2015) Solving the wicked problem of hospital malnutrition. Nutr Diet 72(3):200–204

68. Mathioudakis A et al (2016) How to keep good clinical records. Breathe (Sheffield, England) 12(4):369–373

69. Scott D et al (2016) Health care professionals' experience, understanding and perception of need of advanced cancer patients with cachexia and their families: the benefits of a dedicated clinic. BMC Palliat Care 15(1):100

70. Strebhardt K, Ullrich A (2008) Paul Ehrlich's magic bullet concept: 100 years of progress. Nat Rev Cancer 8(6):473–480

71. Watterson C, Fraser A, Banks M (2009) Evidence based practise guidelines for the nutritional management of malnutrition in adult patients across the continuum of care. Nutr Diet 66:S1–S34

72. National Institute for Health and Clinical Excellence (NICE) (2006) Nutrition support in adults: oral nutrition support, enteral tube feeding and parenteral nutrition (clinical guideline 32)

73. Jensen GL et al (2010) Adult starvation and disease-related malnutrition: a proposal for etiology-based diagnosis in the clinical practice setting from the International Consensus Guideline Committee. J Parenter Enteral Nutr 34(2):156–159

74. Rasmussen HH, Holst M, Kondrup J (2010) Measuring nutritional risk in hospitals. Clin Epidemiol 2:209–216

75. Michie S, van Stralen MM, West R (2011) The behaviour change wheel: a new method for characterising and designing behaviour change interventions. Implement Sci 6:42

76. French SD et al (2012) Developing theory-informed behaviour change interventions to implement evidence into practice: a systematic approach using the Theoretical Domains Framework. Implement Sci 7:38

77. Stevenson J et al (2018) Perspectives of healthcare providers on the nutritional management of patients on haemodialysis in Australia: an interview study. BMJ Open 8(3):e020023

78. Palecek EJ et al (2010) Comfort feeding only: a proposal to bring clarity to decision-making regarding difficulty with eating for persons with advanced dementia. J Am Geriatr Soc 58(3):580–584

79. Druml C et al (2016) ESPEN guideline on ethical aspects of artificial nutrition and hydration. Clin Nutr 35(3):545–556

80. Mon AS, Pulle C, Bell J (2018) Development of an 'enteral tube feeding decision support tool' for hip fracture patients: a modified Delphi approach. Australas J Ageing 37(3):217–223

81. King PC et al (2019) "I wouldn't ever want it": a qualitative evaluation of patient and caregiver perceptions toward enteral tube feeding in hip fracture inpatients. J Parenter Enter Nutr 43(4):526–533

82. Greene GW et al (1999) Dietary applications of the stages of change model. J Am Diet Assoc 99(6):673–678

83. Prochaska JO, Velicer WF (1997) The transtheoretical model of health behavior change. Am J Health Promot 12(1):38–48

84. Wyers CE et al (2018) Efficacy of nutritional intervention in elderly after hip fracture: a multicenter randomized controlled trial. J Gerontol A Biol Sci Med Sci 73(10):1429–1437

85. Golden SD, Earp JA (2012) Social ecological approaches to individuals and their contexts: twenty years of health education & behavior health promotion interventions. Health Educ Behav 39(3):364–372

86. Damschroder LJ et al (2009) Fostering implementation of health services research findings into practice: a consolidated framework for advancing implementation science. Implement Sci 4:50–50

87. Duncan DG et al (2006) Using dietetic assistants to improve the outcome of hip fracture: a randomised controlled trial of nutritional support in an acute trauma ward. Age Ageing 35(2):148–153

88. Curtis K, Wiseman T (2008) Back to basics—essential nursing care in the ED: part one. Australas Emerg Nurs J 11(1):49–53

89. Antoniak AE, Greig CA (2017) The effect of combined resistance exercise training and vitamin D3 supplementation on musculoskeletal health and function in older adults: a systematic review and meta-analysis. BMJ Open 7(7):e014619

Fragility Fracture Audit

19

Cristina Ojeda-Thies, Louise Brent, Colin T. Currie,
and Matthew Costa

19.1 Introduction

Hip fracture is a common, serious and costly injury that presents acutely, requires surgery, carries both residual disability and a high mortality, and is much easier to identify and register than other osteoporotic fractures [1, 2]. It is therefore an ideal index condition for clinical audit and also a tracer condition for the broader fragility fracture pandemic now challenging healthcare systems worldwide. Even though

---

This chapter is a component of Part 5: Cross-cutting issues.
For an explanation of the grouping of chapters in this book, please see Chapter 1: "The multidisciplinary approach to fragility fractures around the world—an overview".

C. Ojeda-Thies (✉)
Department of Traumatology and Orthopaedic Surgery, Hospital Universitario 12 de Octubre, Madrid, Spain

Registro Nacional de Fracturas de Cadera (Spanish National Hip Fracture Registry, RNFC), Madrid, Spain
e-mail: cristina.ojeda@salud.madrid.org

L. Brent
Irish Hip Fracture Database and Major Trauma Audit, National Office of Clinical Audit, Dublin, Ireland

Fragility Fracture Network, Zürich, Switzerland
e-mail: louisebrent@noca.ie

C. T. Currie
Fragility Fracture Network, Zürich, Switzerland

M. Costa
Fragility Fracture Network, Zürich, Switzerland

Orthopaedic Trauma, Nuffield Department of Orthopaedics, Rheumatology and Musculoskeletal Sciences, University of Oxford, Oxford, UK
e-mail: matthew.costa@ndorms.ox.ac.uk

© The Author(s) 2021
P. Falaschi, D. Marsh (eds.), *Orthogeriatrics*, Practical Issues in Geriatrics,
https://doi.org/10.1007/978-3-030-48126-1_19

331

age-adjusted incidence of hip fractures is falling in some regions, population incidence is increasing due to rising life expectancy worldwide, and is estimated to grow
from 1.66 million in 1990 to 6.26 million in 2050, with steep increases throughout
Asia and Latin America [3, 4], potentially placing the healthcare systems of these
regions under considerable stress. Good management of hip fracture demands integration of excellent nursing, surgical, anaesthetic, medical and rehabilitative care.
Furthermore, there is a relatively strong evidence base on key quality standards for
aspects of care in all phases of management, many of which have been implemented
by clinical teams working with hospital management authorities to improve cost-
effectiveness and quality of care [5]; some of these indicators have been used for
international comparisons of care across different healthcare systems [6]. Quality
care of this tracer condition benefits the care of other types of fragility fracture, via
good orthogeriatric care, and access to rehabilitation units and fracture liaison services [7]. Ideally, sustained audit with continuous feedback can deliver continuous
quality improvement by allowing organisations first to ascertain the nature of the
care they provide, including its deficits, then to use data to prompt clinical and service structure improvements and then to assess the impact of these (Fig. 19.1) [8].

19.2   Hip Fracture Audit

Orthopaedic audit as we know it was born in Sweden in the 1970s and began with
elective surgery in the form of the Swedish Knee Arthroplasty Register and Swedish
Hip Arthroplasty Register [9, 10]. The nature of the Swedish healthcare

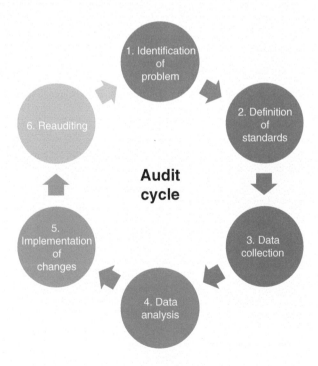

Fig. 19.1 Clinical audit cycle (adapted from: Limb C, Fowler A, Gundogan B, Koshy K, Agha R. How to conduct a clinical audit and quality improvement project. Int J Surg Oncol (N Y). 2017;2(6):e24(8))

system—providing free care at the point of delivery in publicly funded hospitals, and patient traceability since every citizen has a national personal identification number—made implementation of a national registry relatively easy. More national registries developed in the following decades, among them the Swedish Hip Fracture Registry or Rikshöft, initiated in Lund in 1988 by Professor Karl-Göran Thorngren [11]. Rikshöft differed from previously existing orthopaedic registries in that, besides data regarding fracture type and treatment, it also collected data on patients' functional level and residential status.

This was followed by the Scottish Hip Fracture Audit (SHFA) [12], based on Rikshöft and initiated in 1993, and the Standardised Audit of Hip Fracture in Europe (SAHFE) initiative (1994–1998) [13], with participation from 15 European nations, with the goals of (1) devising a standard data set for documentation of treatment and outcome for hip fractures; (2) piloting the use of such a dataset within Europe; (3) promoting Europe-wide comparisons of demographic features, surgical techniques and rehabilitation methods; (4) determining the practicalities of collecting and disseminating this information on a Europe-wide basis; (5) evaluating the effectiveness and differences of hip fracture care throughout Europe and (6) facilitating the dissemination of the best practice of hip fracture surgery and rehabilitation throughout Europe.

As a result of these initiatives, several other national audits emerged in Europe in the following decade, the most important of which was the National Hip Fracture Database (NHFD) which covered England, Wales and Northern Ireland, and is currently the registry with the highest number of cases collected [14]. National hip fracture audits were however mainly limited to Scandinavia, Great Britain and Ireland. The Fragility Fracture Network (FFN), a global not-for-profit organisation founded in 2011, sets out to promote the wider establishment of hip fracture audit—as a way to assess the effectiveness of national fragility fracture networks—and latterly has directed its efforts towards creating regional and national alliances.

Its Hip Fracture Audit Special Interest Group proposed a Minimum Common Data set (Fig. 19.2)—a concise, practical and cost-effective data set for audit start-ups working within resource constraints—that also served to facilitate large-scale international comparisons of case-mix, care and mortality outcomes [15]. It should be considered a minimum recommended data set, to which other variables can be added at the discretion of each local, regional or national audit. The FFN Hip Fracture Audit Database Pilot Phase included hospitals from Lübeck and Stuttgart, Germany; Celje, Slovenia; Msida, Malta; and Barcelona, Spain; the latter two hospitals discontinuing their participation due to organisational constraints, mainly the heavy reliance on the enthusiasm of individual clinicians. In spite of these issues, the Pilot Phase detected large differences in case-mix, care provided and process measures (Fig. 19.3) and usefully highlighted some of the problems encountered by nascent hip fracture audits.

Several new hip fracture audits have been initiated in the past decade, many in regions far from traditional Anglo-Saxon or Scandinavian influence. While not a national-level system, Kaiser Permanente is the largest managed health care organisation of the United States with over 11 million insured and created a hip fracture

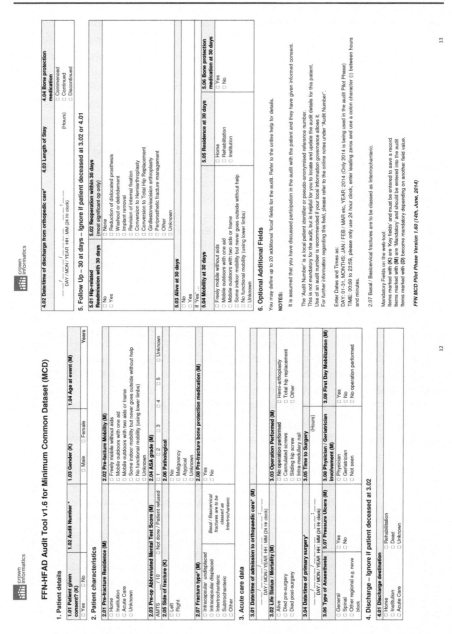

Fig. 19.2 Fragility Fracture Network's Hip Fracture Audit Special Interest Group Minimum Common Dataset (FFN MCD)

a

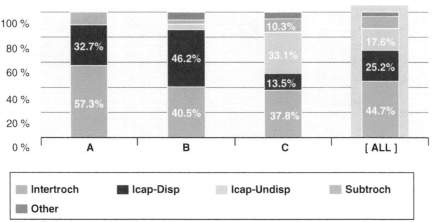

2.07 Fracture Type 2016

FFN Hip Fracture Audit Database - Patients Admitted Jan 2015-July 2016

Fragility Fracture Network 2014 - Technology by Crown Audit (www.CrownAudit.com) (ID: 207)

b

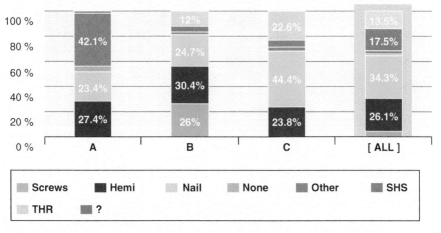

3.03 Operation Performed 2016

FFN Hip Fracture Audit Database - Patients Admitted Jan 2015-July 2016

Fragility Fracture Network 2014 - Technology by Crown Audit (www.CrownAudit.com) (ID: 303)

Fig. 19.3 Results of the FFN Hip Fracture Audit Database Pilot Phase (Data extracted from: Bunning T, Currie, CT. Final Report of the Hip Fracture Audit Database (HFAD) Pilot Phase. Crown Informatics Limited; 2017 [15]). (**a**) Fracture type; (**b**) operation performed; (**c**) time to surgery and (**d**) discharge destination

c

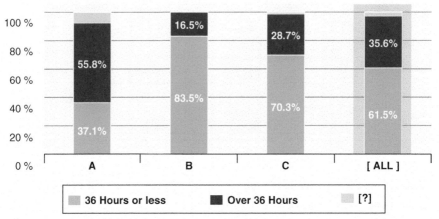

3.05 Time To Surgery 2016

FFN Hip Fracture Audit Database - Patients Admitted Jan 2015-July 2016

Fragility Fracture Network 2014 - Technology by Crown Audit (www.CrownAudit.com) (ID: 305)

d

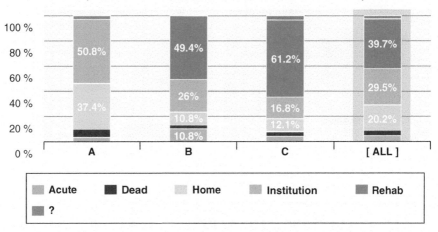

4.01 Discharge Destination 2016

FFN Hip Fracture Audit Database - Patients Admitted Jan 2015-July 2016

Fragility Fracture Network 2014 - Technology by Crown Audit (www.CrownAudit.com) (ID: 401)

Fig. 19.3 (continued)

registry in 2009 as part of its National Implant Registries to track implants in patients insured by the company. Its 2017 report includes over 44.000 patients. Other national audits have been created in Norway [16], Denmark [17], Ireland [18], Australia and New Zealand [19], Germany [20], the Netherlands [21, 22], Italy [23], Spain [24] and France (see Box 19.1). There are, however, marked differences across the health care economies in which they function and in how they are organised and financed. Such factors account for considerable differences in their growth and continuity; their differing ascertainment and follow-up rates and the wide variability documented in Table 19.1. A large majority of the countries with established audits have publicly funded healthcare systems, which seem to offer a more favourable environment for clinical audit and comparison among hospitals.

Box 19.1 List of National Hip Fracture Registries and Their Web Addresses, When Available. Audits Marked with Asterisk Are Currently in Their Pilot Phases

- Sweden (Rikshöft)—https://rikshoft.se/
- Scotland, Scottish Hip Fracture Registry (SHFA)—https://www.shfa.scot.nhs.uk
- Demnark, Dansk Tværfagligt Register for Hoftenære Lårbensbrud (DTRHL)—https://www.rkkp.dk/om-rkkp/de-kliniske-kvalitetsdatabaser/hoftenaere-laerbensbrud/
- Finland (PERFECT)—http://thl.fi/fi/tutkimus-ja-kehittaminen/tutkimuk-set-ja-hankkeet/perfect/osahankkeet/lonkkamurtuma/perusraportit
- Norway, Nasjonalt Hoftebruddregister (NHR)—http://nrlweb.ihelse.net/
- England, Wales & Northern Ireland (National Hip Fracture Database, NHFD)—https://nhfd.co.uk/
- United States (Kaiser Permanente Hip Fracture Registry)—https://national-implantregistries.kaiserpermanente.org/
- Ireland (Irish Hip Fracture Database, IHFD)—https://www.noca.ie/audits/irish-hip-fracture-database
- Australia, New Zealand; Australian and New Zealand National Hip Fracture Registry (ANZHFR)—https://anzhfr.org/
- Germany, Alterstraumaregister (DGU-ATR)—http://www.alterstrau-maregister-dgu.de
- Netherlands, Dutch Hip Fracture Audit (DHFA)—https://dica.nl/dhfa/home
- Italy, Gruppo Italiano di Ortogeriatria (GIOG)*—https://www.sigg.it/gruppo-di-studio/gruppo-italiano-di-ortogeriatria-giog-sigg-aip-sigot/
- Spain, Registro Nacional de Fracturas de Cadera (RNFC)—http://rnfc.es/
- France, Groupe d'étude en traumatologie ostéo-articulaire (GETRAUM)*—http://www.getraum.fr/

Table 19.1 Comparison of national Hip Fracture Audit organisation and Healthcare System structures

Country/region, name of registry	Healthcare system [25]	Hip fracture audit organisation and financing	Year established	Number of patients included (last report)
Sweden, Rikshöft [26]	Government-funded, decentralised mainly to county councils, financed primarily through taxes	Financed through the Swedish Association of Local Authorities and Regions together with the National Board of Health and Welfare	1988	13,272

(continued)

Table 19.1 (continued)

Country/region, name of registry	Healthcare system [25]	Hip fracture audit organisation and financing	Year established	Number of patients included (last report)
Scotland, Scottish Hip Fracture Registry (SHFA) [27]	National Healthcare System (NHS Scotland), providing healthcare to all permanent residents, financed through general taxation	Local Audit Coordinators, Coordinated by the Scottish Government Directorate of Heath	1993	6669
Denmark, Dansk Tværfagligt Register for Hoftenære Lårbensbrud (DTRHL) [17]	Health care is mainly provided by hospitals owned and run by the regions, financed primarily by income taxes	Mandatory reporting through the National Patient Register	2003	6679
Finland (PERFECT) [28]	Decentralised public healthcare system, depending on the municipalities	Under direction of the Department of Health and Welfare	2004	4458
Norway, Norwegian Hip Fracture Registry (Nasjonalt Hoftebruddregister, NHR) [29]	Hospitals are run by regional Health Authorities and publically funded by the public as part of the national budget. Adults must pay a deductible for health care each year	Part of the Norwegian Arthroplasty Register initiated in 1987 by the Norwegian Orthopaedic Association; approved as national medical quality register in 2009	2005	8321
England, Wales and Northern Ireland (National Hip Fracture Database, NHFD) [14]	Provided through their own systems of publicly funded healthcare, National Healthcare Service (NHS), and financed through general taxation	Initially a joint venture of the British Geriatrics Society (BGS) and the British Orthopedic Association (BOA), currently commissioned by the Healthcare Quality Improvement Partnership (HQIP) and managed by the Royal College of Physicians (RCP)	2007	65,958

Table 19.1   (continued)

Country/region, name of registry	Healthcare system [25]	Hip fracture audit organisation and financing	Year established	Number of patients included (last report)
United States (Kaiser Permanente Hip Fracture Registry) [30]	Healthcare coverage is provided through a combination private health insurance and public health coverage (Medicare, Medicaid), without universal coverage	Managed by Kaiser Permanente, the largest integrated managed care consortium in the United States, with over 11 million health plan members, it only includes patients insured by Kaiser Permanente.	2009	44,221
Ireland (Irish Hip Fracture Database, IHFD) [31]	Public health care system, which is managed by the Health Service Executive and funded by general taxation	Joint venture of the Irish Gerontological Society and the Irish Institute for Trauma and Orthopedic Surgery, developed in partnership with the Health Service Executive (HSE), under governance of the National Office of Clinical Audit (NOCA)	2012	3497
Australia, New Zealand (Australian and New Zealand National Hip Fracture Registry, ANZHFR) [19]	Australia's health care is provided publicly through a universal health care system, Medicare, financed through the Medicare levy of at least 2% of a resident's taxable income. New Zealand Healthcare is provided through publicly funded District Health Boards, which provide services at government-owned facilities and purchase others from privately owned providers. Funding is derived mainly from general taxation	Collaborative project between the Australian and New Zealand Society for Geriatric Medicine (ANZSGM), the Australian Orthopedic Association (AOA) and the New Zealand Orthopedic Association (NZOA), funded by several public and private grants	2016	7117 (Australia) 2291 (New Zealand)

(continued)

Table 19.1 (continued)

Country/region, name of registry	Healthcare system [25]	Hip fracture audit organisation and financing	Year established	Number of patients included (last report)
Germany (Alterstraumaregister, DGU-ATR) [20]	Universal multi-payer health care system paid for by a combination of statutory health insurance and private health insurance	Coordinated by the German Society for Trauma Surgery (Deutsche Gesellschaft für Unfallchirurgie (DGU)), it also includes several Swiss hospitals	2016	6137
Netherlands (Dutch Hip Fracture Audit, DHFA) [21, 22]	Dual-level system. Primary and curative care (i.e. the family doctor service and hospitals and clinics) is financed from private mandatory insurance. Long term care for the elderly, the dying, the long term mentally ill etc. is covered by social insurance funded from taxation	Coordinated through the Dutch Institute for Clinical Auditing (DICA), overseen by a multidisciplinary clinical audit Board in which medical associations involved in the hip fracture Care process in the Netherlands	2016	11,086
Italy (Gruppo Italiano di Ortogeriatria, GIOG) [23]	Healthcare is provided by a mixed public-private system. The public part is the Servizio Sanitario Nazionale (SSN), which is organised under the Ministry of Health and is administered on a regional basis	The Gruppo Italiano di Ortogeriatria is an inter-society study group established in 2012, that uses a web-based audit	2016	2557
Spain (Registro Nacional de Fracturas de Cadera, RNFC) [24]	Universally accessible, public health care system funded indirectly through taxes, decentralised and managed by Autonomous Regions through their own institutions, coordinated by the Spanish Ministry of Health	Multidisciplinary group of clinicians, endorsed by over 20 national and regional scientific societies. Financed through private industry sponsorship and public research grants offered by private foundations	2017	11,431

Other start-ups have been reported in the last decade, most notably Hong Kong [32, 33], Malaysia [34] Lebanon [35] and Iran [36, 37], but detailed continuing information about their survival and impact is, to our knowledge, not in the public domain. Other countries such as France, Mexico [38] and Japan [15] are in the pilot phase of national hip fracture audit development. Two are of special interest on account of their size and demography. Japan has the highest life expectancy worldwide [39], and Spain has the highest life expectancy in Europe [6] and is predicted to overtake Japan by 2040, with both countries forecast to exceed 85 years of life expectancy by 2040 [40].

Regional initiatives including those from British Columbia [41] and the Baltic Region [42] should also be mentioned. Several other countries are using large clinical databases to analyse hip fracture management. In the United States, the Nationwide Inpatient Sample (NIS) collects retrospective data from patients admitted using the ICD-9 codes. Other examples include the American College of Surgeons prospective National Surgical Quality Improvement Program (NSQIP) and the Trauma Quality Improvement Project (TQIP) using data obtained directly from the medical records by trained surgeons. Though not specific to hip fracture, they include much hip fracture data and are a source of research studies [43, 44] due to their large numbers of patients and available data. Other studies have, however, shown significant variation in data inclusion and completeness, which could jeopardise the validity of conclusions reached in evaluating the care provided [45, 46].

Other countries with quality analyses based on general clinical or national databases are Germany, with its impressive external quality assurance programme for orthogeriatric care [47, 48]; Canada with the Canadian Institute for Health Information [49, 50] and South Korea using data from the Health Insurance Review and Assessment Service [51, 52].

19.3 Obstacles to Hip Fracture Audit and International Comparison

Several authors have recently compared national hip fracture audits, showing important differences in inclusion criteria, follow-up, variables included and coverage [22, 24, 53, 54]. For example, the minimum age at which hip fracture patients are included ranges from all adults in the Netherlands to patients 75 years old or older in Spain. Follow-up ranges from 30 days for many registries such as Scotland, Ireland and Spain to 120 days for Sweden, Norway, the UK, Germany and Australia and New Zealand. Others, such as Denmark and Italy, have several cut-off points for follow-up. Data collected on function also vary between registries: while some collect the ability to walk assisted or unassisted indoors or outdoors, others use scores such as the cumulative ambulation score (e.g. Denmark) and a new mobility score (e.g. in Ireland) [18]. Functional and residential status data are more difficult to collect than discrete hard data such as re-operation rates or mortality, but it can be argued that the former is just as, if not more, relevant for the patient than the latter [55]. Very few registries include data regarding quality of life, with Germany and the NHFD collecting EQ-5D data.

However, collection of data after discharge can be more resource intensive—and loss of follow-up can pose a threat to the integrity of an overly ambitious audit data set. Some registries, such as the Kaiser Permanente and Norwegian hip fracture registry, are incorporated into larger administrative databases analysing joint implants, but largely lack clinical follow-up. For these reasons, we believe that an international consensus defining a limited but robust core data set—to be included by all interested audits, whatever other data they collect, and judiciously adapted in the light of emerging evidence—is paramount, and accordingly is proposed by the FFN. In terms of coverage, the UK NHFD and the Danish audit capture practically all occurring hip fractures. Other still nascent audits such as those in Australia, New Zealand, Spain and Holland include between one-quarter and one-half of estimated yearly hip fracture numbers. Since hospitals already interested in improving hip fracture care and providing orthogeriatric care are more likely to be early adopters of a voluntary hip fracture audit, concerns arise for possible inclusion bias. Fracture care and outcomes in such settings are better than average, so the overall reported quality of care may deteriorate as later adopters join the audit.

Some audits require individual patient consent to inclusion, as is the case in Spain [24], Italy [23] and Norway [16, 56]. The need for informed individual patient consent to store routinely collected healthcare data is debatable. In the European Union, a new framework known as the General Data Protection Regulation (GDPR) [57] came into force across the EU on 25 May 2018. The GDPR requires that processing of personal data is fair, lawful and transparent. Currently there is nothing in the legislation that prevents clinical audit being carried out locally or nationally. Health data are defined under the GDPR via a special category of personal data and can be processed in situations where it is necessary to do so for reasons of public health. Regarding the conditions for lawful processing of personal data (Article 6), clinical audit fulfils GDPR Articles 6(1)(c), "processing necessary for performance of contract" with the data subject, or Article 6(1)(e), "processing is necessary for the performance of a task carried out in the public interest or in the exercise of official authority vested in the controller", and Article 6(1)(f), "processing is necessary for the purposes of legitimate interests". With reference to conditions for processing special categories of personal data (Article 9), "processing is necessary for the purpose of preventative... medicine... the provision of health or social care or treatment or the management of health or social care systems and services..." (Article 9(2)(h)) and "processing is necessary for reasons of public interest in the area of public health, such as... ensuring high standards of quality and safety of health care..." (Article 9(2)(h)). The Irish National Office for Clinical Audit has recently analysed the relevance of the GDPR and patient consent for national clinical audit [58], and has concluded that (1) for national clinical audit, all patients meeting the criteria of the audit should be included, so that a full national picture can be collected; (2) consent would not be appropriate because the patient could decline to give their consent or subsequently withdraw their consent at any time. Both of these individual rights would prevent collection of a full national picture; (3) national clinical audit should not rely on consent as the lawful basis but should instead

justify such audit on the public health lawful basis as applicable e.g. Articles 6(1)
(e), 6(1)(f). Finally, (4) the collection of data, validation of data, review of outliers
for national clinical audit does not require consent and (5) patients should, however,
be informed that their data may be used as part of a national clinical audit e.g.
through information leaflets.

Patients with cognitive impairment—occurring in up to 30% of patients with hip
fracture—are excluded when consent is required, which greatly limits the practical
utility of audit findings. Validity of consent from a patient's family varies across
jurisdictions, may be time-consuming and may thus increase preoperative delay. In
some jurisdictions, a supplementary explanation about audit and its value may be
provided during consent to surgery—with opt-out where feelings are strong.
However, the evidential value of findings from an audit that includes all, or almost
all, cases is such that all reasonable and sympathetic measures available should
endeavour to achieve universal coverage.

19.4 Hip Fracture Audit and the Improvement of Care

Since improving care is the main purpose of audit, the acquisition, ownership, analysis and use of data are of vital importance. Audit data can be collected by individual units and used by clinicians and management for internal quality reporting and
continuous improvement or for external monitoring by health authorities and
national governments for purposes of accountability for sanction or reward [59].
Data can be collected in an automated fashion through hospital administrative databases and coding by non-clinical staff, but the reliability of these data is relatively
low, with median values for diagnostic accuracy around 80% [60, 61]. Electronic
health records may be expected to improve the reliability of this data, again with the
above proviso.

It should be noted that using outcome data for sanction or reward can lead to
perverse incentives—such as targeting inclusion and treatment to the patients with
the best prognosis or assigning patients to more serious risk categories. To avoid
such "gaming", responsible clinician involvement to defend data reliability is vital.
Where possible, data linkage with centralised national statistics, using patient iden-
tifiers such as national personal identification numbers, is of great value in tracking
both inclusion rates and survival. Data protection laws vary between jurisdictions,
and may complicate achieving data linkage, but uploading to national level may be
facilitated by a process of pseudo-anonymisation of bulked annual data.

Clinical outcomes such as mortality and residential status depend on many factors not related to quality of care. A systematic review showed that, though significant, the correlation between the quality of clinical practice and hospital mortality
was low [62]. Risk adjustment would account only for the variables that have been
measured and these could have a different effect across groups. Other outcomes
such as quality of life or change in residential status are also relevant, especially for
patients and their families, while healthcare systems should also consider readmission and reoperation rates.

Measures of clinical process are, however, easier to collect and compare. These should be quality- and evidence-based, and the effort required to improve the processes analysed should be proportionate to the contingent gains; improvement should also not come at the expense of other variables not monitored. The combination of audit, guidelines and standards constitutes the basis of clinical governance for hip fracture care, and good hip fracture audit has been shown to improve process indicators such as reduction in surgical delay, as well as outcome indicators such as 30-day mortality, with some reports estimating over a 1000 lives saved by the NHFD since its inception in 2007 [63, 64].

Most hip fracture registries and their governing agencies have implemented national standards which address similar quality goals, such as geriatrician involvement, surgical delay, early mobilisation and prevention of new fractures [14, 19, 31, 65–67]. Some of these quality standards are summarised in Table 19.2. The NHS's National Institute for Health and Care Excellence (NICE) defined quality standards for hip fracture care in 2012 and updated them in 2016 [69]. Building upon these, the British Orthopaedic Association, together with the British Geriatrics Society, the NHFD and FFN-UK have recently updated the "BOA Standard of Care (BOAST) for the older or frail orthopaedic trauma patient", adding detail for fragility fracture patients beyond hip fracture [70].

In addition, the Best Practice Tariff (BPT), an individual patient-level payment made to hospitals when they deliver care which meets all of the quality standards in the audit, was introduced in England in 2010 and relied heavily on NHFD data [14]. Criteria were updated in 2017 to include delirium, nutrition and early physiotherapy. Achievement of BPT criteria has been shown to lead to improved survival following hip fracture, both in single-centre cohort studies [68] and when comparing results in England and Scotland, with over 1000 deaths avoided per year in England that could be attributed to these interventions [71]. The UK NHFD incorporates standards from all three criteria as benchmarks that are publicly available on their website, with BPT criteria achieved for 57.1% of all NHFD patients in 2017.

Quality standards are regularly updated and modified, and while initial standards focused mainly on acute care, they now incorporate achievement of rehabilitation and post-acute care goals and more. All registries studied include secondary fracture prevention among their quality standards [31, 65–67]. The Irish Hip Fracture Database has also implemented a BPT since 2018 and in the initial 12-month period there has been a significant improvement in data quality seen in the Irish Hip Fracture Care Standards and hospital governance arrangements [18]. The most notable improvement has been the development of an orthogeriatric service in almost every hospital.

Clinical audits must be sustained in order to maintain continuous improvement and benchmarking standards should be updated to close the quality improvement circle. Interruption of the Scottish Hip Fracture Audit showed a deterioration of process indicators such as time to theatre, which recovered when the audit was re-introduced 5 years later [72].

Finally, national registries have been the source for further research regarding hip fracture care both for comparison of local results with other international

Table 19.2 Comparison of quality standards for hip fractures

Standard	Standards organisation						
	NICE [60]	BPT [14]	NHFD benchmarks [68]	Ireland (NOCA/IHFD) [57]	Australia/New Zealand (ANZHFR) [58] [64]	Spain (RNFC) [59]	Scotland (SHFA) [66]
Time to surgery	<36 h[a]	<36 h	<36 h[a]	<48 h	<48 h	<48 h	<36 h
Time in the Emergency Department	–	–	<4 h	<4 h	–	–	<4 h
Evidence of local arrangements for the management of patients with hip fracture in the emergency department	–	–	–	–	Included	–	Included
Admission under consultant-led joint orthopaedic–geriatric care	Hip fracture Programme	Substituted 2017	–	–	Included	–	Included
Documented assessment of pain within 30 min of presentation to the emergency department; either receive analgesia within this time or do not require it, according to the assessment	Throughout hospitalisation (discontinued 2016)	–	–	–	Included	–	Included
Multidisciplinary assessment protocol on admission agreed on by geriatric, orthopaedics and anaesthesia	Included	Substituted 2017	Included	–	–	–	Included
Geriatrician assessment within 72 hours of admission	–	Included	–	Included	–	–	Included
Receiving a bone health assessment	Discontinued 2016	Included (as a single point)	Included	Included	Included[b]	Included[c]	Included
Receiving a specialist falls assessment	Discontinued 2016	Included	Included	Included	–	–	Included[d]
Geriatrician-directed multiprofessional rehabilitation	–	Substituted 2017	–	–	–	–	–
Cognitive assessment (abbreviated mental test) performed before and after surgery	Discontinued 2016	Introduced 2011; since 2017 only preop	Included	–	Included	–	Included[d]

(continued)

Table 19.2 (continued)

	Standards organisation						
Nutritional assessment during admission	–	Introduced 2017	Included	–	Included	–	Included^d
Delirium assessment using the 4AT screening tool during the admission	–	Introduced 2017	Included	–	Included	–	Included^d
Avoidance of repeated fasting; clear fluids up to 2 h before surgery	Included						Included
Assessment by a physiotherapist the day of or day following surgery	Included	Introduced 2017	Included	–	Included	–	Included
Assessment b occupational therapist by day 3 post admission							Included
New Stage II or higher pressure injury during their hospital stay	–	–	Included	Included	Included	Included	
Mobilisation on day one post hip fracture surgery	Included	–	Included	–	Included	Included	Included
Unrestricted weight-bearing status immediately post hip fracture surgery	–	–		–	Included	–	
Return to pre-fracture mobility	–	–		–	Included	–	
Proportion of patients with independent mobility at 30 days	–	–		–		Included	
Evidence of local arrangements for the development of an individualised care plan for hip fracture patients prior to the patient's separation from hospital	Discontinued 2016	–		–	Included	–	
Return to private residence within 120 days post separation from hospital (for those living in private residence before fracture)	–	–	Included	Included	Included	–	Included (30 days)
Re-operation of hip fracture patients within follow-up	–	–	Included^e		Included^f	–	
Survival at 30 days post-admission for surgery	–	–		–	Included	–	

People with displaced intracapsular fracture should have a total hip replacement if clinically eligible, rather than hemiarthroplasty	Included (updated 2017)	–	Included	–	–	–
Use of extramedullary implants for trochanteric fractures above and including the lesser trochanter (AO types A1 and A2)	Included	–	Included	–	–	–
Use of intramedullary nail for subtrochanteric fractures	New in 2016	–	Included	–	–	–

[a]Defined as "surgery scheduled on a planned trauma list, with consultant or senior staff supervision on the day of, or the day after, admission"

[b]Proportion of patients with a hip fracture receiving bone protection medicine prior to separation from the hospital at which they underwent hip fracture surgery

[c]Includes three separate standards (a) bone protection medication, (b) calcium intake, and (c) vitamin D intake

[d]Within 24 h of admission

[e]120 day follow-up

[f]30-day follow-up

registries [46, 47, 66] and for studies adding on national registry data to address specific questions. An excellent example is the UK Anaesthesia Sprint Audit of Practice (ASAP-2) [73], a large NHFD-based prospective study including 11,085 cases. This highlighted the critical importance of maintaining intra-operative systolic normo-tension and identified the associated risks of higher dosages of subarachnoid local anaesthetic. Together with its predecessor ASAP-1 [74], this has transformed the evidence base for hip fracture anaesthesia, which had previously consisted of a number of small trials from one or two hospitals, which often excluded patients with cognitive impairment (typically c. 30%) and were thus of limited impact in terms of the care of the typical hip fracture casemix. Another Anaesthesia Sprint Audit of Practice, ASAP-3, aimed at studying the anaesthetic management of periprosthetic fractures, is set to commence in 2020.

Many published single-hospital NHFD reports have documented care quality improvements such as improved pain control, reductions in peri-operative medical and surgical complications, and more rapid recovery, and reduced length of stay, sometimes with substantial reductions in bed days. More recently, the World Hip Trauma Evaluation (WHiTE) initiative has been set up to measure outcome in a cohort of hip fracture patients within the framework of the NHFD [75]. Under individual patient consent or family agreement where appropriate, WHiTE has recruited over 20,000 patients with hip fracture and collected patient-reported outcome measurement in more than 80% of participants. Studies such as WHiTE provide reliable observational outcome data, but also act as a platform for virtual clinical trials which can assess single interventions such as new forms of surgery and also serves as a framework to assess innovations throughout the hip fracture journey of care from pre-hospital pain relief to community rehabilitation [76].

Though good evidence can be obtained from both registries and clinical trials, registry studies are not equivalent to formal clinical trials. In orthopaedic surgery, knowledge usually advances from individual case series of a new operative technique or care process to case–control studies and then randomised trials. However, even these trials usually show results under optimal conditions in academic or specialised centres, with a high risk for publication bias. National guidelines are usually based on systematic reviews of randomised investigations, while these are excellent in compensating for confounding factors, they present problems in addition to selection and publication bias. Clinical trials are cost-intensive and often limited to a short observation period. Ethical issues arise when studying controversies such as surgical delay or weight-bearing after hip fractures.

National registries, however, pose the advantage of covering all incident cases within a country, reflecting the breadth of experience and training across a whole healthcare system, rather than specialist academic centres. They therefore offer a truer picture of everyday practice and regional variability. Another advantage of national registries is their large case numbers, allowing for collection of data of uncommon patient features and adverse events, such as surgical delay of patients with double anticoagulation, or fat embolism syndrome. They also allow for analysis of patient-centred outcome variables such as patient quality of life, social living situation and functional capacity from a representative group of patients, though trials are more likely to collect good quality outcome data especially during follow-up, largely as a result of better funding.

Finally, continuous data collection allows for identification of time trends in hip fracture epidemiology and the effects of measures implemented by healthcare practitioners or healthcare systems. Interestingly, the BMJ recently pointed out that "observational research using Big Data can explore the effect of disease and care on many patients… at a low cost per question. Big Data are more representative of the 'real world' than Little Science trials that recruit a few patients from referral centres. Clinical trialists can often use Big Data to design more efficient and useful trials…" [77]. The implications of this for audit-based clinical research in hip fracture care appear to be clear—with Big Data abundantly available now and for the foreseeable future.

19.5 Audit of Other Fragility Fractures and Fracture Liaison Services (FLS)

While hip fracture audit is relatively established in many regions worldwide, other fragility fractures are audited much less commonly. This is in large part due to the difficulty of identifying cases that frequently do not require hospital admission; as a matter of fact, many vertebral fractures go clinically undetected [78, 79]. As noted above, nearly all hip fractures are diagnosed acutely, hospitalised and managed surgically, making them easier to identify and register. In the United Kingdom, the Royal College of Physicians (RCP) is leading a 2020 Sprint Audit to investigate vertebral fracture identification [80]. Sweden has developed a Fracture Registry including all types of fractures (fragility and non-fragility) starting in 2011, covering 80% of orthopaedic departments in 2018. It has to date collected more than 400,000 fracture cases, including patient-reported outcome measures [81, 82]. Many hip fracture registries already include non-hip femoral fractures or plan to do so: while the German registry includes periprosthetic fractures and peri-implant fractures, the NHFD and ANZHFR are planning to add distal femoral fractures, and several arthroplasty registries are performing sub-analyses of periprosthetic fractures. These, while they study intraoperative factors and issues related to prosthetic design, often lack data regarding patient outcomes [83–85].

Further audit research is now focussing on Fracture Liaison Services (FLS) databases, for example that in England under the RCP, as part of the same Falls and Fragility Fracture Audit Programme (FFFAP) together with the NHFD [86], and in Canada, with 45 FLSs in 2018 [87]. Spain is currently piloting a fragility fracture and FLS audit, the REFRA-FLS-registry, with over a dozen hospitals participating [88]. The international development of FLS programs has previously been extensively studied in the book by Seibel and Mitchell [89]. These FLS registries, however, are more centred on secondary prevention than on acute multidisciplinary care and post-acute care and rehabilitation, and do not report on individual fracture types apart from ad hoc research studies such as the proposed RCP Vertebral Fracture Sprint Audit mentioned above. Finally, FLS registries appear to work best where they are integrated with other fracture registries (e.g. hip fracture audit), rather than when they are standalone registries.

19.6   Expansion of Hip Fracture Registries in Other Regions

Healthcare administrators have an interest in not only providing quality care but also cost-effective care. As the Blue Book published by the British Orthopaedic Association and British Geriatrics Society states, "Looking after hip fracture patients well is a lot cheaper than looking after them badly" [90]. In many countries, open comparisons between hospitals and regions have become commonplace; this however requires a certain cultural sensitivity. Press coverage of registry reports can be misleading, because journalists may not understand the importance of case-mix and random variation, since low-volume hospitals are more likely to show poorer figures due to statistically non-significant adverse events. Participation of healthcare professionals in the evaluation and communication of audit reports is important. Emphasis should be placed on overall changes in outcomes or process, rather than on outliers, and on targeting the particular strengths and weaknesses of organisations. Over time, small marginal gains of only 1% can amount to large improvements [91–93]. Delaunay states "registries are a manifestation of the evaluation culture. Thus, their widespread development in some countries (such as Scandinavian, Australia, UK) and their virtual absence in others (such as southern European countries) highlights the impact of cultural differences on healthcare evaluation" [94]. Though newer registries such as those from Spain, Germany, the Netherlands and Italy do not yet offer publicly available data comparing hospitals, other established registries, such as the NHFD, the IHFD and the ANZHFR, do, though they did not do so in their early stages.

Public recognition of registry participation such as in Germany—in which participation is a prerequisite of being recognised as a "Geriatric Trauma Centre", or of achievement of standards or improvement, such as the SHFA's "Golden Hip Award" can help raise awareness and raise the enthusiasm of healthcare professionals and administrators initially not aware of issues regarding the hip fracture care process. At a global level, the recent award in a world-wide WHO competition to the Spanish RNFC hip fracture audit as the best healthcare initiative to benefit elderly patients did much to raise the profile of hip fracture care internationally [95]. Though the reality of fragility fracture management can be very different in regions such as Southeast Asia and Latin America in comparison to Northern Europe, the same general principles apply for registry implementation. It is important, while maintaining a minimum common dataset, to tailor audit data sets to each country's particular social and healthcare characteristics, as small local gains can lead to significant improvements and healthcare savings over time, especially in regions with rapidly growing elderly populations.

Several nascent registries arose as collaborative initiatives by scientific societies, as in Australia and New Zealand, Spain, Italy, France and Germany. The number of disciplines actively participating in these registries is variable, with some depending almost exclusively on orthopaedic surgeons and/or geriatricians, and others more widely inclusive. It is important for the healthcare providers and governments to recognise the importance of these registries as instruments for assessment of variability, benchmarking and quality improvement. The cost of maintaining a national registry is a small fraction of the overall expense of hip fractures on a healthcare system; the care of 3.5 million fragility fractures which occurred in the European Union in 2010 was estimated to have cost 37 billion euros [96]. Meanwhile, the UK NHFD has been estimated to cost approximately 0.5% per case of the total cost of hip fracture care [7]. Improvements in care processes and outcomes of good audits allow for cost savings many times higher than the cost of maintaining the audit itself. It is much more expensive to ignore current information when deciding policy than it is to invest in obtaining that information through audits. Audit provides information with the potential to deliver care that is both better and cheaper, which translates into a brief but effective formulation: "If you think information's expensive, try ignorance".

19.7 New Developments in Fracture Audit

Electronic health records (EHR) may make manual entry of many of the variables such as time of admission or surgery superfluous. However, the large number and variability of providers of EHRs and operating systems make automated data difficult, and healthcare administrations should consider automated data extraction for registry analysis when choosing one EHR system over another.

Automation of data reporting allows for real-time data evaluation and communication: prompt recognition of changes in the care process or adverse effects allows for quick responses by healthcare professionals and a more direct sense of their participation in audit. This is in contrast to the often cumbersome and sterile annual reports in which it is difficult to establish connections between actions and their results.

The UK NHFD webpage is exemplary in that sense [97], with online charts updated every 2 months comparing individual hospital, regional and national overall performances and their evolution over time, as well as performance in relation to different standards, including the quartiles achieved for each indicator. With increasing numbers of web-based registries, automation of these reports is feasible, with the Baltic Fracture Consortium using the R programming language to offer real-time statistical reports (including analyses such as Fisher's test to assess for significance of complication rates) to participants [42].

In line with the regionalisation strategy promoted by the FFN, establishment of new fragility fracture audits should be encouraged and supported, especially in regions likely to be most seriously affected by the fragility fracture pandemic, such as Asia and Latin America. Pilot studies have revealed the reality of surgical delay in countries such as India [98], Mexico [99], Peru [100]—with only 30, 10.5 and 5.3% receiving surgery within 48 h of hospital admission, respectively—or the Mediterranean region, with Portugal, Italy and Spain among the four countries of the OECD with the lowest proportion of hip fractures operated on in less than 48 h [6]. This is far from what is considered standard in Western countries with longer established hip fracture audit, and the scope for improvement is large. But with clinically led, web-based hip fracture audit established as a mature technology supporting the substantial international expansion of effective quality improvement in hip fracture care in recent years, there are now grounds for cautious optimism about facing up to the challenge of care for the impending global pandemic of fragility fractures. With continuing international collaboration and the support of scientific societies such as the FFN, there is promise too for large-scale clinical and epidemiological research to improve the evidence-base for hip fracture care, and thus to create a virtuous cycle of continuing improvement in care, outcomes and cost-effectiveness over the coming decades.

References

1. Cummings SR, Melton LJ (2002) Epidemiology and outcomes of osteoporotic fractures. Lancet 359(9319):1761–1767
2. Kanis JA, Odén A, McCloskey EV, Johansson H, Wahl DA, Cooper C et al (2012) A systematic review of hip fracture incidence and probability of fracture worldwide. Osteoporos Int 23(9):2239–2256
3. Cooper C, Campion G, Melton LJ (1992) Hip fractures in the elderly: a world-wide projection. Osteoporos Int 2(6):285–289
4. Cooper C, Cole Z, Holroyd C, Earl S, Harvey N, Dennison E et al (2011) Secular trends in the incidence of hip and other osteoporotic fractures. Osteoporos Int 22(5):1277–1288
5. Voeten SC, Krijnen P, Voeten DM, Hegeman JH, Wouters MWJM, Schipper IB (2018) Quality indicators for hip fracture care, a systematic review. Osteoporos Int 29(9):1963–1985
6. OECD (2017) Health at a Glance 2017: OECD indicators. OECD Publishing, Paris
7. Currie C (2018) Hip fracture audit: creating a "critical mass of expertise and enthusiasm for hip fracture care"? Injury 49(8):1418–1423
8. Limb C, Fowler A, Gundogan B, Koshy K, Agha R (2017) How to conduct a clinical audit and quality improvement project. Int J Surg Oncol (N Y) 2(6):e24
9. Kärrholm J (2010) The Swedish Hip Arthroplasty Register (https://www.shpr.se). Acta Orthop 81(1):3–4
10. Robertsson O, Ranstam J, Sundberg M, W-Dahl A, Lidgren L (2014) The Swedish Knee Arthroplasty Register. Bone Joint Res 3(7):217–222
11. Thorngren K-G (2009) National registration of hip fractures in Sweden. In: European Instructional Lectures. Springer. pp 11–18
12. Currie CT, Hutchison JD (2005) Audit, guidelines and standards: clinical governance for hip fracture care in Scotland. Disabil Rehabil 27(18–19):1099–1105
13. Parker MJ, Currie CT, Mountain JA, Thorngren K-G (1998) Standardised Audit of Hip Fracture in Europe (SAHFE). Hip Int 8(1):10–15
14. The Royal College of Physicians (2017) National Hip Fracture Database annual report 2018. eISBN 978-1-86016-736-2 [Internet]. https://nhfd.co.uk/20/hipfractureR.nsf/docs/2018Report
15. Bunning T, Currie CT (2017) Final report of the Hip Fracture Audit Database (HFAD) Pilot Phase [Internet]. Crown Informatics Limited. https://fragilityfracturenetwork.org/wp-content/uploads/2018/03/hfad_final_report_2017.pdf
16. Gjertsen J-E, Engesæter LB, Furnes O, Havelin LI, Steindal K, Vinje T et al (2008) The Norwegian hip fracture register: experiences after the first 2 years and 15,576 reported operations. Acta Orthop 79(5):583–593
17. Röck ND, Hjetting AK (2017) Dansk Tværfagligt Register for Hoftenære Lårbensbrud Dokumentalistrapport [Internet]. https://www.sundhed.dk/content/cms/62/4662_hofte-fraktur-årsrapport_2017.pdf

18. Irish Hip Fracture Database National Report 2018 (2019) National Office of Clinical Audit. [Internet]. National Office of Clinical Audit, Dublin. https://www.noca.ie/publications

19. Australian and New Zealand National Hip Fracture Registry (2018) ANZHFR bi-national annual report of hip fracture care 2018. ISBN 978-0-7334-3824-0 [Internet]. http://anzhfr. org/wp-content/uploads/2018/08/2018-ANZHFR-Annual-Report-FULL-FINAL.pdf

20. Arbeitsgemeinschaft Alterstraumatologie der Deutschen Gesellschaft für Unfallchirurgie e.V (2018) AUC—Akademie der Unfallchirurgie GmbH. Jahresbericht 2018— AltersTraumaRegister DGU® für den Zeitraum 2017 [Internet]. http://www.alter-straumaregister-dgu.de/fileadmin/user_upload/alterstraumaregister-dgu.de/docs/Allgemeiner_ATR_Jahresbericht.pdf

21. Dutch Hip Fracture Audit (2018) DHFA Jaarrapportage 2017 [Internet]. https://dica.nl/jaarrapportage-2017/dhfa

22. Voeten SC, Arends AJ, Wouters MWJM, Blom BJ, Heetveld MJ, Slee-Valentijn MS, et al (2019) The Dutch Hip Fracture Audit: evaluation of the quality of multidisciplinary hip fracture care in the Netherlands. Arch Osteoporos [Internet]. 2019 [cited 2019 Aug 25];14(1). https://www.ncbi.nlm.nih.gov/pmc/articles/PMC6397305/

23. Zurlo A, Bellelli G (2018) Orthogeriatrics in Italy: the Gruppo Italiano di Ortogeriatria (GIOG) audit on hip fractures in the elderly. Geriatric Care 4(2):7726

24. Ojeda-Thies C, Sáez-López P, Currie CT, Tarazona-Santalbina FJ, Alarcón T, Muñoz-Pascual A et al (2019) Spanish National Hip Fracture Registry (RNFC): analysis of its first annual report and international comparison with other established registries. Osteoporos Int 30(6):1243–1254

25. Thomson S, Osborn R, Squires D, Reed SJ (2011) International profiles of health care systems 2011: Australia, Canada, Denmark, England, France, Germany, Iceland, Italy, Japan, the Netherlands, New Zealand, Norway, Sweden, Switzerland, and the United States

26. Rikshöft Årsrapport 2017 [Internet] (2018) RIkshöft. https://rikshoft.se/wp-content/uploads/2018/10/rikshoft_rapport2017_kompl181002.pdf

27. Scottish Hip Fracture Audit (2018) Hip fracture care pathway report 2018 [Internet]. https://www.shfa.scot.nhs.uk/Reports/_docs/2018-08-21-SHFA-Report.pdf

28. PERFECT project (2016) Perusraportit—THL [Internet]. Terveyden ja hyvinvoinnin laitos. http://thl.fi/fi/tutkimus-ja-kehittaminen/tutkimukset-ja-hankkeet/perfect/osahankkeet/lonkkamurtuma/perusraportit

29. Nasjonalt Register for Leddproteser. Nasjonalt Hoftebruddregister. Nasjonalt Korsbåndregister. Nasjonalt Barnehofteregister. Rapport 2017. ISSN 1893-8914 [Internet]. http://nrlweb.ihelse.net/Rapporter/Rapport2018.pdf

30. Kaiser Permanente National Implant Registries. 2017 annual report [Internet]. Kaiser Permanente. https://national-implantregistries.kaiserpermanente.org/Media/Default/documents/2017%20Implant%20Registry%20FINAL%20v2.pdf

31. Irish Hip Fracture Database National Report 2016 (2017) Dublin: National Office of Clinical Audit. ISSN 2565-5388 [Internet]. https://www.noca.ie/wp-content/uploads/2015/04/Irish-Hip-Fracture-Database-National-Report-2016-FINAL.pdf

32. Chow SK-H, Qin J-H, Wong RM-Y, Yuen W-F, Ngai W-K, Tang N et al (2018) One-year mortality in displaced intracapsular hip fractures and associated risk: a report of Chinese-based fragility fracture registry. J Orthop Surg Res 13(1):235

33. Leung KS, Yuen WF, Ngai WK, Lam CY, Lau TW, Lee KB et al (2017) How well are we managing fragility hip fractures? A narrative report on the review with the attempt to setup a Fragility Fracture Registry in Hong Kong. Hong Kong Med J 23(3):264–271

34. Abdullah MAH, Abdullah AT (2009) National Orthopaedic Registry of Malaysia (NORM)— Hip Fracture Registry. Kuala Lumpur, Malaysia: abd

35. Sibai AM, Nasser W, Ammar W, Khalife MJ, Harb H, Fuleihan GE-H (2011) Hip fracture incidence in Lebanon: a national registry-based study with reference to standardized rates worldwide. Osteoporos Int 22(9):2499–2506

36. Keshtkar A, Khashayar P, Etemad K, Dini M, Ebrahimi M, Mohammadi Z, et al (2013) Iranian Hip Fracture Registry (IHFR): a basic framework for improving quality of care in patients with osteoporotic fracture. S60 p

37. Meybodi HA, Heshmat R, Maasoumi Z, Soltani A, Hossein-nezhad A, Keshtkar AA et al (2008) Iranian osteoporosis research network: background, Mission and its role in osteoporosis. Management 1:1–6

38. Viveros-García J, Robles-Almaguer E, Albrecht-Junghanns R, López-Cervantes R, López-Paz C, Olascoaga-Gómez de León A et al (2019) Mexican Hip Fracture Audit (ReMexFC): objectives and methodology. MOJ Orthop Rheumatol 11(3):115–118

39. World Health Organization (2019) World health statistics overview 2019: monitoring health for the SDGs, sustainable development goals. 2019 [cited 2019 Aug 25]; https://apps.who.int/iris/handle/10665/311696

40. Foreman KJ, Marquez N, Dolgert A, Fukutaki K, Fullman N, McGaughey M et al (2018) Forecasting life expectancy, years of life lost, and all-cause and cause-specific mortality for 250 causes of death: reference and alternative scenarios for 2016–40 for 195 countries and territories. Lancet 392(10159):2052–2090

41. BC Hip Fracture Redesign Project [Internet]. [cited 2019 Aug 25]. http://www.hiphealth.ca/research/research-projects/Hip-Fracture-Redesign/

42. Registry—BFCC [Internet]. https://www.bfcc-project.eu/registry.html

43. Sathiyakumar V, Greenberg SE, Molina CS, Thakore RV, Obremskey WT, Sethi MK (2015) Hip fractures are risky business: an analysis of the NSQIP data. Injury 46(4):703–708

44. Ottesen TD, McLynn RP, Galivanche AR, Bagi PS, Zogg CK, Rubin LE et al (2018) Increased complications in geriatric patients with a fracture of the hip whose postoperative weight-bearing is restricted: an analysis of 4918 patients. Bone Joint J 100-B(10):1377–1384

45. Shelton T, Hecht G, Slee C, Wolinsky P (2019) A comparison of geriatric hip fracture databases. J Am Acad Orthop Surg 27(3):e135–e141

46. Bohl DD, Basques BA, Golinvaux NS, Baumgaertner MR, Grauer JN (2014) Nationwide Inpatient Sample and National Surgical Quality Improvement Program give different results in hip fracture studies. Clin Orthop Relat Res 472(6):1672–1680

47. Smektala R, Endres HG, Dasch B, Maier C, Trampisch HJ, Bonnaire F et al (2008) The effect of time-to-surgery on outcome in elderly patients with proximal femoral fractures. BMC Musculoskelet Disord 9:171

48. Smektala R, Hahn S, Schräder P, Bonnaire F, Schulze Raestrup U, Siebert H et al (2010) Medial hip neck fracture: influence of pre-operative delay on the quality of outcome. Results of data from the external in-hospital quality assurance within the framework of secondary data analysis. Unfallchirurg 113(4):287–292

49. Sobolev B, Guy P, Sheehan KJ, Kuramoto L, Sutherland JM, Levy AR et al (2018) Mortality effects of timing alternatives for hip fracture surgery. CMAJ 190(31):E923–E932

50. Sheehan KJ, Filliter C, Sobolev B, Levy AR, Guy P, Kuramoto L et al (2018) Time to surgery after hip fracture across Canada by timing of admission. Osteoporos Int 29(3):653–663

51. Lee Y-K, Yoon B-H, Nho J-H, Kim K-C, Ha Y-C, Koo K-H (2013) National trends of surgical treatment for intertrochanteric fractures in Korea. J Korean Med Sci 28(9):1407–1408

52. Lee Y-K, Ha Y-C, Park C, Koo K-H (2013) Trends of surgical treatment in femoral neck fracture: a nationwide study based on claim registry. J Arthroplast 28(10):1839–1841

53. Johansen A, Golding D, Brent L, Close J, Gjertsen J-E, Holt G et al (2017) Using national hip fracture registries and audit databases to develop an international perspective. Injury 48(10):2174–2179

54. Sáez-López P, Brañas F, Sánchez-Hernández N, Alonso-García N, González-Montalvo JI (2017) Hip fracture registries: utility, description, and comparison. Osteoporos Int 28(4):1157–1166

55. Griffiths F, Mason V, Boardman F, Dennick K, Haywood K, Achten J et al (2015) Evaluating recovery following hip fracture: a qualitative interview study of what is important to patients. BMJ Open 5(1):e005406

56. Parker MJ (2008) Databases for hip fracture audit. Acta Orthop 79(5):577–579

57. Regulation (EU) 2016/679 of the European Parliament and of the Council of 27 April 2016 on the protection of natural persons with regard to the processing of personal data and on the free movement of such data, and repealing Directive 95/46/EC (General Data Protection Regulation) [Internet]. https://eur-lex.europa.eu/legal-content/EN/TXT/?uri=CELEX%3A02016R0679-20160504

58. GDPR (2019) Guidance for Clinical Audit, Version 2 [Internet]. National Office of Clinical Audit. http://s3-eu-west-1.amazonaws.com/noca-uploads/general/NOCA_GDPR_Guidance_for_Clinical_Audit_version_2_Updated_June_2019.pdf

59. Lilford RJ, Brown CA, Nicholl J (2007) Use of process measures to monitor the quality of clinical practice. BMJ 335(7621):648–650

60. Burns EM, Rigby E, Mamidanna R, Bottle A, Aylin P, Ziprin P et al (2012) Systematic review of discharge coding accuracy. J Public Health (Oxf) 34(1):138–148

61. Dalal S, Roy B (2009) Reliability of clinical coding of hip facture surgery: implications for payment by results? Injury 40(7):738–741

62. Pitches DW, Mohammed MA, Lilford RJ (2007) What is the empirical evidence that hospitals with higher-risk adjusted mortality rates provide poorer quality care? A systematic review of the literature. BMC Health Serv Res 7:91

63. Neuburger J, Currie C, Wakeman R, Tsang C, Plant F, De Stavola B et al (2015) The impact of a national clinician-led audit initiative on care and mortality after hip fracture in England: an external evaluation using time trends in non-audit data. Med Care 53(8):686–691

64. Wise J (2015) Hip fracture audit may have saved 1000 lives since 2007. BMJ 351:h3854

65. Condorhuamán-Alvarado PY, Pareja-Sierra T, Muñoz-Pascual A, Sáez-López P, Ojeda-Thies C, Alarcón-Alarcón T et al (2019) First proposal of quality indicators and standards and recommendations to improve the healthcare in the Spanish National Registry of Hip Fracture. Rev Esp Geriatr Gerontol 54(5):257–264

66. Scottish Hip Fracture Audit (2018) Scottish standards of care for hip fracture patients 2018 [Internet]. https://www.shfa.scot.nhs.uk/_docs/2018/Scottish-standards-of-care-for-hip-fracture-patients-2018.pdf

67. Australian Commission on Safety & Quality in Health Care (2016) Hip fracture care: clinical care standard [Internet]. http://www.safetyandquality.gov.au/our-work/clinical-care-standards/hip-fracture-care-clinical-care-standard/

68. Whitaker SR, Nisar S, Scally AJ, Radcliffe GS (2019) Does achieving the "Best Practice Tariff" criteria for fractured neck of femur patients improve one year outcomes? Injury 50(7):1358–1363

69. Quality statements|Hip fracture in adults|Quality standards|NICE [Internet]. https://www.nice.org.uk/guidance/qs16/chapter/Quality-statements

70. British Orthopaedic Association (2019) BOAST—The Care of the Older or Frail Orthopaedic Trauma Patient [Internet]. https://www.boa.ac.uk/resources/boa-standards-for-trauma-and-orthopaedics/boast-frailty.html

71. Metcalfe D, Zogg CK, Judge A, Perry DC, Gabbe B, Willett K et al (2019) Pay for performance and hip fracture outcomes: an interrupted time series and difference-in-differences analysis in England and Scotland. Bone Joint J 101-B(8):1015–1023

72. Ferguson KB, Halai M, Winter A, Elswood T, Smith R, Hutchison JD et al (2016) National audits of hip fractures: are yearly audits required? Injury 47(2):439–443

73. White SM, Moppett IK, Griffiths R, Johansen A, Wakeman R, Boulton C et al (2016) Secondary analysis of outcomes after 11,085 hip fracture operations from the prospective UK Anaesthesia Sprint Audit of Practice (ASAP-2). Anaesthesia 71(5):506–514

74. Boulton C, Currie C, Griffiths R, Grocott M, Johansen A, Majeed A, et al (2014) Anaesthesia Sprint Audit of Practice 2014. p 64

75. Metcalfe D, Costa ML, Parsons NR, Achten J, Masters J, Png ME et al (2019) Validation of a prospective cohort study of older adults with hip fractures. Bone Joint J 101-B(6):708–714

76. Costa ML, Griffin XL, Achten J, Metcalfe D, Judge A, Pinedo-Villanueva R, et al (2016) World Hip Trauma Evaluation (WHiTE): framework for embedded comprehensive cohort studies. BMJ Open [Internet]. 6(10). https://bmjopen.bmj.com/content/6/10/e011679

77. Montori VM (2017) Big Science for patient centred care. BMJ [Internet]. 359. https://www.bmj.com/content/359/bmj.j5600

78. Cooper C, Atkinson EJ, O'Fallon WM, Melton LJ (1992) Incidence of clinically diagnosed vertebral fractures: a population-based study in Rochester, Minnesota, 1985–1989. J Bone Miner Res 7(2):221–227

79. Pizzato S, Trevisan C, Lucato P, Girotti G, Mazzochin M, Zanforlini BM et al (2018) Identification of asymptomatic frailty vertebral fractures in post-menopausal women. Bone 113:89–94

80. Vertebral Fracture Sprint Audit [Internet] (2019) RCP London. https://www.rcplondon.ac.uk/projects/vertebral-fracture-sprint-audit

81. Wennergren D, Möller M (2018) Implementation of the Swedish Fracture Register. Unfallchirurg 121(12):949–955

82. Svenska Frakturregistret [Internet]. https://sfr.registercentrum.se/

83. Thien TM, Chatziagorou G, Garellick G, Furnes O, Havelin LI, Mäkelä K et al (2014) Periprosthetic femoral fracture within two years after total hip replacement: analysis of 437,629 operations in the nordic arthroplasty register association database. J Bone Joint Surg Am 96(19):e167

84. Palan J, Smith MC, Gregg P, Mellon S, Kulkarni A, Tucker K et al (2016) The influence of cemented femoral stem choice on the incidence of revision for periprosthetic fracture after primary total hip arthroplasty: an analysis of national joint registry data. Bone Joint J 98-B(10):1347–1354

85. Kristensen TB, Dybvik E, Furnes O, Engesæter LB, Gjertsen J-E (2018) More reoperations for periprosthetic fracture after cemented hemiarthroplasty with polished taper-slip stems than after anatomical and straight stems in the treatment of hip fractures: a study from the Norwegian Hip Fracture Register 2005 to 2016. Bone Joint J 100-B(12):1565–1571

86. Fracture Liaison Service Database (FLS-DB) [Internet] (2015) RCP London. https://www.rcplondon.ac.uk/projects/fracture-liaison-service-database-fls-db

87. Osteoporosis Canada (2018) Report from Osteoporosis Canada's first national FLS audit [Internet]. https://fls.osteoporosis.ca/wp-content/uploads/Report-from-Osteoporosis-Canadas-first-national-FLS-audit.pdf

88. Registro REFRA [Internet]. Seiomm. https://seiomm.org/registro-refra/

89. Seibel MJ, Mitchell P (2018) Secondary fracture prevention: an international perspective. Academic Press, New York

90. British Orthopaedic Association (2007) The care of patients with fragilty fracture [internet]. British Orthopaedic Association, London. http://www.bgs.org.uk/pdf_cms/pubs/Blue%20Book%20on%20fragility%20fracture%20care.pdf

91. Lemer C, Cheung R, Klaber R, Hibbs N (2016) Understanding healthcare processes: how marginal gains can improve quality and value for children and families. Arch Dis Childhood Educ Pract 101(1):31–37

92. Yousri TA, Khan Z, Chakrabarti D, Fernandes R, Wahab K (2011) Lean thinking: can it improve the outcome of fracture neck of femur patients in a district general hospital? Injury 42(11):1234–1237

93. Sayeed Z, Anoushiravani A, El-Othmani M, Barinaga G, Sayeed Y, Cagle P et al (2018) Implementation of a hip fracture care pathway using lean six sigma methodology in a level I trauma center. J Am Acad Orthop Surg 26(24):881–893

94. Delaunay C (2015) Registries in orthopaedics. Orthop Traumatol Surg Res 101(1 Suppl):S69–S75

95. Executive Board 144 (2019). His highness Sheikh Sabah Al-Ahmad Al-Jaber Al-Sabah prize for research in health care for the elderly and in health promotion [Internet]. World Health Organization, Geneva. https://extranet.who.int/iris/restricted/handle/10665/327207

96. Hernlund E, Svedbom A, Ivergård M, Compston J, Cooper C, Stenmark J et al (2013) Osteoporosis in the European Union: medical management, epidemiology and economic burden. A report prepared in collaboration with the International Osteoporosis Foundation

(IOF) and the European Federation of Pharmaceutical Industry Associations (EFPIA). Arch Osteoporos 8(1–2):136

97. The National Hip Fracture Database [Internet]. https://www.nhfd.co.uk/
98. Rath S, Yadav L, Tewari A, Chantler T, Woodward M, Kotwal P et al (2017) Management of older adults with hip fractures in India: a mixed methods study of current practice, barriers and facilitators, with recommendations to improve care pathways. Arch Osteoporos 12(1):55
99. Viveros-García J, Robles-Almaguer E, Albrecht-Junghanns R, López-Cervantes R, López-Paz C, Olascoaga-Gómez de León A, et al (2019) Mexican hip fracture audit: results from the pilot phase. In: 8th FFN global congress 2019. p 116
100. Palomino L, Ramírez R, Vejarano J, Ticse R (2016) Fractura de cadera en el adulto mayor: la epidemia ignorada en el Perú. Acta Méd Peruana 33(1):15–20

Printed by Printforce, United Kingdom